CANCER ETIOLOGY, DIAGNOSIS AND TREATMENTS

HEPATOCELLULAR CARCINOMA

A GLOBAL CHALLENGE

CANCER ETIOLOGY, DIAGNOSIS AND TREATMENTS

Additional books in this series can be found on Nova's website under the Series tab.

Additional E-books in this series can be found on Nova's website under the E-book tab.

CANCER ETIOLOGY, DIAGNOSIS AND TREATMENTS

HEPATOCELLULAR CARCINOMA

A GLOBAL CHALLENGE

ISABELLE CHEMIN
EDITOR

Nova Science Publishers, Inc.
New York

For permission to use material from this book please contact us:
Telephone 631-231-7269; Fax 631-231-8175
Web Site: http://www.novapublishers.com

LIBRARY OF CONGRESS CATALOGING-IN-PUBLICATION DATA

Hepatocellular carcinoma : a global challenge / editor, Isabelle Chemin.
p. ; cm.
Includes bibliographical references and index.
ISBN 978-1-61470-644-1 (hardcover)
1. Liver--Cancer. I. Chemin, Isabelle, 1965-
[DNLM: 1. Carcinoma, Hepatocellular. WI 735]
RC280.L5H453 2011
616.99'436--dc23

2011024910

Published by Nova Science Publishers, Inc. † New York

Contents

Preface

Primary human liver cancer, of which hepatocellular carcinoma (HCC) is by far the predominant type, is a major cause of cancer death worldwide, accounting for 700,000 deaths per year. The epidemiology of HCC is particular with both geographic and temporal patterns of incidence paralleling exposure to viral etiologic factors. The highest HCC incidence rates are areas endemic for chronic infection with Hepatitis B virus, mainly Asia and Africa. The pathways by which HCC develop are heterogeneous and influenced by a variety of environmental and host factors. This book is dedicated to hepatocellular carcinoma and includes contributions that span various aspects of the disease from epidemiology, mechanisms and viruses, to promising new biomarkers and targets for treatment.

Chapter I - The burden of Hepatocellular Carinoma (HCC) has been increasing in several African countries including Egypt. In Africa, the predominant risk factors for the development of liver cancer, known for over 2 decades, include chronic infection by hepatitis B (HBV), hepatitis C (HCV) and long-term exposure to foodstuffs contaminated with aflatoxin. It has been well documented that Egypt has one of the highest prevalence rates of HCV infection in the world. The natural history of HCV infection and disease progression are influenced by additional factors such as duration of infection, age at infection, sex, co-infection with HBV, the level of HCV viraemia and its genotype. Several studies in Africa indicated the role of exposure to aflatoxins and development of HCC. In Egypt, recent food sampling surveys and population based studies indicated that exposure to aflatoxins in Egypt may have been underestimated in the past. Recent results indicated that both local and imported samples were positive for aflatoxin B1. Prevention and intervention approaches directed to risk factors of HCC can play a critical role in its prevention. HBV vaccination can help effectively. HCV prevention programme can be achieved by changing personal behaviors and/or cultural habits which are risk factors for HCV transmission. Prevention of exposure to aflatoxins can be achieved either at community or individual levels. In this chapter, the authors' goal is to summarize several research studies on the prevalence of HCC, and its risk factors in Africa with special emphasis in Egypt which can help in the development of preventive interventions. In conclusion, due to the alarming increase in the incidence of HCC in Africa, there is a need to investigate the contribution of these emerging risk factors to determine the susceptibility to HCC among high risk groups and to provide these individuals with effective measures for early prevention or intervention.

Chapter II - Hepatocellular Carcinoma (HCC) imposes a growing disease burden in Asia, a region that already shoulders more than 70% of the global load. Analysis of epidemiological data shows regional changes in disease incidence and etiological factors. This chapter examines the epidemiology of HCC in Asia in 4 parts – the burden of disease and its distribution, changing trends in the etiology, the reliability of data and future directions for research and public health initiatives.

Chapter III - Latin America (LA) represents a heterogeneous region in terms of ethnic admixtures and exhibits an intermediate incidence of Hepatocellular carcinoma (HCC). The mains factors associated to HCC development in LA are alcohol consumption, HBV and HCV infection. HCV infection is more frequently found in HCC cases in countries like Argentine, Brazil and Mexico, while in Colombia and Peru, HBV infection seems to be more prevalent. HCV genotype 1 is the most frequent genotype in LA, followed by either genotype 2 or 3. This last genotype has been more frequently found among HCC cases in Brazil. Among the eight HBV genotypes (A–H), the ones most commonly found in LA are the worldwide distributed A and D, and the American F and H The American HBV genotype F has been associated to a rapid development of HCC in Alaska. More studies are needed to analyze if this situation is also frequent in the LA countries where this genotype is frequent. In order to reduce its incidence, more efforts are needed to improve the strategies for prevention and treatment of HCC in the region.

Chapter IV - Hepatocellular carcinoma(HCC), the main form of primary liver cancer, occurs mostly in the setting of cirrhosis. Chronic HCV infection, alcohol consumption, and obesity/diabetes are the main risk factors in Europe. The overall annual incidence of liver cancer in Europe was estimated around 60 000 cases in 2008 (two-third in men) but with a wide spectrum according to different countries. There is an increasing gradient from Northern to Southern Europe, reflecting geographical differences in exposure to risk factors for HCC. Mortality is very close to incidence, reflecting the poor prognosis of patients. Upward trends in incidence and mortality from liver cancer have been reported in several European countries, but with a large pattern of outcomes. In France, in contrast with persistently increasing incidence, a slight decrease in mortality from late-1990s has been recently reported after several decades of continuous increase. Significant improvement in HCC incidence and mortality in the future will require effective control of exposure to the main causes of cirrhosis, promotion of periodic ultrasonographic surveillance and effective antiviral control of HCV and HBV infections in patients with cirrhosis, and further improvements in curative treatments for HCC.

Chapter V - A number of risk factors appear to play a role in hepatocellular carcinoma (HCC), hepatitis B infection being one of the most important. Hepatitis B surface antigen (HBsAg) is the hallmark of hepatitis B virus (HBV) since it is the best and most reliable diagnostic marker. However, since most studies do not rely on longitudinal observations but mostly on cross-sectional studies little is known on time changes in those markers and their incidence. Chronic inflammation and cytokines are key determinants in the development of fibrosis and liver cell proliferation. Integration of HBV DNA into host cellular DNA is crucial during HBV chronic infection by disrupting or promoting expression of cellular genes that are important in cell growth and differentiation. In addition, expression of HBV proteins may have a direct effect on cellular functions, and some of these gene products can promote malignant transformation. Several HBV genes have been found in infected tumoral tissues more frequently than others, including truncated pre-S2/S and hepatitis B X genes. The proteins expressed from these integrated genes have been shown to have intracellular activities that may account for their association with HCC, including effects on cellular growth and apoptosis. A major player involved in this form of viral transactivation is the X protein (HBx) that displays pleiotropic functions and has been implicated in the malignant transformation of chronically-infected liver cells. Occult hepatitis B virus infection is characterized by persistence of HBV DNA in HBsAg-negative individuals. There are evidences that occult HBV constitutes a risk factor for the development of HCC and that the mechanisms whereby overt HBV might induce tumor formation are maintained in those atypical HBV infections.

Chapter VI - HCC represents the first primary malignancy of the liver followed by cholangiocarcinoma. Its incidence is still increasing owe to the increased prevalence of the various risk factors of chronic liver diseases, mainly related to hepatitis infection with hepatitis C and B viruses, and more recently Fatty Liver Diseases which are mostly associated with metabolic syndrome [1]. Indeed, 60 to 90% of HCC occur in the setting of chronic liver diseases leading to cirrhosis. Still now, HCC carries a poor prognosis which is partly explained by its late diagnosis, the clinical context of the patient which may compromise potential therapeutic strategies, and also tumor itself which is prone to display angioinvasion.

Chapter VII - *TP53* encodes a major tumor suppressor protein, which is mutated or otherwise inactivated in the majority of human cancers, including HepatoCellular Carcinoma (HCC). In HCC, the frequency and type of *TP53* mutation show striking geographic variations in relation with etiologic factors. In areas of high endemicity for Hepatitis B Virus (HBV) and of chronic exposure to Aflatoxin B_1 (AFB_1), a single mutation at codon 249 (*R249S*) occurs in at least half of HCC cases. In other etiological contexts (e.g. HCV, alcohol, iron overload, HBV without AFB_1 exposure), *TP53* mutation is less frequent (20-30%) and mutations are distributed throughout the central core domain of the p53 protein. This diversity in mutation patterns highlights the importance of p53 in managing the responses of hepatocytes to various forms of stress. In this chapter, the authors review recent evidence showing that p53 plays an important role as inducer of senescence of liver cells in response to DNA damage, oxidative stress or oncogene activation. The authors also discuss current data and hypotheses regarding how the HBx antigen may interfere or cooperate with wild-type and mutant p53 in hepatocarcinogenesis. Finally, they summarize the evidence implicating the two members of the *TP53* family, *TP73* and *TP63*, in specific mechanisms of responses of hepatocytes to DNA damaging agents. Based on these considerations, they suggest a model of progression to liver cancer in which *TP53* mutation may represent either a primary or a secondary event, depending upon the etiological context.

Chapter VIII - Hepatocellular carcinoma (HCC) is a leading health problem worldwide. It is a poor prognosis tumor ranking third in terms of death by cancer [Parkin 2001]. This can be attributable to a common late diagnosis with advanced cancerous spread at presentation while patients have inoperable HCC. In this setting, therapies are mostly of modest benefit. Among systemic therapies, only sorafenib – i.e. the antiangiogenic and Ras-Raf-MAPK inhibitor - has been shown to significantly improve survival rates [Llovet 2008]. The growing incidence of HCC has generated intense research to understand its cellular and molecular mechanisms, with the hope of developing innovative therapies. Hepatocarcinogenesis is a complex process associating accumulation of genetic and epigenetic changes that occur during initiation, promotion and progression of the disease. Activation of oncogenes and the role of tumor suppressor genes have well been documented, and the signal transduction pathways implicated in HCC are being extensively studied [Hoshida 2008; Merle 2009]. Among these, evidence is accumulating that activation of the Wnt/Frizzled-mediated signaling could play a key role in HCC. The role of the Wnt pathway in liver biology has come to the forefront over the last several years. In the present paper, we'll aim at understanding the Wnt/Frizzled-mediated signaling and highlighting its deregulations encountered in hepatocarciniogenesis.

Chapter IX - The innate immune response detects pathogen associated molecular patterns (PAMPs) via a panel of pattern recognition receptors (PRRs). Binding of PAMPs to PRRs expressed in a variety of cell types, initiates the innate inflammatory immune response. Hepatitis B virus (HBV) infection leads to chronicity in most cases in which inflammatory responses are some how deregulated.This chapter aims to summarize the different PRR currently identified and how HBV regulates their function post infection.

Chapter X - Epigenetic mechanisms can be viewed as an interface between the genome and environmental influences. Aberrant epigenetic events associated with viral infection and various environmental factors are likely to play an important role in the onset and progression of different human cancers, including hepatocellular carcinoma (HCC). At the cellular level, aberrant epigenetic events may deregulate critical cellular events, such as gene expression, DNA damage response and DNA repair, cell cycle checkpoints, and carcinogen detoxification, all of which may contribute to the initiation and progression of liver cancer. In this review, the authors summarize recent progress in the authors' understanding of epigenetic mechanisms by which viral agents and environmental factors may promote hepatocarcinogenesis. Although they focus on epigenetic changes and risk factors involved in liver cancer, similar mechanisms may operate in the development of other cancer types.

Chapter XI - Hepatocellular carcinoma (HCC) is a highly malignant tumor that invariably kills patients not eligible for surgical procedures [1]. This appalling situation is primarily due to the late detection of patients with a locally advanced tumor. Furthermore, hepatocytes, the transformed cells that form the tumor, are specialized in detoxification, an originally beneficial function that makes them almost naturally resistant to anticancer chemotherapy [2]. Since decades, HCC incidence is steadily increasing worldwide and the tumor represents now a serious concern for public health.

Chapter XII - Hepatocellular Carcinoma (HCC) is a complex phenotypically and genetically heterogeneous polyclonal disease caused by a variety of risk factors. For a better understanding of the molecular mechanisms underlying the carcinogenesis, molecular profiling of genes, proteins, metabolites and other molecules are needed. The completion of the Human Genome Project changed the paradigm for large-scale biology projects and was critical for the development of the new era of "omics" research with the aim of understanding the complexity of a cell, tissue, and an organism in its entirety. Today, various physiological and pathological events can systematically be interpreted through the combination of comprehensive measurements of genomics (global gene analysis), epigenetics (global analysis of genetic modifications that are not attributable to changes in the primary DNA sequence), transcriptomics (global gene expression analysis), proteomics (global protein expression analysis), metabolomics (global metabolite expression analysis) and so on. Technological and bio-computing advances in large-scale omics analyses are providing researchers and doctors with an unprecedented capacity to capture and assess complex molecular information from biological samples. And importantly, large repositories of specimens collected in clinical or epidemiological studies are being developed, providing access to series of biospecimens with large statistical power for assessing complex sets of biomarkers. In this chapter, systematic -omics approaches used in the study of HCC in the scales of genomics including chromosomal instability and epigenetic changes, transcriptomics and microRNAs, proteomics and also metabolomics are discussed. What are now needed are major integrative omics and systems biology efforts for a systematic understanding of the pathogenesis and pathophysiology of HCC. This will lead to discovery of new therapeutic targets, prediction of therapeutic response, personalized treatment regimens and ultimately to the prevention of HCC.

Section One: Epidemiology of Hepatocellular Carcinoma

In: Hepatocellular Carcionoma: A Global Challenge
Editor: Isabelle Chemin
ISBN: 978-1-61470-644-1

Introduction to Section One: Global Strategy to Prevent Hepatitis Viruses

Silvia Franceschi
International Agency for Research on Cancer, Lyon, France

Background on Liver Cancer

Liver cancer is an important public health problem worldwide and a major example of inequality across different world populations. According to the most recent estimates from Globocan [Ferlay et al., 2010], approximately 750,000 new liver cancer cases were diagnosed in 2008, representing 7% of all cancers in women and men combined. Less developed countries are hit especially hard by the disease: 85% of liver cancer worldwide occurs in less developed countries, and half of those in China. However, there is also reason for concern in more developed countries because, although liver cancer is relatively rare, upward trends have been reported in the United States and Japan [Tanaka et al., 2002], as well as several European countries [Bosetti et al., 2008] in the last two or three decades.

Globally, approximately 80% of liver cancer is caused by the long-term consequences of infection with two viruses, hepatitis B virus (HBV) and hepatitis C virus (HCV), which are reported to account for 50% and 25%, respectively, of the disease burden. Heavy alcohol consumption is responsible for an important fraction of liver cancer especially in more developed countries where HBV and HCV infections are rare. Tobacco smoking has also been recently associated with increased liver cancer risk [IARC, 2004]. Noteworthy contributions to liver cancer causation derive from aflatoxin contamination of food in some less developed countries [Wild and Gong, 2010], and from dietary and metabolic factors (i.e., obesity, diabetes, and iron overload) in more developed countries [Yuan et al., 2004].

Liver cancer is one of the least curable malignancies and the updated worldwide estimate of yearly deaths from the disease (700,000) is very similar to the number of new cases [Ferlay et al., 2010], thus making liver cancer the third most frequent cause of cancer death worldwide. The possibility of treating liver cancer depends on disease stage at diagnosis, but also on the severity of liver impairment, as liver cancer most often arises within the framework of liver fibrosis and cirrhosis. Complete surgical resection and therapeutic liver transplantation are seldom possible, even in more developed countries. In addition, radiotherapy and chemotherapy show a very low success rate among liver cancer patients [Liang and Heller, 2004]. Palliative treatments (local ethanol injection and radiofrequency ablation) offer some benefits and should be made increasingly available in less developed countries. It is clear, however, that primary prevention is the best strategy to diminish the worldwide liver cancer burden.

Since 1982, about 1 billion people have been vaccinated against HBV. The vaccine is highly effective, safe and cheap enough to be available even in less developed countries. It has been included in national immunisation programmes in 164 countries, and at present reaches two-thirds of the world's children (www.who.int). In some countries in Asia where vertical transmission of HBV is common, additional efforts are necessary to ensure that vaccination is started within 24 hours after birth. There is, however, a real possibility of eradicating HBV within a generation or two.

With respect to HCV infection, however, prevention strategies are more complicated and, for the moment, sorely lacking in many less developed countries. The continued transmission of HCV represents a very real threat to the reduction of the worldwide liver cancer burden. The World Health Organization (WHO) estimates that about 180 million people, some 3% of the world's population, are infected with HCV, of which 130 million are chronic carriers at risk of developing liver cirrhosis and/or liver cancer (www.who.int). At least 3-to-4 million people are newly infected each year. The burden of HCV is, therefore, lower than the burden of HBV (i.e., 350 million people with chronic HBV infection), but there is evidence that HCV incidence and prevalence are substantially underestimated due to different problems: 1) lack of country-specific data, even in more developed countries [Muhlberger et al., 2009]; 2) poor sensitivity of HCV surveillance systems that focus on acute HCV infection, which is rarely symptomatic; 3) tendency of available HCV prevalence surveys not to include the populations with the highest prevalence (i.e., middle-aged and elderly people and, in more developed countries, intravenous drug users).

Point 3, in particular, is a more important cause of underestimation of HCV than HBV infection because hepatitis prevalence surveys are mainly carried out in young populations (e.g., blood donors or pregnant women). By young adulthood, the majority of HBV infections have already occurred because, in populations where HBV vaccination has not yet been introduced, viral transmission occurs at birth (e.g., China), during childhood (e.g., sub-Saharan Africa and India) or after becoming sexually active (e.g., more developed countries). In contrast, HCV is nearly exclusively transmitted through contact with blood and blood products. In countries where routine blood screening for HCV and safe injection practices are not available (or have been only recently introduced), iatrogenic transmission of HCV continues into adulthood and old age [Dondog et al., 2010]. It is also worth noting that, whereas late acquisition of HBV in adulthood is not only rare, but also associated with a substantially lower probability of the infection becoming chronic when compared to early acquisition, the risk of HCV becoming chronic does not decline with age at infection.

HCV epidemics have accompanied the increasing availability of these medical procedures in different countries until safe blood supplies and safe injection practices were implemented [Prati, 2006]. Massive and unsafe injection campaigns took place between the two World Wars in many countries (e.g., anti-schistosomal treatments in Japan and Egypt), and unsafe blood transfusions and medical procedures increased in times of military conflict in Europe (especially Spain and Italy) and Asia (China, Vietnam). By the end of the 1980s, one out of 50 units of blood in more developed countries transmitted HCV [Prati, 2006]. As a result, most chronic transfusion recipients and virtually all patients receiving clotting factor concentrates developed chronic hepatitis. However, the incidence of HCV infection greatly decreased a few years later because of the introduction of anti-HCV tests for blood donors, inactivation procedures for blood derivatives, and disposable needles and syringes. The majority of new HCV infections in more developed countries in the last 15 years have been due to needle sharing by intravenous drug users. Not so, however, elsewhere. Approximately half of less developed countries, mostly in Asia and Africa, but also a few countries in Latin America and the Caribbean, do not systematically screen blood donations for HCV (although blood is generally screened for HBV and HIV). Blood safety in less developed countries is additionally threatened by lack of voluntary non-paid blood donors, inadequate supplies of medical instruments and laboratory reagents, and lack of infrastructure. Furthermore, although the probability of HCV transmission is maximised through contaminated blood transfusions, the use of contaminated injections concerns a much larger number of people of all ages, and is therefore the main cause of unrecognised HCV transmission.

More than 16 billion injections are administered annually in less developed countries. Particularly high rates of injections have been reported in some countries of the former Soviet Union, Mongolia, Pakistan [Ahmad, 2004], and in some African countries [Attia, 1998]. The most frequently injected medications include antibiotics, vitamins, and analgesics or treatments for non-specific symptoms, such as headache, fatigue, or fever that could be taken orally. In poorly funded healthcare systems avoidable injections represent an important source of revenue for the providers and are encouraged by the popular belief that injections are more effective than oral administration. Insufficient hygiene, inappropriate use of multiple-dose medication vials, and sharing of bottles of intravenous solution for multiple patients also contribute to the spread of HCV in overcrowded hospitals in less developed countries. In addition, transmission occurs through traditional medicine (e.g., acupuncture and scarring) and outside health care settings (e.g., tattooing).

The release of a special resolution on HBV and HCV by the 63th Session of the World Health Assembly is therefore a very timely action and includes plans to add viral hepatitis to the portfolio of the Global Fund to Fight AIDS, Tuberculosis and Malaria [Burki, 2010; World Health Organization Sixty-Third World Health Assembly, 2010]. Indeed, the new resolve to tackle hepatitis viruses will strengthen many aspects of health systems (including immunisation programmes, and safety of blood and injections) that are essential also to the prevention and management of the other most important infections. It would also represent one of the most cost-effective ways to curb cancer mortality in less developed countries.

References

Ahmad, K. (2004). Pakistan: a cirrhotic state? *Lancet, 364,* 1843-1844.

Attia, M. A. (1998). Prevalence of hepatitis B and C in Egypt and Africa. *Antivir Ther, 3,* 1-9.

Bosetti, C.; Levi, F.; Boffetta, P.; Lucchini, F.; Negri, E. & La Vecchia, C. (2008). Trends in mortality from hepatocellular carcinoma in Europe, 1980-2004. *Hepatology, 48,* 137-145.

Burki, T. (2010). New resolve to tackle viral hepatitis. *Lancet Infect Dis, 10,* 450-451.

Dondog, B.; Lise, M.; Dondov, O.; Baldandorj, B. & Franceschi, S. (2011). Hepatitis B and C virus infections in hepatocellular carcinoma and cirrhosis in Mongolia. *Eur J Cancer Prev, 20,* 33-39.

Ferlay, J.; Shin, H. R.; Bray, F.; Forman, D.; Mathers, C.; & Parkin DM. (2010). GLOBOCAN 2008, Cancer Incidence and Mortality Worldwide: IARC CancerBase No. 10 [Internet]. Lyon, France: International Agency for Research on Cancer; Available from: http://globocan.iarc.fr.

IARC (2004). *Monographs on the Evaluation of Carcinogenic Risks to Humans, Volume 83: Tobacco Smoke and Involuntary Smoking.* Lyon, IARC Press.

Liang, T. J. & Heller, T. (2004). Pathogenesis of hepatitis C-associated hepatocellular carcinoma. *Gastroenterology, 127,* S62-S71.

Muhlberger, N.; Schwarzer, R.; Lettmeier, B.; Sroczynski, G.; Zeuzem, S. & Siebert, U. (2009). HCV-related burden of disease in Europe: a systematic assessment of incidence, prevalence, morbidity, and mortality. *BMC Public Health, 9*, 34.

Prati, D. (2006). Transmission of hepatitis C virus by blood transfusions and other medical procedures: a global review. *J Hepatol, 45,* 607-616.

Raza, S. A.; Clifford, G. M. & Franceschi, S. (2007). Worldwide variation in the relative importance of hepatitis B and hepatitis C viruses in hepatocellular carcinoma: a systematic review. *Br J Cancer, 96,* 1127-1134.

Tanaka, Y.; Hanada, K.; Mizokami, M.; Yeo, A. E.; Shih, J. W.; Gojobori, T. & Alter, H. J. (2002). Inaugural Article: A comparison of the molecular clock of hepatitis C virus in the United States and Japan predicts that hepatocellular carcinoma incidence in the United States will increase over the next two decades. *Proc Natl Acad Sci U S A, 99,* 15584-15589.

Wild, C. P.; Gong, Y. Y. (2010). Mycotoxins and human disease: a largely ignored global health issue. *Carcinogenesis*, *31*, 71-82.

World Health Organization Sixty-Third World Health Assembly (2010) Viral hepatitis. Report by the Secretariat. Provisional Agenda item 11.12. World Health Organization, Geneva. Available from: http://apps.who.int/gb/ebwha/pdf_files/WHA63/A63_15-en.pdf

Yuan, J. M.; Govindarajan, S.; Arakawa, K. & Yu, M. C. (2004). Synergism of alcohol, diabetes, and viral hepatitis on the risk of hepatocellular carcinoma in blacks and whites in the U.S. *Cancer, 101,* 1009-1017.

In: Hepatocellular Carcionoma: A Global Challenge
Editor: Isabelle Chemin
ISBN: 978-1-61470-644-1

Chapter I

Hepatocellular Carinoma in Africa with Special Overview in Egypt

Wagida A. Anwar*

Community, Environmental and Occupational Medicine; Faculty of Medicine, Ain Shams University, Egypt

Abstract

The burden of Hepatocellular Carinoma (HCC) has been increasing in several African countries including Egypt. In Africa, the predominant risk factors for the development of liver cancer, known for over 2 decades, include chronic infection by hepatitis B (HBV), hepatitis C (HCV) and long-term exposure to foodstuffs contaminated with aflatoxin. It has been well documented that Egypt has one of the highest prevalence rates of HCV infection in the world. The natural history of HCV infection and disease progression are influenced by additional factors such as duration of infection, age at infection, sex, co-infection with HBV, the level of HCV viraemia and its genotype. Several studies in Africa indicated the role of exposure to aflatoxins and development of HCC. In Egypt, recent food sampling surveys and population based studies indicated that exposure to aflatoxins in Egypt may have been underestimated in the past. Recent results indicated that both local and imported samples were positive for aflatoxin B1. Prevention and intervention approaches directed to risk factors of HCC can play a critical role in its prevention. HBV vaccination can help effectively. HCV prevention programme can be achieved by changing personal behaviors and/or cultural habits which are risk factors for HCV transmission. Prevention of exposure to aflatoxins can be achieved either at community or individual levels. In this chapter, our goal is to summarize several research studies on the prevalence of HCC, and its risk factors in Africa with special emphasis in Egypt which can help in the development of preventive interventions. In **conclusion**, due to the alarming increase in the incidence of HCC in Africa, there is a need to investigate the contribution of these emerging risk factors to determine the susceptibility to HCC

* E-mail: wagidaanwar@yahoo.com.

among high risk groups and to provide these individuals with effective measures for early prevention or intervention.

Keywords: Hepatocellular carcinoma (HCC), Africa, Egypt, Risk factors, HBV, HCV, Aflatoxins, Prevention

Introduction

Hepatocellular Carcinoma (HCC) is a major cause of cancer death worldwide, accounting for over half a million deaths per year, (Parkin et al, 2001, and Kirk, Bah, and Montesano, 2006). It is a rapidly lethal cancer, with life expectancy after diagnosis rarely exceeding 3 years in developed countries, and 3 months elsewhere (Scheff, 2007). HCC is endemic in China, Taiwan, Korea and Africa, where the incidence is between 20 and 100 cases per 100,000 humans (El-Serag and Rudolph, 2007). The geographic pattern of HCC incidence is parallel to exposure to etiologic factors. According to recent reports, the incidence of HCC has increased sharply in the last 5-10 years (Bruix et al, 2001; El-Serag, 2002; Velazquez et al, 2003), with an especially high incidence in Egypt (Anwar et al, 2008).

Hepatocellular Carinoma (HCC) occurs commonly in the Black population of sub-Saharan Africa. It carries a particularly grave prognosis, average survival times from the onset of symptoms being as short as 14 weeks (Kew and Geddes, 1985, and Ndububa, et al, 2001) and, with very few exceptions, all of the patients surviving for less than one year (annual fatality ratio 0.97). Approximately 46,000 new cases of the tumour are reported to occur each year in the sub-continent (Boyle, 2002). According to Kew, (2010), the growth patterns and pathological features of HCC in Black Africans differ in a number of ways from those in other populations. The tumours are far larger and more likely to be of the expanding (massive) variety. HCC occurs in a non-cirrhotic liver more often than is the case in HCCs in other populations.

The great majority of the population live in rural areas where the incidence of the tumour is higher than it is in urban areas and where facilities for diagnosing and treating HCC are least adequate. HCC often occurs at a relatively young age in Black Africans, and men are affected far more often than are women (Kew and Geddes 1985).

Chronic infections with HBV or HCV have both been recognized as human liver carcinogens with a combined attributable fraction of at least 75% of all HCC cases (Boyle, 2002). HBV is considered as a major risk factor for the progression to liver cirrhosis and HCC (Ohata et al, 2004). The relative risk of developing HCC for HBV carriers may be 100-200-fold higher than that for non-carriers (Xiong et al, 2003). HCV is also an important etiologic factor for HCC, with an estimated attributable fraction of 23% (Pisani et al, 1997). Yates et al. (1999) reported that 67% of HCC patients were HCV seropositive compared to 30% of the controls. Several lines of evidence indicate a strong causal association between HCV and HCC, as shown by the raised prevalence of anti-HCV (El-Zayadi et al 2001; Velazquez et al, 2003) and/or HCV-RNA (Liang et al, 1993) in patients with HCC. The role of HBV infection in pathogenesis of HCC differs from that of HCV infection; HBV-DNA genome integrates in hepatocyte chromosomes (El-Nady, Ling, and Harrison, 2003). The fundamental mechanism by which HCV is related to HCC is not definitely known. Most researchers believe that HCV plays an indirect role in hepatocarcinogenesis through production of cirrhosis with chronic inflammation leading to severe liver damage (Bosch, Ribes, Borras, 1999 and Colombo, 1999). More recently, however, some reports suggest a direct role of HCV in hepatocarcinogenesis, due to the possible carcinogenic action of the HCV core protein in inducing liver cell proliferation (El-Nady, Ling, and Harrison, 2003, Szab et al, 2004). However, it seems that cirrhosis is the common pathway by which several risk factors exert their carcinogenic effect (Fattovich, 1998).

The pathways by which HCC develop are influenced by a variety of environmental and host factors such as the age or gender of the infected person and the genetic characteristics of the virus in cases of HBV or HCV infections. The role of other carcinogens, such as aflatoxin exposure, despite evidence elsewhere that such exposures may damage the DNA in liver cells and lead to mutations in the p53 tumor suppressor gene (Szab et al, 2004) requires further studies

With recognized etiologic factors and improved mechanistic understanding, rational interventions to reduce the incidence and morbidity associated with HCC can be designed and implemented. Vaccination against HBV in infancy is the most effective approach to prevent HBV related HCC, particularly in developing countries. Antiviral drug therapies may prevent virus-associated liver cancer by reducing or eliminating viral replication, if treatment starts before the liver is compromised (Kao and Chen, 2002). Aflatoxin contamination may be eliminated through safe farming and food storage practices, although these practices have yet to be implemented in most of Africa.

Hepatocellular Carinoma (HCC) in Africa

From 1993 to 1997 in Africa, the highest age-standardized incidence rates of HCC were found in sub-Saharan Africa in The Gambia with a rate of 48.9 per 100,000 humans. By comparison, during the same period, the two populations ranked in the middle of the distribution had very different rates: In Harare, Zimbabwe, the rate was 27.9, and the next lowest rate was in Kyadondo, Uganda (6.5). Algeria had the lowest incidence rate of liver cancer at 0.9 per 100,000 humans (Parkin et al, 2002, Scheff, 2007).

The combination of chronic HBV and exposure to aflatoxin B1 appears to be the dominant risk for HCC in sub-Saharan Africa, although HCV infection may be a confounding factor (Kirk, Bah and Montesano, 2006).

Cirrhosis, whatever its cause, is a premalignant condition. In most parts of the world 80% to 90% of HCCs occur in patients with underlying cirrhosis. The proportion of African Black patients in whom the HCC arises in a cirrhotic liver is generally less than that in other populations but is still high. Of the major risk factors for HCC in sub-Saharan Africa, HBV, HCV, and dietary iron overload are all capable of causing cirrhosis. Short-term heavy dietary exposure to AFB1 causes severe acute hepatic necrosis (acute aflatoxicosis), which is often complicated by acute hepatic failure and a fatal outcome. However, long-term exposure to the fungal toxin has not been thought to cause chronic necroinflammatory hepatic disease in the form of chronic hepatitis or cirrhosis. Cirrhosis has therefore not been incriminated in contributing to the pathogenesis of AFB1-induced HCC (Kew, 2010).

Epidemiology of Liver Cancer in Egypt

The National Cancer Registry (NCR) data confirmed the high incidence of HCC in Egypt and the change in the trends during the last decade. The National Cancer Institute Pathology Registry indicated that liver cancer formed 11.75% of the malignancies of all digestive organs and 1.68% of total malignancies (Anwar et al, 2008).

Statistics provided by Middle East Cancer Consortium (MECC) registries showed that Liver cancer's relative frequency was below 2.0% in the other MECC registries and in the US SEER population. In Egypt, liver cancer accounted for 12.7% of male cancers, 3.4% of female cancers, and 8.1% of both sexes together. Male predominance was marked in Egyptians, with a 3.8:1 male-to-female ratio. It is important to note that the sex ratios for the MECC registries other than Egypt are based on small numbers; therefore, they are subject to considerable uncertainty (Ibrahim, 2004). The Age-standardized Incidence Rates (ASR) for Egypt was 20.6 for males, 5.2 for females, and 12.8 for both sexes together. The rate for Egyptian males was more than 3 times the corresponding US SEER rate. For females, the rate for Egyptians was more than twice the US SEER rate (Figure 1).

Liver cancer ASRs showed a progressive increase with age. Below the age of 50 years, the incidence was generally low. Egyptian males had the highest rate (3.4), which is 5 times the rates in the other MECC registries and 2.5 times the US SEER rate.

From 1992 to 2005, 1,012 cases of HCC were diagnosed at Egypt's Gastroenterology Center, Mansoura University. The number of humans with HCC increased yearly from 9 in 1992 to 80 in the first 5 months of 2005. Previous treatment for chronic HCV infection in these patients was 76.6%; schistosomiasis was present in 37.6% of the HCC observed; HBV accounted for 3.3%; and HBV/HCV accounted for 3.6% (Abdel-Wahab et al, 2007; and Darwish et al, 1997).

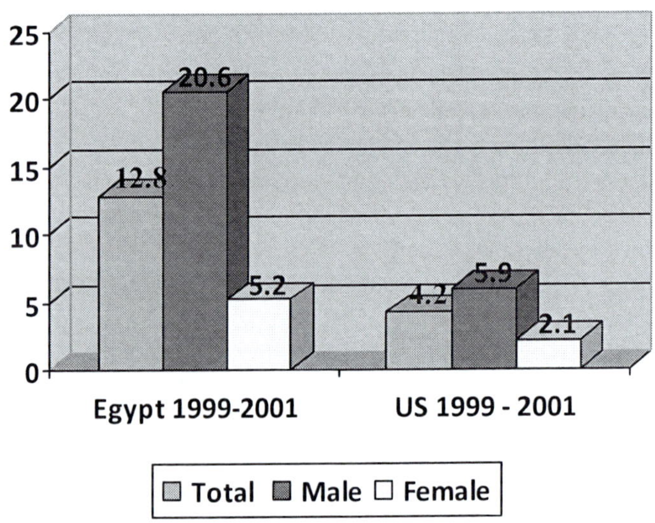

Figure 1. Age-Standardized Incidence Rates (ASR) of Liver Cancer/100,000 MECC Registries, Both Sexes.

In El Zayadi's study in 2005, the trends and pattern changes of HCC in Egypt over the past decade, as well as the possible risk factors were studied. The duration of the study was divided into two periods of 5 years each; period I (1993-1997) and period II (1998-2002). Over this decade, 1,328 HCC patients (5.9%) out of 22,450 chronic liver disease (CLD) patients were diagnosed. The annual proportion of HCC showed a significant rising trend from 4.0% in 1993 to 7.2% in 2002. HCC was significantly more prevalent in rural residents, and patients with a history of schistosomiasis and/or blood transfusion. There was a significant decline of HBsAg from 38.6% to 20.5%, and a slight increase of HCV-Ab from 85.6% to 87.9% in periods I and II respectively. HBV conferred a higher risk to develop HCC more than HCV in period and period II, but the relative contribution of HBV for development of HCC declined in period II compared to period I (El-Zayadi et al, 2005).

In Egypt, Hassan, et al, 2008 indicated in their study that the total mortality rates related to liver diseases and the number of YLL showed little variations during the period (1986-1999) then started to increase from year 2000 up to year 2005. The study addressed the magnitude of liver diseases (HBV infection, HCV infection, liver cancer and liver cirrhosis) in Egypt over the period (1986-2005). Death records of Egypt during the period (1986-2005) were obtained from Central Agency of Public Mobilization and Statistics (1986-1999, using ICD-9 coding system) and National Information Center of Ministry of Health (2000-2005, using ICD-10 coding system). It was reported that the total mortality rates and YLL for liver diseases are steadily increasing with time with higher mortality from liver diseases among males than females all through the study period. Mortality rates and number of YLL due to liver cancer showed a gradual increase from 1986 to 2005 (from 15 to 65 /100000). From year 2000, there was an upward trend for mortality rates and number of YLL due to hepatitis C infection. The mortality was higher in old age groups than young ones (Hassan, et al, 2008).

Lehman et al, (2008) calculated age- and sex-specific and age- and sex-standardized HCC incidence rates for the eight districts in Gharbiah. They also compared rates from Gharbiah with the USA (US Surveillance Epidemiology and End Results [SEER] database). The incidence rate of HCC in Gharbiah was 3.5 times higher than that reported in the USA. Similar findings for a longer period suggest that variation in rates truly reflect different risk factor profiles of these two populations. The analysis revealed a higher incidence in males than in females, significant geographic variations among districts, and a higher incidence in Gharbiah than that reported by SEER. A satisfactory biologic interpretation has yet to be demonstrated. Several hypotheses have been investigated, including the interaction of sex hormones with HBV, leading to a different natural history depending on the sex of the individual or the impact of sex specific exposure. The most notable finding of this study, however, was the statistically significant geographic variation in incidence of HCC among districts within Gharbiah Province. The incidence ranged from 12.9/100 000 PY (Kotour) to less than half that rate at 6.1/100 000 PY (Samanoud). Districts were similar with respect to age distribution and sex ratios, suggesting that the at-risk populations were fairly homogeneous. Consequently, this observed heterogeneity was likely attributable to variations in local risk factors that future studies may investigate. Another interesting finding demonstrated that HCC incidence among urban individuals was nearly twice that of rural residents.

HBV in Africa

According to Professor Kramwis, Africa has 12% of the world's population, and approximately 18% of its HBV infections. Sixty-five million HBV chronically infected humans live in Africa (Kramvis and Kew, 2007). Of the 1.3 million deaths attributed to HBV-related diseases recorded annually worldwide, approximately 250,000 occur in Africa, almost 1 in every 5. Recent studies have examined variation in the natural history of HCC in predominantly HBV-endemic regions, such as Asia and Africa. In these areas, males are 8 times more likely to develop HCC than females, whereas the male to female ratio is 2:1 in North America and Europe (Parkin, Bray and Devesa, 2001). Viral replication declines steeply after adolescence in sub-Saharan Africa, with almost no persistent replication detected in individuals over 25 years of age. This is according to data presented over time by the Gambia Hepatitis Intervention Study (GHIS), which in 1986 was the first program in Africa designed to assess the efficacy of HB vaccination in the prevention of chronic liver disease and HCC (GHIS, 1987; Kirk et al 2004; WHO, 2004,). In 2006, Kirk, Bah and Montesano suggested that this variation may be attributable to the variation in routes of HBV transmission (Kirk, Bah and Montesano, 2006).

In Africa, most primary HBV infections are transmitted either perinatally (around the time of childbirth), or horizontally before the age of 10 years by HBV-infected humans living in the same household. Perinatal transmission occurs at a low rate, however, and is high only when mothers are HBeAg positive HBV carriers (Allain et al, 2003; Okoth et al 1991; Yamanaka et al 1991; Triki et al, 1997; Bile et al, 1992). Most Africans become infected with HBV during childhood, and 8% to 10% of humans in the general population become chronically infected (Hepatitis B fact sheet, 2000). The Baka pygmies of eastern Cameroon have the highest exposure to HBV(Chiaramonte et al, 1991). Ninety percent of children are infected during the first year of life and 30% to 50% of children between 1 and 4. The risk of death from HBV- related cirrhosis or liver cancer in Africa has been estimated at approximately 25% for humans who become chronically infected during childhood (State of the World's Children, 2003). Thus 1 in 4 children infected with HBV die of it in Africa's developing countries.

Medical procedures, including tonsillectomy, indiscriminate injections and the reuse or use of nonsterilized syringes have been shown to increase the risk of HBV infection, as has sexual activity (Belo, 2000; Jacobs et al, 1997; Jombo et al, 2005; Otegbayo, Fasola, and Abja, 2003; Pido and Kagimu, 2005).

Chronic carriage of HBV is indicated by the persistence of HBsAg (the hepatitis B "s" antigen) 6 months after exposure. After decades of chronic infection, HBsAg carriers go on to develop HCC. It has been hypothesized that, since the hepatocarcinogenic process involves a complex interplay between the virus and host hepatocytes, both genomes contribute to the final pathogenic outcomes, either individually or synergistically (Liu and Kao, 2007).

HBV may be grouped into 8 genotypes based on genetic variation in HbsAg. Globally, there is significant geographic variation in the prevalence of HBV genotypes (Bjornsdottir et al, 2005; Chu et al, 2003; Ganne-Carrié et al, 2006; Kato et al, 2004; Westland et al, 2003). There is also growing evidence that different HBV genotypes may result in different clinical outcomes, including variation in persistent infection, viral replication and HCC risk. For example, the relative risk of developing HCC is 4.5 (95% CI, 1.86 to 10.90) times higher in black Africans living south of the Sahara who are infected with genotype A (subgenotype B1) compared with those infected with non-A genotypes (Kew et al, 2005).

Most African genotype A isolates appear to belong to subgenotype B1 as a consequence of trade and travel along the eastern coast of Africa by Asians. This subgenotype is mainly found in the southern and eastern regions of Africa, including South Africa, Malawi, Tanzania, Uganda, the Congo and Somalia. Subgenotype A2 or the 'European' subgenotype of A has been isolated from South African carriers of the virus. It has been suggested that this subgenotype originated in southern Africa and was introduced to Europe by European (Portuguese) sailors who travelled to South Africa in the 15th century,(Hannoun e al, 2005).

HCV in Africa

Although HBV is the predominant risk factor for HCC in Africa, HCV has an estimated attributable fraction of 23% in The Gambia. These attributable risk estimates of the burden of HCC resulting from hepatitis viruses are comparable with IARC estimates of 60% and 20% of HCC cases attributable to HBV and HCV respectively throughout sub- Saharan Africa (Kirk, Bah and, Montesano, 2006, Parkin, Bray and Devesa, 2001). In contrast to HBV, most humans infected with HCV become chronic carriers. However, confounding this issue is the difficulty of differentiating liver cancer originating from HBV and HCV infection. The cyclical process of hepatocyte destruction, regeneration and development of fibrosis and eventually cancer requires decades of chronic infection and in many ways is the same with either virus (Brechot, 2004; Brechot et al, 2000; Chu, 2000; Kirk et al 2004, Liang and Heller 2004).

Other studies have estimated the HCV prevalence in sub-Saharan Africa at 3%, although HCV prevalence data in Africa are not as reliable as the data on HBV infections (Madhava, Burgess, and Drucker, 2002). Kirk, Bah and Montesano, (2006) suggest that this is due to the variability and selectivity of the populations studied, inconsistent HCV testing methods, and a lack of data regarding mode of transmission (Kirk, Bah and Montesano, 2006).

WHO estimates that up to 40% of medically related injections given in subSaharan Africa may be unsterile and that HCV transmission through re-use of contaminated syringes and medical equipment appears plausible (Simonsen et al, 1999; Drucker, Alcabes, and Marx, 2001). There is strong epidemiologic evidence that the HCV prevalence observed in Egypt is explained by widespread parenteral transmission during an antischistosomiasis campaign conducted in the 1960s (Frank et al, 2002).

HCC develops only after 2 or more decades of HCV infection, and the increased risk is restricted largely to patients with cirrhosis or advanced fibrosis. The likelihood of development of HCC among HCV-infected persons is estimated to be 1%-3% after 30 years. Once cirrhosis is established, however, HCC develops at an annual rate of 1% to 4% (El Serag, 2002b).

Viral Hepatitis and HCC in Egypt

The rising incidence of HCC in Egypt may be explained by the increasing prevalence of risk factors such as the emergence of Hepatitis C virus (HCV) over the same period of time (Anwar et al, 2008; Mohamed, 2004). Several small-scale hospital-based studies have been conducted to examine the etiologic significance of the primary HCC risk factors in Egypt. These studies have shown the increasing importance of HCV in liver cancer, estimated to account for 40–50% of liver cancer cases, and the declining influence of HBV and HBV/HCV infection, 25% and 15%, respectively (El-Zayadi et al, 2005; Hassan et al, 2001; Strickland et al, 2002).

Lehman and Wilson, (2009) carried out a systematic search of MEDLINE, ISI Web of Science, ScienceDirect and World Health Organization databases which was undertaken for relevant articles regarding HBV and HCV prevalence in Egypt among healthy populations and HCC cases. They calculated weighted mean prevalences for HBV and HCV among the populations of interest and examined differences in prevalence by descriptive features, including age, year and geographic region. Prevalences for HBV and HCV were 6.7% and 13.9% among healthy populations, and 25.9% and 78.5% among HCC cases. Adults had higher prevalences of both infections (Adult HBV= 8.0%, Child HBV =1.6%; Adult HCV =15.7%, Child HCV= 4.0%). Geographically, HBV was higher in the south, whereas HCV was greater in the north (North HBV = 4.6%, South HBV= 11.7%; North HCV = 15.8%, South HCV= 6.7%). Among HCC cases, HBV significantly decreased over time ($p = 0.001$) while HCV did not, suggesting a shift in the relative influences of these viruses in HCC etiology in Egypt.

The contribution of HBV infection, and improvements in screening programmes and diagnostic tools (El-Serag, 2001), as well as the increased survival rate among patients with cirrhosis allowing time for some of them to develop HCC. In part to assess the relative contributions of all these risk factors, Hassan and colleagues (Hassan et al, 2001) studied the attributable risk of HCV in Egyptian patients with HCC. Thirty-three patients with HCC and 35 healthy controls who had a similar socioeconomic status were prospectively enrolled at the University of Cairo National Cancer Institute. Anti-HCV antibodies were present in 75.8% of the patients and in 42.9% of the controls; HBsAg was present in 15.2% of the patients and in 2.9% of the controls. They estimated the attributable fraction of HCC to HCV to be 64% in this study population and 48% in the general Egyptian population. The study concluded that both HCV and HBV infection increase the risk of HCC in Egyptian patients, whereas isolated Schistosomal infection does not. A much larger case-control study with over 200 patients in each group recently reported similar findings (Ezzat et al, 2005) but with an even higher estimate of the attributable fraction (around 90%) of current HCC due to chronic HCV infection. This likely represents the current status of HCV as the predominant and increasing cause underlying the epidemic of HCC in Egypt.

The prevalence of HBV infection in Egypt has been declining over the last two decades (El-Zayadi et al, 2005), while HCV has increased (El-Serag, 2002). Egypt has possibly the highest HCV prevalence worldwide (WHO Global surveillance, 1999) estimated among the general population to be around 14% (Heintges and Wands, 1997).

Overall prevalence of antibody to HCV in the general population is around 15%-20% (Frank et al, 2000). In 1997, the Egyptian Ministry of Health initiated the National Hepatitis C Research Laboratory at the National Tropical Diseases Institute, which was designed to assess the prevalence of HCV infection and evaluate intervention programmes, with the main goal of preventing chronic liver disease and HCC. According to a report from this programme in 2004 (Mohamed, 2004; Pisani et al, 1997), high HCV rates were observed among rural residents, reaching up to 20%. Estimates of national prevalence of HCV and HBV infections were derived from two large community-based surveys in 1996 for estimation of viral hepatitis B and C prevalence in Egypt. In the first study, serum HCV antibody was analyzed for 5000 individuals in a survey of Egyptian workers tested in pre-employment health examination. In the second national survey, serum HCV antibody and HBsAg were analyzed for 7357 individuals in a cluster household study design of representative Egyptian communities in 10 selected governorates representing the four major regional areas of Egypt: metropolitan areas, Lower Egypt, Upper Egypt, and seashore and border areas. The overall anti-HCV prevalence was 18%. The overall adjusted prevalence of anti-HCV and HBsAg was 13.5% and 4.5 respectively. Rural areas had higher age and gender adjusted prevalence (17.2% and 5.5%) than urban areas (7.8% and 3.8%) of these markers respectively. In the same study (Pisani et al, 1997), individuals living in rural areas had significantly more anti-HCV seropostivity than those in urban areas (36.1% and 24.7% respectively). Also individuals living in Cairo and seashore governorates had lower HCV seropostivity (14.7% and 12.7% respectively) than those living in governorates of Upper Egypt and Lower Egypt (29.3% 36.3% respectively).

At the same time that the above prevalence surveys were carried out, studies of the HCV genome confirmed a uniquely high proportion of genotype 4 (over 90%) in Egypt (Ray et al, 2000; Tanaka et al, 2004) and have traced back the genomic mutation for HCV RNA in different samples in Egypt analyzed by both restriction fragments length polyphorism (RFLP) and phylogenic tree construction. To further explore the genetic diversity of HCV in Egypt, sera from 131 Egyptians (56 from community studies, 37 chronic hepatitis patients, 28 HCC (HCC) patients and 10 patients with non-Hodgkin's lymphoma) were examined (Hamid, et al 2007). The majority of the viruses (83 of 131; 63 %) were of subtype 4a, but five other subtypes within genotype 4 were also observed, as well as three genotype 1b, five genotype 1g and one genotype 3a samples. Interestingly, subtype 4o, which was easily identifiable in all three genomic regions, showed an association with HCC, which merits further investigation.

Other surveys conducted during this same time period were designed to assess the modes of HCV transmission in Egypt. The major identified risk factors for acquisition of HCV in Egypt include intravenous injection, body piercing and invasive health care practice (surgeries catheterization dental practice etc.) and occupational exposure (El Gaafary et al, 2005). For many individual cases, however, there is no identifiable risk factor, highlighting the critical need for further research on this issue. Due to the large reservoir in this population, HCV is likely to remain prevalent in Egypt for several decades (Pybus et al, 2003).

The HCV epidemic in Egypt is unique. Egypt developed the world's highest rates of HCV infection over a short period of time, largely due to a massive public health campaign.

The vast majority of infections among individuals aged 30 years and older can be explained by parenteral anti-Schistosomal therapy (PAT) and other iatrogenic exposures. The anti-Schistosomiasis campaign extended from the 1950's to the 1980's, with peak transmission probably occurring during the 1960s and 1970s. In 1982, praziquantal, an oral treatment for Schistosomiasis, was introduced, and the use of PAT declined. Since Schistosomiasis was a greater problem in rural regions, these populations were more affected by the PAT campaign, and consequently, HCV transmission. With iatrogenic infections nearly eliminated, person-to-person transmission is presently the dominant route, which should preserve the urban/rural disparity. Higher rates of HCV infection should manifest as higher rates of HCC.

Earlier research efforts to discover the causes of HCC in Egypt focused on a variety of tropical diseases, including schistosomiasis and its relation to HCV infection. The changes in prevalence of HCV is very well correlated in time and geographical regions to the mass treatment injection campaigns for Schistosomiasis during the years 1950-1980 (Frank, et al 2000; Ghaffar et al, 1991; Mohamed, 2004). It was hypothesized that the risk factor for HCV transmission that specifically sets Egypt apart from other countries is a personal history of parenteral anti-schistosomal therapy (PAT). A review of the Egyptian PAT mass-treatment campaigns, discontinued only in the 1980s, shows a very high potential for transmission of bloodborne pathogens. A cohort-specific HCV prevalence was lower in children and young adults than in older cohorts. These lower prevalence rates coincided with the gradual and final replacement of PAT with oral anti-schistosomal drugs at different points in time. Egypt's mass campaigns of PAT may represent the world's largest iatrogenic transmission of bloodborne pathogens (Frank et al, 2000).

Schistosomiasis also induces immune suppression, which could result in increased persistence viremia, following acute infection of either hepatitis B or C (Ezzat et al, 2005). The combination of Schistosomiasis and HCV infection was found to have more severe effects on liver pathology and progression into worsening complications than HCV infection alone. Fortunately, recent epidemiologic surveys have reported a declining prevalence of Schistosoma infection (El Khoby, 2000).

Aflatoxin (AFB1) in Africa

Many agricultural products are vulnerable to attack by a group of fungi that produce toxic metabolites called mycotoxins, which includes aflatoxin. Aflatoxins are toxic and carcinogenic metabolites of moulds, mainly *Aspergillus flavus* and *parasiticum* that contaminate a variety of agricultural commodities, particularly peanuts, maize and cottonseed, in countries with hot and humid climates. Aflatoxin B1 (AFB1) is the major metabolite produced by these moulds. Aflatoxins are classified as human carcinogens based on sufficient evidence of carcinogenicity (IARC, 1987). In Africa, food products contaminated with aflatoxin B1 include cereal (maize, groundnuts [peanuts], sorghum, pearl millet, rice, wheat), oilseeds (groundnut, soybean, sunflower, cotton), spices (chilies, black pepper, coriander, turmeric, zinger), tree nuts (almonds, pistachio, walnuts, coconut) and milk. Early epidemiologic studies showed a clear association between exposure to aflatoxin B1 contaminated foods and risk of HCC (Jackson and Groopman, 1999).

The identification of aflatoxin B1 biomarkers in molecular epidemiological studies has permitted a better understanding of aflatoxin in HCC pathogenesis (Garner, Dvorackova and Tursi 1988; Groopman 1999, Groopman, Cain and Kensler 1988; Sabbioni et al, 1987; Wild et al 1990; Wild et al, 1993; Wild CP, et al, 1986; Sizaret et al, 1982).

The p53 gene, TP53, is known as the "tumor-suppressing gene and "the guardian of the genome," because it delivers a message to cancerous cells to program their own self-destruction. A molecular-centered review of ~1,000 HCC tumors data taken from the IARC p53 mutation database demonstrate a clear association between a particular kind of mutation (249ser mutation), exposure to AFB1, and incidence of HCC (Hainaut and Hollstein, 2000). The data suggest that the 249ser mutation may represent past exposure to AFB1 and prove useful in epidemiologic studies to predict HCC risk, target preventive interventions, or serve as an intermediate endpoint in chemoprevention trials (Kirk, Bah and Montesano, 2006).

Aflatoxins and HCC in Egypt

In Egypt, while HBV and HCV may account for the majority of HCC, there is suggestive evidence for an additional etiologic role of aflatoxin in hepatocarcinogenesis. Methods of grain storage are not controlled, and there is lack of awareness of the dangers of improper storage. A study was conducted in 2 districts in Upper Egypt to measure the presence of fungal population in silage. Aflatoxins showed the highest incidence rates of occurrence in 22.5% of all samples analyzed. Other mycotoxins were detected in all samples (El Shanawany et al, 2005). Mohamed et al. (1999) detected a significant higher percent of aflatoxins in the serum of Egyptian patients with HCC compared to their controls; with two fold increased risk. Aflatoxins may cause mutations in the tumor suppressor gene p53 that act as initiating agents leading to liver cell hyperplasia and HCC. In support of this hypothesis, El- Kafrawy et al. (2005) documented the presence of p53 codon 249 mutations associated with aflatoxin exposure in a sample of HCC tumor tissues analyzed by gene chip analysis in Egypt.

Hifnawy et al, 2004 suggested that the progressive nature of HCV-related liver diseases was influenced by aflatoxin exposure. The quantitative identification of the possible aflatoxins contamination in six urban and eleven rural areas using high performance liquid chromatography technique, revealed that the prevalence of AFB1 contamination in corn, wheat, peanut, lupine, white rice, cowpea, fava bean and brown rice was 64.7%, 53%, 53%, 47%, 47%, 41%, 29.4% and 29.4% respectively. A positive correlation was found between aflatoxin and positive HCV-PCR together with liver disease progression to stage G3S3, that was indicative of HCC.

Several studies were carried out to evaluate the level of aflatoxins in food products in different governorates in Egypt (Amra et al, 2007). From Qaluobia and Kafr El- Sheikh Governorates, one hundred samples of imported and local wheat grains were collected (*Triticum sativum*) and examined for the natural occurrence of aflatoxins during 2000-2001. Results indicated that both local and imported samples were positive for aflatoxin B1 (17.5 % and 20% respectively), and the concentration ranged from 3-25 μg/kg. The level of aflatoxins was dependant on the area of collection as well as the season of the year.

During 2004, samples were collected from Menofeya Governorate (4 different districts: Mnuf, Quisna, Shibin El-Kom and Tala) to survey the natural occurrence of aflatoxins in local and imported corn grains and some corn products. The results showed that the local and imported corn grains were naturally infected with fungi belonging to genera of *Aspergillus*. The concentrations of aflatoxin B1 ranged between 5.8 and 7.5 μg/kg corn grains, while the concentration of aflatoxin B2 varied from 2.7 to 4.1 μg/kg corn grains.

In a study to screen for biomarkers of aflatoxin exposure in Egypt, Polychronaki et al, 2006 assessed the level and frequency of breast milk AFM1 as a biomarker of maternal exposure. Breast milk samples were collected from a selected group of 388 Egyptian lactating mothers of children attending the New El-Qalyub Hospital, Qalyubiyah governorate, Egypt, during May-September 2003. Approximately 36% of mothers tested positive for AFM1. Non-working status, obesity, high corn oil consumption, number of children, and early lactation stage (<1 month), contributed to the occurrence of AF in breast milk.

The same research group continued their study (Polychronaki et al, 2007), following up with fifty of those women who were AFM1 positive at baseline; they were revisited monthly for 12 months to assess the temporal variation in breast milk AFM1. In a multilevel regression model of the data there was a highly significant ($p<0.001$) effect of month of sampling on the frequency of AFM1 detection with summer months having the highest frequency (>80%) and winter months the lowest frequency (<20%) of detection. The duration of lactation and peanut consumption also contributed to the model. The identification and understanding of factors determining the presence of toxicants in human milk is important and may provide a knowledge driven basis for controlling the transfer of chemicals to infants.

Hassan, et al 2006 assessed the presence of aflatoxin (AFM1) in both mothers' milk and the infants' sera. Fifty healthy breast lactating mothers and their infants who were exclusively breast fed for at least 4 months were included. Twenty-four mothers (48%) and their infants had detectable levels of aflatoxin with the following mean contamination levels (ng/ml); mothers' serum of 8.9+/-4.2, mothers' milk of 1.9+/-0.6 and infants' serum of 1.8+/-0.9.

Role of Pesticides in the Etiology of HCC

Occupational exposure pesticides may have a contributory role in the etiology or progression of HCC. According to Ezzat et al. (2005), a major segment of the Egyptian population is employed in agriculture and uses pesticides routinely to control insects, weeds, rodents, and fungal infections of crops and livestock. A case-control study was carried out to investigate pesticides as environmental risk factors for HCC while taking into account viral risk factors. 236 subjects with confirmed HCC were recruited from the National Cancer Institute, Cairo University, Egypt, and 236 controls matched on sex, age group and urban-rural status recruited from the Orthopaedic Department, Cairo University Hospital, Egypt. Among rural males, the adjusted odds ratio (OR) for organophosphorus compounds was 2.7 and for carbamates it was 2.9. No statistically significant associations between HCC and household application of pesticides were observed for urban males or for females. As expected, the strongest risk factors for HCC in this study were HCV RNA and current HBV infection. This study therefore suggested that exposures to organophophorus and carbamate pesticides are additive risk factors to current HCV and HBV infection among rural males. Future investigation should address the possible hepatocarcinogenicity of pesticides using biomarkers of exposure and other techniques to better estimate dose-response relationships.

Hepatitis C Comorbidities

Several studies have demonstrated that the outcome of chronic hepatitis C infection is profoundly influenced by a variety of comorbidities. Many of these comorbidities have a significant influence on the response to antiviral therapy and the outcome of liver disease, often reducing the chance of achieving a sustained virological response. The most important comorbidities include hepatitis B virus coinfection, metabolic syndrome, and intestinal bacterial overgrowth, schistosomiasis, iron overload, alcohol abuse, and excessive smoking (El-Zayadi, 2009).

Dietary Iron Overload in Africans and HCC

More recently, another important cause of HCC has been recognized. The liver is the main organ of iron storage and high hepatic iron concentrations, comparable with those in the genetically determined iron storage disease, Hemochromatosis gene (HFE). In African Blacks hemochromatosis, result from the consumption over time of large volumes of home-brewed beer rich in iron. Over time, the resulting hepatic iron overload may be complicated by HCC development (Kew, 2010).

Alcohol and HCC

There is compelling epidemiologic data, supported by animal experiments, confirming the increased risk of cancer associated with alcohol consumption. Cancer of the liver associated with alcohol usually occurs in the setting of cirrhosis (Voigt, 2005).

Interactions among Risk Factors

Sylla et al.m 1999 expressed the importance of interactions between HBV infection and exposure to aflatoxins in the development of HCC. There is evidence from both epidemiological studies and animal models that the 2 factors can act synergistically to increase the risk of HCC (Sylla et al, 1999). Co-infection with HBV and HCV could be considered a potential HCC risk, higher than the risk attributed to infection with either type of virus alone. A multivariate analysis done by Benvegnu and Alberti shows that the risk of HCC is significantly higher in HBV and HCV co-infected patients, compared with those with single HBV surface antigen or anti-HCV positivity. These results indicate different patterns of risk factors, morphogenesis, and incidence of HCC development in HBV- and HCV-associated cirrhosis, suggesting different mechanisms of carcinogenesis (Benvegnu and Alberti, 2001). Alcohol may act as a co-carcinogen, and it has strong synergistic effects with other risk factors, including HBV, HCV, aflatoxin, vinyl chloride, obesity, and diabetes mellitus. Alcohol enhances the effects of environmental carcinogens directly; it also enhances them indirectly by contributing to nutritional deficiency and impairing immunological tumor surveillance. Acetylaldehyde, the main metabolite of alcohol, causes hepatocellular injury and is an important factor in causing increased oxidant stress, which damages DNA (Voigt, 2005).

Human immunodeficiency virus (HIV) is also endemic in sub-Saharan Africa and co-infection between this virus and HBV occurs in 17% of the Black population. Since the introduction of highly active antiretroviral therapy (HAART) for HIV/AIDS, increasing numbers of patients co-infected with HIV and HCV or HBV have been reported to develop HCC. One possible explanation for this observation is that the considerably longer survival of patients allows sufficient time for hepatitis virus-induced HCC to develop. Another explanation is that the immune deficiency caused by HIV infection results in higher HBV viral loads, which are known to increase the risk of malignant transformation of hepatocytes. Alternatively, co-infection with HIV may directly enhance the hepatocarcinogenic potential of the hepatitis viruses (Kew, 2010).

Approaches to HCC Prevention

Molecular epidemiology studies may develop early detection markers and provide a better understanding of the occurrence of genetic and epigenetic alterations in the natural history of liver carcinogenesis which are vital in designing strategies to reduce HCC mortality (Montesano, Hainaut and Wild, 1997; Wild, Law, and Roman, 2002 and Hussain and Harris, 1998).

Most interventions in developing countries are aimed at preventing exposure to carcinogens or treating viral infections. Treatment of HCV with antiretrovirals has resulted in sustained viral response (SVR), or nondetectable virus 6 months after end of treatment (EOT) about 19 to 29% of the time. When there is no virus at EOT, the virus will relapse after treatment has stopped, with 90% of relapses occurring in the first 12 weeks. If the virus remains undetectable for 24 weeks after EOT, the relapse rate is 1 or 2 % in patients that have been followed up to 7 years. The case is different with HBV which can and does "hide," while still being present in a non-replicative state, although antiviral therapy in the treatment of HBV has also been proven effective. Although these drugs appear to reduce the incidence of HCC, they are expensive and unavailable in most developing countries. Even in developed countries where resources are available, less than 10% of humans with chronic HBV and HCV have received antiviral therapy and the incidence of liver cancer is doubling (Dooley et al, 1986; Hoofnagle et al, 1988; Wong et al, 1993; Shaw and Locarnini, 2004;.Lai et al, 1997; Dienstag et al, 1999; Liaw et al, 2000; Janssen et al 2005; Cooksley et al, 2005; Cooksley et al, 2003).

Anti-viral treatment against HBV or HCV may interrupt or delay progression to HCC. The lengthy asymptomatic period prior to HCC diagnosis at advanced stages provides opportunities for earlier HCC detection. Key to the success of these secondary preventive interventions will be identifying the target groups for which antivirals or screening are appropriate. The quantitative plasma 249ser p53 mutation is a prototypical example of a marker of both exposure and HCC risk. Screening and prevention strategies could be tailored to individuals based on 249ser p53 levels. Similarly, recent data on the predictiveness of HBV DNA levels for HCC suggest that appropriate management should be tailored to the specific levels and persistence of HBV viral load. Analysis of multiple markers can result in a 'molecular profile' of each stage of progressive liver disease from chronic viral infection to significant fibrosis/ cirrhosis to HCC. These 'molecular profiles' may further delineate individuals for whom aggressive monitoring may be the most beneficial. Unfortunately, once advanced HCC is diagnosed, limited options exist for limiting complications or reducing mortality from HCC.

Prevention of chronic HBV infection could be achieved by the universal inclusion of the HBV vaccine in the Expanded Programme of Immmunization in all sub-Saharan countries. WHO/UNICEF reported that by 2005, 45% of children in Africa had received safe and effective HB vaccinations, (Hall and Smith, 1999; WHO/UNICEF, 2006). WHO estimates that approximately 60% of all Black African infants are now receiving the vaccine. This approach gives promise of the eventual elimination of HBV infection and, at a suitable interval thereafter, HBV-induced HCC.

Vaccination against HBV in infancy appears to be the most effective approach to prevent HCC in developing countries (Kao and Chen, 1982). A safe, effective HBV vaccine has been available since the early 1980s (Blumberg and London, 1982 and Muraskin, 1995). After a decade of follow-up in The Gambia, the GHIS reported HB vaccine efficacy in children at 9 and 4 years of age (Viviani, et al, 1999; Fortuin et al, 1993; Kirk, 1997). Chronic HBV carriage prevalence was 10% among unvaccinated children compared with <1% among vaccinated children. Protection against HBV infection was over 80% and protection against chronic carriage over 90%.

Since then, the HB vaccine has been given to millions of humans worldwide and has been found to be one of the safest and most efficacious vaccines in use (Whittle et al, 2002 and Kirk, 2003). While questions remain about the need to ensure protection using booster doses, efficacy against chronic HBV infection remains high for up to 15 years (Liao et al, 1999; Lin et al, 2003; Wu et al, 1999; Kane and Brooks, 2002). However, prevention of chronic HCV infection is a far more difficult problem since vaccines for prevention of HCV are not available. General public health measures to minimise the spread of the virus, including detecting asymptomatic infection in high risk individuals, need to be introduced.

Prevention programmes can also be implemented against HCV infection by changing personal behavioural patterns and/or cultural habits which are considered as risk factors for HCV such as injection with contaminated syringes, blood transfusion, surgical operations, venous catheterization, use of common syringes, dental treatment and circumcision at home.

In parallel, reduction of exposure to AFB1, may also prove an effective primary prevention measure. This can be achieved either at community (via good agriculture practices) or individual levels (treatment or dietary interventions). Easier methods for field detection and quantification of aflatoxin contamination of foodstuffs could aid epidemiologic studies of exposure and behavioral intervention trials aimed at reducing contamination (Carlson, et al, 2000).

Heavy lifetime exposures to aflatoxin B1 continue in West Africa, according to GHIS data. In high exposure environments, community interventions aimed at modifying post-harvest practices may have the greatest impact on lowering aflatoxin contamination levels in groundnuts and other subsistence crops. However, because groundnuts are the primary income source for many Gambians, the practice of selling the least visibly contaminated groundnuts and keeping contaminated groundnuts for personal consumption continues (Kirk, Bah and Montesano, 2006). Behavioral interventions, such as modification of food storage practices, require minimal direct expenditures; however, the difficulty in changing cultural practices also must be recognized (Turner et al, 2005). A community intervention study in rural Guinea, West Africa, of post-harvest interventions demonstrated a reduction in aflatoxin B1 contamination of food stores. At the other end of the technology spectrum, genetic engineering could produce aflatoxin resistant crops, however, there are significant scientific, ethical and environmental barriers to this approach (Wild and Hall, 2000).

Prevention of dietary exposure to aflatoxin B_1 should also be possible in the long-term. It has already been shown that simple, low-technology, and inexpensive practices can result in a striking decrease in dietary exposure to the fungal toxin (Kuniholm et al, 2008). However, for these interventions to be successful on a wide scale in resource-poor countries will require training of subsistence farmers in the handling of the responsible crops and providing the appropriate storage facilities required.

Amra, et al, 2007 studied the effect of processing steps of corn products on the destruction of aflatoxins for popcorn and porridge. The results of the trial indicated that the process of popcorn and porridge preparation had a significant effect on aflatoxins' destruction. The temperature of preparing and treatment with 5% salt (Sodium Chloride) yielded the highest destruction rates (ranging from 90 to 97% depending on the specific compound measured). Such effects of processing of corn grains on the fate of residual aflatoxins should stimulate more trials aiming at prevention of aflatoxins health hazards.

Several probiotic bacteria are able to bind AFB1 in vitro, including *Lactobacillus rhamnosus* LC-705 and *Propionibacterium freudenreichii subsp. shermanii* JS (Gratz, Mykkanen and El-Nezami, 2005). A mixture of these two probiotics is used by the food and feed industry as biopreservative (Bioprofit), making it a promising candidate for future applications. Consequently, ongoing studies in Egypt and elsewhere are investigating the *in vitro* and *ex vivo* ability of this probiotic mixture to bind AFB1. In vitro experiments, 57 to 66% of AFB1 was removed from the solution by the probiotic mixture, but only 38 to 47% could be extracted from the bacterial surface. In ex vivo experiments, only up to 25% of AFB1 was bound by bacteria, and tissue uptake of AFB1 was significantly reduced when probiotic bacteria were present in the duodenal loop. Furthermore, the effect of intestinal mucus on the bacterial binding ability was investigated in vitro and was found to significantly reduce AFB1 binding by the probiotic mixture. Such probiotic supplementation reduces the biologically effective dose of aflatoxin exposure, and may thereby offer an effective dietary approach to prevent the development of liver cancer.

El-Zayadi et al, 2010 carried out a retrospective study to evaluate the effect of surveillance on early detection of HCC among cirrhotic patients from 2003 to 2008. Patients examined every 6 months using ultrasound and α-fetoprotein (α-FP) (group A) and those diagnosed for the first time symptomatically or incidentally (group B). Groups were compared for α-FP level, tumour characteristics, severity of liver disease; tumour staging was evaluated, in addition to the potential therapeutic options. Group A comprised 122 HCC cases and group B 473 cases. Surveillance improved HCC detection: at the stage of single nodule in 62.3% in group A versus 52.2% in group B, ($P = 0.046$) and reduced the percentage of HCC with portal vein thrombosis in 16.4 versus 33.8%, ($P = 0.000$) and the percentage of α-FP >400 ng/ml in 19.5 versus 32.6%, ($P = 0.006$) in groups A and B, respectively. Surveillance doubled the detection of HCC at early stage of BCLC (25.4 vs. 11.9% $P = 0.000$) and doubled the patients' chance for loco-regional ablation (12.3 vs. 5.9%, $P = 0.015$) and liver transplantation (10.7 vs. 3.2%, $P = 0.001$) in groups A and B, respectively. The authors concluded that HCC surveillance increases early detection of HCC and doubled the chances for curative options.

Conclusion

Studies have indicated that the high incidence of HCC in sub-Saharan Africa resulted from childhood HBV infection and longterm exposure to aflatoxin B1, as well as the high percentage of chronic HCV infection in some areas of Africa. The ASR for Egyptians was 20.6 for males, 5.2 for females, and 12.8 for both sexes together. The Egyptian rates for males were 7 times the highest MECC rate, and more than 3 times the corresponding US SEER rate. For Egyptian females, the rate was more than 3 times the highest MECC rate and more than twice the US SEER rate. Compared with rates reported in *Cancer Incidence in Five Continents*, Egypt ranked next to East and Southeast Asian countries and 3 African countries. In Egypt, extensive research over the past decade has documented high and increasing HCC incidence resulting from chronic HBV and HCV infections, and possibly augmented by agricultural pesticide exposures and dietary aflatoxin exposure. Studies worldwide have shown that interventions aimed at preventing or limiting exposure to HBV, HCV, and aflatoxin B1 are effective at lowering the incidence of new cases of liver cancer. Antiviral therapies hold promise for interrupting the effects of infection by HBV and HCV, although these are expensive and unavailable to most in resource-limited countries. It is clearly shown that HB vaccination can be implemented in the national immunization programmes and that immunization is highly effective in the preventing chronic HBV infection. Vaccination for HBV has been available for 2 decades, and data from The Gambia Hepatitis Intervention Study (GH IS), as well as studies worldwide, suggest that this vaccination is highly effective in preventing HBV infection. In the absence of vaccination for HCV, further investigation of the risk factors and modes of transmission of HCV is required to reduce infection rates and to prevent future cases of HCC. Using population-based sampling of markers of HBV, HCV and AFB1 exposure could provide useful data in formulating reasoned, cost-effective and country-specific intervention strategies to reduce HCC.

References

Abdel-Wahab M: El-Ghawalby N; Mostafa M; Sultan A; ElSadany M; Fathy O; Salah T; Ezzat F. (2007). Epidemiology of hepatocellular carcinoma in lower Egypt, Mansoura Gastroenterology Center. *Hepato-Gastroenterology.;* 54:157-62.

Allain JP; Candotti D; Soldan K; Sarkodie F; Phelps B; Giachetti C; Shyamala V; Yeboah F; Anokwa M; Owusu-Ofori S; Opare-Sem O (2003). The risk of hepatitis B virus infection by transfusion in Kumasi, Ghana. *Blood.;* 101:2419-25.

Anwar WA, Khaled HM. Amra HA, El-Nezami H, Loffredo CA. Changing Pattern of Hepatocellular Carcinoma (HCC) and its Risk Factors in Egypt: Possibilities for Prevention, *Mutation Research,*Volume 659, Issues 1-2, July-August 2008, Pages 176-184 (2008).

Amra HA.; Masheal SF; Ebba MM; Bakr, A.A; Nogaim, Q.A and Anwar WA (2007). Aflatoxins level in some Egyptian Crops collected from different governorates: Possibilities for Detection and Prevention (Poster No. 26 *) 5th International Conference on Environmental Mutagens in Human Populations*: "Identification of Environmental Hazards and Promotion of Health", Antalya, Turkey, May 20 – 24.

Belo AC (2000) Prevalence of hepatitis B virus markers in surgeons in Lagos, Nigeria. East Afr Med J.; 77:283-5.

Benvegnu L, & Alberti A. (2001) Patterns of hepatocellular carcinoma development in hepatitis B virus and hepatitis C virus related cirrhosis. *Antiviral Res*; 52:199-207.

Bile K, Mohamud O, Aden C, Isse A, Norder H, Nilsson L, Magnius L. (1992) The risk for hepatitis A, B, and C at two institutions for children in Somalia with different socioeconomic conditions. *Am J Trop Med Hyg.;* 47:357-64.

Blumberg BS, & London WT. (1982) Hepatitis B virus: pathogenesis and prevention of primary cancer of the liver. *Cancer.;* 50:265765.

Brechot C. (2004). Pathogenesis of hepatitis B virus-related hepatocellular carcinoma: old and new paradigms. *Gastroenterology.;* 127:S56-61.

Brechot C, Gozuacik D, Murakami Y, Paterlini-Brechot P. (2000). Molecular bases for the development of hepatitis B virus (HBV) related hepatocellular carcinoma (HCC). *Semin. Cancer Biol.;* 10:211-231.

Bjornsdottir TB, Stanzeit B, Sallberg M, Love A, Hultgren C. (2005). Changing prevalence of hepatitis B virus genotypes in Iceland. *J Med Virol.;* 77:481-5.

Bosch FX, Ribes J, Borras J. (2002). Epidemiology of primary liver cancer. *Semin Liver Dis;* 19: 271-285 (1999).

Boyle P. The globalization of cancer. *Lancet;* 368: 629-630

Bruix J, Sherman M, Llovet JM, Beaugrand M, Lencioni R, Burroughs AK, Christensen E, Pagliaro L, Colombo M, Rodes J. EASL (2001). Panel of Experts on HCC. Clinical management of hepatocellular carcinoma. Conclusions of the Barcelona-2000 EASL Conference. *J Hepatol;* 35: 421-430.

Carlson,M.A., Bargeron,C.B., Benson,R.C., Fraser,A.B., Phillips,T.E., Velky,J.T., Groopman,J.D., Strickland,P.T and Ko,H.W. (2000). An automated, handheld biosensor for aflatoxin. *Biosens. Bioelectron.,* 14, 841–848

Chiaramonte M, Stroffolini T, Ngatchu T, Rapicetta M, Lantum D, Kaptue L, Chionne P, Conti S, Sarrecchia B, Naccarato R. (1991). Hepatitis B virus infection in Cameroon: a seroepidemiological survey in city school children. *J Med Virol.;* 33:95-9.

Chu CM. (2000). Natural history of chronic hepatitis B virus infection in adults with emphasis on the occurrence of cirrhosis and hepatocellular carcinoma. *J. Gastroenterol. Hepatol.;* 15:E25-30.

Chu CJ, Keeffe EB, Han SH, Perrillo RP, Min AD, Soldevila-Pico C, Carey W, Brown RS Jr, Luketic VA, Terrault N, Lok AS. (2003). Hepatitis B virus genotypes in the United States: results of a nationwide study. *Gastroenterology.;* 125:444-51.

Colombo M. (1999).Hepatitis C virus and hepatocellular carcinoma. *Semin Liver Dis;* 19: 263-269.

Cooksley WG, Piratvisuth T, Lee SD, Mahachai V, Chao YC, Tanwandee T, Chutaputti A, Chang WY, Zahm FE, Pluck N. (2003). Peginterferon alpha-2a (40 kDa): an advance in the treatment of hepatitis B e antigen-positive chronic hepatitis B. *J Viral Hepatol;*10:298-305.

Cooksley G, Manns M, Lau G K K, Liaw Y F, Marcellin P, Chow W C. (2005). Effect of genotype and other baseline factors on response to peginterferon alfa-2a (40 KD) (Pegasys) in HBeAg-positive chronic hepatitis B: results from a large, randomized study. *J Hepatol;*42:30.

Darwish MA, Amer AF, El-Moeity AA, Darwish NM. (1997) Association of hepatitis C virus with liver cirrhosis and hepatocellular carcinoma compared with hepatitis B virus in Egyptian patients. *Journal of the Egyptian Public Health Association;* 72:569-89.

Dienstag JL, Schiff ER, Wright TL, Perrillo RP, Hann HW, Goodman Z, Crowther L, Condreay LD, Woessner M, Rubin M, Brown NA. (1999). Lamivudine as initial treatment for chronic hepatitis B in the United States. *N Engl J Med.;* 341:1256-63.

Dooley JS, Davis GL, Peters M, Waggoner JG, Goodman Z, Hoofnagle JH. (1986). Pilot study of recombinant human alpha-interferon for chronic type B hepatitis.*Gastroenterology.;* 90:150-7.

Drucker,E., Alcabes,P.G and Marx,P.A. (2001). The injection century: massive unsterile injections and the emergence of human pathogens. *Lancet;* 358:1989-92.

El Gaafary MM, Rekacewicz C, Abdel-Rahman AG, Allam MF, El Hosseiny M, Abdel Hamid M, Colombani F, Sultan Y, El-Aidy S, Fontanet A, Mohamed MI (2005). Surveillance of acute hepatitis C in Cairo, Egypt. J *Med Virol;* 76:520-5.

El-Kafrawy SA, Abdel-Hamid M, El-Daly M, Nada O, Ismail A, Ezzat S, Abdel-Latif S, Abdel-Hamid A, Shields PG, Loffredo C (2005). P53 mutations in hepatocellular carcinoma patients in Egypt. *Int J Hyg Environ Health;* 208(4):263-70

El Khoby T, (2000). Schistosomiasis in Egypt. *Amer J Trop Med & Hygiene volume* 62:88-99.

El-Nady GM, Ling R, Harrison TJ. (2003). Gene expression in HCV-associated hepatocellular carcinoma-upregulation of a gene encoding a protein related to the ubiquitin-conjugating enzyme. *Liver Int;* 23: 329-337

El-Serag HB. (2001). Epidemiology of hepatocellular carcinoma. *Clin Liver Dis;* 5: 87-107.

El-Serag HB (2002). Hepatocellular carcinoma: an epidemiologic view. *J Clin Gastroenterol;* 35 (Suppl 2): S72-78.

El Serag HB (2002b). Hepatocellular carcinoma and hepatitis C in the United States. *Hepatology;* 36:S74-S83.

El-Serag HB, and Rudolph KL (2007). Hepatocellular carcinoma: epidemiology and molecular carcinogenesis. *Gastroenterology.;* 132:2557-76.

El Shanawany AA, Mostafa ME, Barakat A (2005). Fungal populations and mycotoxins in silage in Assiut and Sohag governorates in Egypt, with a special reference to characteristic Aspergilli toxins. *Mycopathologia;* 159:281-9.

El-Zayadi AR, Badran HM., Shawky S, Emara S, El-Bareedy A, and Sobhi,M. (2010). Effect of surveillance for hepatocellular carcinoma on tumor staging and treatment decisions in Egyptian patients, *Hepatol IntJune;* 4(2): 500–506.

El-Zayadi AR, Abaza H, Shawky S, Mohamed MK, Selim OE, Badran HM. (2001). Prevalence and epidemiological features of hepatocellular carcinoma in Egypt-a single center experience. *Hepatol Res;* 19: 170-179.

El-Zayadi AR, Badran HM, Barakat EMF, Attia MED, Shawky S, Mohamed MK, Selim O, Saeid A (2005). Hepatocellular carcinoma in Egypt: A single center study over a decade. *World J Gastroenterol;* 11(33): 5193-5198.

El-Zayadi AR (2009), Hepatitis C comorbidities affecting the course and response to therapy, *World J Gastroenterol* October 28; 15(40): 4993-4999.

Ezzat S, Abdel-Hamid M, Eissa SA, Mokhtar N, Labib NA, El-Ghorory L, Mikhail NN, Abdel-Hamid A, Hifnawy T, Strickland GT, Loffredo CA (2005). Associations of pesticides, HCV, HBV, and hepatocellular carcinoma in Egypt *Int J Hyg Environ Health.;* 208(5):329-39.

Fattovich G. (1998). Progression of hepatitis B and C to hepatocellular carcinoma in Western countries. *Hepatogastroenterology;* 45 (Suppl 3): 1206-1213.

Fortuin M, Chotard J, Jack AD, Maine NP, Mendy M, Hall AJ, Inskip HM, George MO, Whittle HC. Efficacy of hepatitis B vaccine in The Gambian expanded programme on immunisation. *Lancet.* 1993; 341:1129-31.

Frank C, Mohamed MK, Strickland GT, Lavanchy D, Arthur RR, Magder LS, et al. (2000). The role of parenteral antischistosomal therapy in the spread of hepatitis C virus in Egypt. *Lancet;* 355:887-91.

Frank C, Mohamed MK, Strickland GT, Lavanchy D, Arthur RR, Magder LS, El Khoby T, Abdel-Wahab Y, Aly Ohn ES, Anwar W, Sallam I (2002). The role of parenteral antischistosomal therapy in the spread of hepatitis C virus in Egypt. *Lancet.* 355:887-891.

Ganne-Carrié N, Williams V, Kaddouri H, Trinchet JC, DziriMendil S, Alloui C, Hawajri NA, Dény P, Beaugrand M, Gordien E (2006). Significance of hepatitis B virus genotypes A to E in a cohort of patients with chronic hepatitis B in the Seine Saint Denis District of Paris (France*). J Med Virol.;* 78:335-40.

Garner RC, Dvorackova I, Tursi F (1988). Immunoassay procedures to detect exposure to aflatoxin B1 and benzo(a)pyrene in animals and man at the DNA level. *Int. Arch. Occup. Environ. Health.;* 60:145-50.

Ghaffar YA, Fattah SA, Kamel M, Badr RM, Mahomed FF, Strickland GT (1991). The impact of endemic schistosomiasis on acute viral hepatitis. *Am J Trop Med Hyg;* 45: 743-750

GHIS. The Gambia Hepatitis Intervention Study (1987). The Gambia Hepatitis Study Group. *Cancer Res.;*47:5782-7.

Gratz S, Mykkanen H, El-Nezami H. (2005). Aflatoxin B1 binding by a mixture of Lactobacillus and Propionibacterium: in vitro versus ex vivo, *J Food Prot.* Nov; 68(11):2470-4.

Groopman JD. Molecular dosimetry methods for assessing human aflatoxin exposures. In D. Eaton and JD Groopman (eds). (1999). *The Toxicology of Aflatoxins: Human Health, Veterinary and Agricultural Significance.* Academic Press, Inc., San Diego, CA, pp. 259-79.

Groopman JD, Cain LG, Kensler TW (1988). Aflatoxin exposure in human populations: measurements and relationship to cancer. *Crit. Rev. Toxicol.;* 19:113-45.

Hainaut P, Hollstein M (2000). p53 and human cancer: the first ten thousand mutations. *Adv. Cancer Res.*; 77:81-137.

Hall AJ, Smith PG (1999). Prevention of hepatocellular cancer: one of the most cost-effective ways to reduce adult mortality? *Br. J. Cancer.;* 81:1097-8.

Hamid MA, Mai El-Daly,Vilma Molnegren, Sherif El-Kafrawy,1,4 Sohair Abdel-Latif, Gamal Esmat, G. Thomas Strickland, Christopher Loffredo, Jan Albert and Anders Widell. (2007). Genetic diversity in hepatitis C virus in Egypt and possible association with hepatocellular carcinoma. *Journal of General Virology*, 88, 1526–1531.

Hannoun C, Soderstrom A, Norkrans G, Lindh M. (2005). Phylogeny of African complete genomes reveals a West African genotype A subtype of hepatitis B virus and relatedness between Somali and Asian A1 sequences. *J Gen Virol.* 86:2163-7.

Hassan MM, Zaghloul AS, El-Serag HB, Soliman O, Patt YZ, Chappell CL, Beasley RP, Hwang LY (2001). The role of hepatitis C in hepatocellular carcinoma: a case control study among Egyptian patients.*J Clin Gastroenterol. Aug;33*(2):123-6.

Hassan AM, Sheashaa HA, Abdel Fatah MF, Ibrahim AZ, Gaber OA (2006). Does aflatoxin as an environmental mycotoxin adversely affect the renal and hepatic functions of Egyptian lactating mothers and their infants? A preliminary report. : *Int Urol Nephrol.;* 38(2):339-42

Heintges T, Wands JR (1997). Hepatitis C virus: epidemiology and transmission. *Hepatology;* 26: 521-526.

Hepatitis B fact sheet no. 204 (2000). Geneva: World Health Organization, Oct.

Hifnawy MS, Mangoud AM, Eissa MH, Nor Edin E, Mostafa Y, Abouel-Magd Y, Sabee EI, Amin I, Ismail A, Morsy TA, Mahrous S, Afefy AF, el-Shorbagy E, el-Sadawy M, Ragab H, Hassan MI, el-Hady G, Saber M (2004). The role of aflatoxin-contaminated food materials and HCV in developing hepatocellular carcinoma in Al-Sharkia Governorate, Egypt. *J Egypt Soc Parasitol.*;34 (1 Suppl):479-88.

Hoofnagle JH, Peters M, Mullen KD, Jones DB, Rustgi V, Di Bisceglie A, Hallahan C, Park Y, Meschievitz C, Jones EA (1988). Randomized, controlled trial of recombinant human alpha-interferon in patients with chronic hepatitis B. *Gastroenterology.;* 95:1318-25.

Hussain,S.P and Harris,C.C. (1998). Molecular epidemiology of human cancer. *Toxicol. Lett.,* 102-103, 219–225.

Ibrahim AS, Liver and Intrahepatic Bile Duct Cancer, MEEC Monograph51, Chapter 51 -61, *seer.cancer.gov/publications/mecc/mecc_liver.pdf.* September, 2004.

International Agency for Rescarch on Cancer. IARC '(1987). S7.Monographs on the Evaluation of Careinogenie Risks to Humans. Overall Evaluations of Careinogenicity. 440 pp. Lyon, France.

Jackson PE, Groopman JD (1999). Aflatoxin and liver cancer. *Baillieres Best Pract. Res. Clin. Gastroenterol.;* 13:545-555.

Jacobs B, Mayaud P, Changalucha J, Todd J, Ka-Gina G, Grosskurth H, Berege ZA (1997). Sexual transmission of hepatitis B in Mwanza, Tanzania. *Sex Transm Dis.;* 24:121-6.

Janssen HL, van Zonneveld M, Senturk H, Zeuzem S, Akarca US, Cakaloglu Y, Simon C, So TM, Gerken G, de Man RA, Niesters HG, Zondervan P, Hansen B, Schalm SW (2005). Pegylated interferon alfa-2b alone or in combination with lamivudine for HBeAg-positive chronic hepatitis B: a randomised trial. *Lancet;* 365:1239.

Jombo GT, Egah DZ, Banwat EB (2005). Hepatitis B virus infection in a rural settlement of northern Nigeria. *Niger J Med.;* 14:425-8.

Kane MA, Brooks A (2002). New immunization initiatives and progress toward the global control of hepatitis B. *Curr. Opin. Infect. Dis.;* 15:465-9.

Kao, J.H and Chen, D.S. (2002). Global control of hepatitis B virus infection. *Lancet Infect. Dis.,* 2, 395–403

Kato H, Gish RG, Bzowej N, Newsom M, Sugauchi F, Tanaka Y, Kato T, Orito E, Usuda S, Ueda R, Miyakawa Y, Mizokami M (2004). Eight genotypes (A-H) of hepatitis B virus infecting patients from San Francisco and their demographic, clinical, and virological characteristics. *J Med Virol.;* 73:516-21.

Kew MC (2010). Hepatocellular carcinoma in African Blacks: Recent progress in etiology and pathogenesis, *World J Hepatol,* 27; 2(2): 65-73

Kew MC, and Geddes EW (1985). Hepatocellular carcinoma in rural southern African Blacks. *Medicine (Balt);* 61; 98-108.

Kew MC, Kramvis A, Yu MC, Arakawa K, Hodkinson J (2005). Increased hepatocarcinogenic potential of hepatitis B virus genotype A in Bantu-speaking sub-Saharan Africans. *J Med Virol.* 75:513-21.

Kirk, G.D (2003). Hepatitis B vaccination and liver cancer. In Stewart, B.W. and Kleihues, P. (eds) *World Cancer Report.* IARC Press, Lyon, pp. 144–147.

Kirk, GD., Bah, E. and Montesano R. (2006) *Molecular epidemiology of human liver cancer: insights into etiology, pathogenesisand prevention from The Gambia,* West Africa, Carcinogenesis vol.27 no.10 pp.2070–2082).

Kirk GD, Lesi OA, Mendy M, Akano AO, Sam O., Goedert JJ, Hainaut P, Hall AJ, Whittle H, Montesano R (2004). The Gambia Liver Cancer Study: Infection with hepatitis B and C and the risk of hepatocellular carcinoma in West Africa. *Hepatology.;*39:211-9.

Kramvis A, Kew MC. (2007). Epidemiology of hepatitis B virus in Africa, its genotypes and clinical associations of genotypes. *Hepatology Research.,* 37:S9.

Kuniholm MH, Lesi OA, Mendy M, et al. (2008). Aflatoxin exposure and viral hepatitis in the etiology of cirrhosis in The Gambia, west Africa. *Environ. Health Perspect* ; 116: 1553-1557.

Lai CL, Ching CK, Tung AK, Li E, Young J, Hill A, Wong BC, Dent J, Wu PC (1997). Lamivudine is effective in suppressing hepatitis B virus DNA in Chinese hepatitis B surface antigen carriers: a placebo-controlled trial. *Hepatology.;*25:241-4.

Lehman EM., Amr S. Soliman, Kadry Ismail, Ahmed Hablas, Ibrahim A. Seifeldin, Mohamed Ramadan, Hesham El-Hamzawy, Christiana S. Shoushtari and Mark L. Wilson (2008), Patterns of hepatocellular carcinoma incidence in Egypt from a population-based cancer registry, *Hepatology Research*; 38: 465–473.

Lehman EM and Wilson ML. (2009). Epidemiology of hepatitis viruses among hepatocellular carcinoma cases and healthy people in Egypt: A systematic review and meta-analysis, *Int. J. Cancer:* 124, 690–697

Liang TJ, Heller T (2004). Pathogenesis of hepatitis C-associated hepatocellular carcinoma. *Gastroenterology.;* 127:S62-71.

Liang TJ, Rustgi V, Galun E, Blum HE (1993). Viral pathogenesis of hepatocellular carcinoma in the United States. *Hepatology;* 18: 1326-1333

Liao SS, Li RC, Li H, Yang JY, Zeng XJ, Gong J, Wang SS, Li YP, Zhang KL (1999). Long-term efficacy of plasma-derived hepatitis B vaccine: a 15-year follow-up study among Chinese children. *Vaccine.;* 17:2661-6.

Liaw YF, Leung NW, Chang TT, Guan R, Tai DI, Ng KY, Chien RN, Dent J, Roman L, Edmundson S, Lai CL (2000). Effects of extended lamivudine therapy in Asian patients with chronic hepatitis B. *Gastroenterology;* 119:172-80.

Lin YC, Chang MH, Ni YH, Hsu HY, Chen DS (2003). Long-term immunogenicity and efficacy of universal hepatitis B virus vaccination in Taiwan. *J. Infect. Dis.;* 187:134-8.

Liu CJ, Kao JH (2007). Hepatitis B Virus-related Hepatocellular Carcinoma: Epidemiology and Pathogenic Role of Viral factors. *J Clin Med Assoc.;* 70:141-5.

Madhava V, Burgess C, Drucker E (2002). Epidemiology of chronic hepatitis C virus infection in sub-Saharan Africa. *Lancet Infect. Dis.;*2:293-302.

Mohamed MK. and El Zayadi AR. Anoun SA. Abaza H. Selim OE. Badran HM. Strickland GT (1999).-Trend of hepatocellular carcinoma and associated risk factor in Egypt In the Pan Arab Association of Gastroentrology 12-16 Sept. *Egypt (Abstract).*

Montesano,R., Hainaut,P and Wild,C.P (1997). Hepatocellular carcinoma: from gene to public health. *J. Natl Cancer Inst.,* 89, 1844–1851

Mohamed MK (2004). Epidemiology of HCV in Egypt. *The Afro-Arab Liver Journal,* Vol 3, No.2 (July), pp 41-52

Muraskin,W. (1995). *The War Against Hepatitis B.* University of Pennsylvania Press, Philadelphia, PA.

Ndububa DA, Ojo DS, Adeodu OO, et al. (2001). Primary hepatocellular carcinoma in Ile-Ife, Nigeria: A prospective study of 154 cases. *Niger Med J;* 10: 59-63.

Ohata K, Hamasaki K, Toriyama K, Ishikawa H, Nakao K, Eguchi K (2004). High viral load is a risk factor for hepatocellular carcinoma in patients with chronic hepatitis B virus infection. *J Gastroenterol Hepatol.;* 19: 670-675

Okoth FA, Kobayashi M, Kaptich DC, Kaiguri PM, Tukei PM, Takayanagi T, Yamanaka T (1991). Seroepidemiological study for HBV markers and anti-delta in Kenya. *East Afr Med J.;* 68:515-25.

Otegbayo JA, Fasola FA, Abja A. (2003). Prevalence of hepatitis B surface and e antigens, risk factors for viral acquisition and serum transaminase among blood donors in Ibadan, Nigeria. *Trop Gastroenterol.;* 24:196-7.

Parkin, DM., Bray, FI and Devesa, SS (2001). Cancer burden in the year 2000: The global picture. *Eur. J. Cancer,* 37 (suppl. 8), S4–66.

Parkin DM, Whelan SL, Ferlay J, Teppo L, editors. (2002). Cancer incidence in five continents, volume VIII. IARC Scientific Publication No. 155. Lyon (France): *International Agency for Research on Cancer;*

Pido B, Kagimu M (2005). Prevalence of hepatitis B virus (HBV) infection among Makerere University medical students. *Afr Health Sci.;* 5:93-8.

Pisani,P., Parkin,D.M., Munoz,N and Ferlay,J. (1997) Cancer and infection: estimates of the attributable fraction in. Cancer Epidemiol. *Biomarkers Prev.,* 6, 387–400.

Polychronaki N, C Turner P, Mykkanen H, Gong Y, Amra H, Abdel-Wahhab M, El-Nezami H. (2006). Determinants of aflatoxin M1 in breast milk in a selected group of Egyptian mothers. *Food Addit Contam.* Jul; 23(7):700-8

Polychronaki N, West RM, Turner PC, Amra H, Abdel-Wahhab M, Mykkanen H, El-Nezami H. (2007). A longitudinal assessment of aflatoxin M (1) excretion in breast milk of selected Egyptian mothers. *Food Chem Toxicol.* Jul; 45(7):1210-5

Pybus O. G., Drummond A. J., Nakano T., Robertson B. H. and Rambaut A(2003). The Epidemiology and Iatrogenic Transmission of Hepatitis C *Virus in Egypt: A Bayesian Coalescent Approach Mol. Biol. Evol.* 20(3):381-387.

Ray SC, Arther RR, Carella A, Bukh J., Thomas DL (2000)., Genetic Epidemiology of Hepatitis C virus throughout Egypt. *J. Infect Dis* 182 (3): 698.

Sabbioni G, Skipper PL, Buchi G, Tannenbaum SR. (1987). Isolation and characterization of the major serum albumin adduct formed by aflatoxin B1 in vivo in rats. *Carcinogenesis.* 8:819-24.

Scheff N (2007). Liver cancer in africa, *Medical Journal of Therapeutics Africa* Vol 1, No 3 Page 236- 243

Shaw T (2004), Locarnini S. Entecavir for the treatment of chronic hepatitis B. *Expert Rev Anti Infect Ther.;* 2:853-71.

Simonsen L, Kane A, Lloyd J, Zaffran M, Kane M. (1999). Unsafe injections in the developing world and transmission of bloodborne pathogens: a review. *Bull World Health Organ.* 77:789-800.

Sizaret P, Malaveille C, Montesano R, Frayssinet C (1982). Detection of aflatoxins and related metabolites by radioimmunoassay. *J. Natl Cancer Inst.;* 69:1375-81.

State of the World's Children (2003). *United Nations Children's Fund* (UNICEF).

Strickland GT, Elhefni H, Salman T *et al (*2002). Role of hepatitis C infection in chronic liver disease in Egypt. *Am J Trop Med Hyg*; 67: 436–42.

Sylla A, Diallo MS, Castegnaro J, Wild CP (1999). Interactions between hepatitis B virus infection and exposure to aflatoxins in the development of hepatocellular carcinoma: a molecular epidemiological approach. *Mutat Res;* 428:187-96.

Szab E, Paska C, Kaposi Novak P, Schaff Z, Kiss A (2004). Similarities and Differences in Hepatitis B and C Virus Induced Hepatocarcinogenesis. *Pathol Oncol Res;* 1: 5-11.

Tanaka Y., Agha S., Saudy N., Kubanov F., Orito E., Kato T., Abo-Zeid M., Khalaf M., Miyakawa Y., Mizokami M (2004). Exponential spread of Hepatitis C virus Genotype 4a in Egypt. *J. Mol Evol* 58 (2): 191.

Triki H, Said N, Ben Salah A, Arrouji A, Ben Ahmed F, Bouguerra A, Hmida S, Dhahri R, Dellagi K (1997). Seroepidemiology of hepatitis B, C and delta viruses in Tunisia. *Trans R Soc TropMed Hyg;* 91:11-4.

Turner PC, Sylla A, Gong YY, Diallo MS, Sutcliffe AE, Hall AJ, Wild CP (2005). Reduction in exposure to carcinogenic aflatoxins by postharvest intervention measures in west Africa: a community based intervention study. *Lancet.;* 365:1950-6.

Yamanaka T, Takayanagi N, Nakao T, Kobayashi M, Baba K. (1991). *Seroepidemiological study of hepatitis B virus (HBV) infection in the rural community in Kenya - changing pattern of transmission model of HBV in Kenya.* Kansenshogaku Zasshi.; 65:26-34.

Yates, S.C., Hafez, M., Beld, M., Lukashov, VV., Hassan, Z., Carboni, G., Khaled, H., McMorrow, M., Attia, M. & Goudsmit, J (1999). Hepatocellular carcinoma in Egyptians with and without a history of hepatitis B virus infection: association with hepatitis C virus (HCV) infection but not with (HCV) RNA level. *Am. J. Trop. Med. Hyg.,* 60, 714-720

Velazquez RE, Rodriguez M, Navascues CA, Linares A, Perez R, Sotorrios NG, Martinez I, Rodrigo L. (2003). Prospective analysis of risk factors for hepatocellular carcinoma in patients with liver cirrhosis. *Hepatology;* 37: 520-527

Viviani S, Jack A, Hall AJ, Maine N, Mendy M, Montesano R, Whittle HC (1999). Hepatitis B vaccination in infancy in The Gambia. *Vaccine.;* 17:2946-50.

Voigt MD (2005). Alcohol in hepatocellular cancer. *Clin Liver Dis;* 9:151-69.

Westland C, Delaney W 4th, Yang H, Chen SS, Marcellin P, Hadziyannis S, Gish R, Fry J, Brosgart C, Gibbs C, Miller M, Xiong S. (2003). Hepatitis B virus genotypes and virologic response in 694 patients in phase III studies of adefovir dipivoxil. *Gastroenterology.;*125:107-16.

Whittle H, Jaffar S, Wansbrough M, Mendy M, Dumpis U, Collinson A, Hall A (2002). Observational study of vaccine efficacy 14 years after trial of hepatitis B vaccination in Gambian children. *BMJ.;* 325:569.

WHO. Hepatitis B vaccines. (2004). *Wkly Epidemiol Rec.;* 79:25563.

WHO Global surveillance, control of hepatitis C (1999). Report of a WHO Consultation organized in collaboration with the Viral Hepatitis Prevention Board, Antwerp, Belgium. *J. Viral. Hepat.,* 6, 35–47.

WHO/UNICEF. *Global Immunization* 1989-2005.

Wild CP, and Hall AJ (2000). Primary prevention of hepatocellular carcinoma in developing countries. *Mutat. Res.;* 462:381-93.

Wild, C.P., Law, G.R and Roman, E (2002). Molecular epidemiology and cancer: promising areas for future research in the post-genomic era. *Mutat. Res.,* 499, 3–12.

Wild CP, Jiang YZ, Allen SJ, Jansen LA, Hall AJ, Montesano R (1990). Aflatoxin-albumin adducts in human sera from different regions of the world. *Carcinogenesis.;* 11:2271-4.

Wild CP, Jansen LA, Cova L, Montesano R (1993). Molecular dosimetry of aflatoxin exposure: contribution to understanding the multifactorial etiopathogenesis of primary hepatocellular carcinoma with particular reference to hepatitis B virus. *Environ. Health Perspect.* 99:115-22.

Wild CP, Garner RC, Montesano R, Tursi F (1986). Aflatoxin B1 binding to plasma albumin and liver DNA upon chronic administration to rats. *Carcinogenesis.;* 7:853-8.

Wong DK, Cheung AM, O'Rourke K, Naylor CD, Detsky AS, Heathcote J (1993). Effect of alpha-interferon treatment in patients with hepatitis B e antigen positive chronic hepatitis B. A meta-analysis. *Ann Intern Med.;*119:312-23.

Wu JS, Hwang LY, Goodman KJ, Beasley RP (1999). Hepatitis B vaccination in high-risk infants: 10-year follow-up. *J. Infect. Dis.;* 179:1319-25.

Xiong J, Yao YC, Zi XY, Li JX, Wang XM, Ye XT, Zhao SM, Yan YB, Yu HY, Hu YP (2003). Expression of hepatitis B virus X protein in transgenic mice. *World J Gastroenterol;* 9: 112-116.

In: Hepatocellular Carcionoma: A Global Challenge
Editor: Isabelle Chemin
ISBN: 978-1-61470-644-1

Chapter II

Hepatocellular Carcinoma in Asia

***Fahad J. Siddiqui*[1,2], *Edwin S. Y. Chan*[1,2], *Say-Beng Tan*[1,2,4] and *Pierce K. H. Cho*[2,3,4]**

[1]Department of Epidemiology, Singapore Clinical Research Institute, Singapure
[2]Centre for Quantitative Medicine, Office of Clinical Sciences, Duke-NUS Graduate Medical School, Singapure
[3]Department of Surgery, Singapore General Hospital, Singapore
[4]National Cancer Center, Singapore

Abstract

Hepatocellular Carcinoma (HCC) imposes a growing disease burden in Asia, a region that already shoulders more than 70% of the global load. Analysis of epidemiological data shows regional changes in disease incidence and etiological factors. This chapter examines the epidemiology of HCC in Asia in 4 parts – the burden of disease and its distribution, changing trends in the etiology, the reliability of data and future directions for research and public health initiatives.

Epidemiology

Primary liver cancer is one of the most commonly occurring cancers in the world and Hepatocellular Carcinoma (HCC) constitutes over 85 - 90% of all primary liver cancers, hence we will use the terms interchangeably. [1] A wide variation in HCC disease burden and changing trends in etiology encourages a closer look at the differences among countries in various global regions with regards to risk, modifying factors and methods of surveillance. To achieve this purspose this chapter is organized in 4 parts: *Part 1* describes the burden of disease starting with a brief description of the global situation before moving on to the regional burden in East-Asia (EA) and South-east Asia (SEA) and ending with country-specific commentaries. *Part 2* will discuss etiology and risk factors and changing trends at the global, regional and country levels. *Part 3* will review the general reliability of the surveillance data from which these burdens and trends are derived. *Part 4* will comment on future directions for research and public health initiatives.

In this chapter, the reported incidence and mortality rates are all age-standardized using the World Health Organization (WHO) world population 2000 [2].

Burden of Disease

The Global Burden

HCC is the 7th most commonly occurring cancer in the world with 748,271 incident cases recorded in 2008 [3]. This comprises 6% of the total number of cancer cases in the world. The estimated age-standardized incidence rate is more than 10 per 100,000 person years (ht pyrs) worldwide. Men and women differ in their susceptibility to HCC [3]. It is the 5th most frequent cancer in men but the 7th most frequent in women, with incidence rates of 16/ht pyrs and 6/ht pyrs in men and women respectively [3]. The vast majority of HCC (70%) occurred in men with the developing world shouldering 85% of the total global burden.

Even with current improved treatment regimens, mortality is high with a case fatality rate of 93% making it the 3rd deadliest cancer in the world [3]. In 2008, the global burden of death was 695,900 (487,000 men and 217,000 women) [3]. The Global mortality rate was 10/ht pyrs (men: 14.6/ht pyrs women: 5.7/ht pyrs) [3]. HCC deaths made up 9.2% (men: 11.3; women: 6.5) of all cancer deaths.

Asia bears a disproportionate amount of this burden and so this chapter focuses on HCC in Asian countries where it is the 3rd most common cancer and the variation in incidence is extremely wide. This could be due to the diversity of health care systems, cultures and varied levels of economic development; hence there is a need to take a more granular overview.

For the purpose of this discussion we will adopt the classification of the GLOBOCAN 2008 report [4]. This report divides Asia into 4 regions, namely Eastern Asia (EA), South-eastern Asia (SEA), South-central Asia (SCA), Western Asia (WA) [4]. Most of the population is concentrated in the first three regions. India is within the SCA region and as it is covered in another chapter of this book, this chapter focuses on the EA and SEA regions.

East Asia and South-east Asia

EA includes China, Japan, Democratic People's Republic of Korea (North Korea), South Korea, Taiwan & Mongolia [4, 5]. SEA comprises of Malaysia, Singapore, Indonesia, Thailand, Philippines, Cambodia, Vietnam, Brunei Darussalam, Laos, Myanmar (Burma) [4, 6]. It should be noted that the Hong Kong Special Administrative Region (SAR) of China has been considered in previously published articles as a separate geographic entity. There are no published estimates for small countries such as Timor-Leste. Hence these countries will only be discussed very briefly.

Morbidity

These two regions appear on the top of the list of regions with the highest incidence of HCC. Combined, the two regions added over half a million new cases of HCC in 2008, 73% of the estimated global number [7]. Of these half a million HCC cases, 72% occurred in men and 28% in women [7]. The male to female ratio was 3:1 as in all high incidence areas. No combined incidence rates estimates are available for the two regions. Of all new cancer cases in the regions combined, a little over 12% were of HCC (male: 15.8%; female: 7.9%), this was twice the global proportion [7].

The EA region had the highest number of incident cases in 2008 (47,2287), and comprised 63.1% of the global burden. Over 72% of these cases occurred in men and 27% in women. The overall incidence rate was 24/ht pyrs (men: 35.5/ht pyrs; women: 12.6/ht pyrs). Of all new cancer cases, 12.7% cases were HCC (men: 16%; women 8.3%).

SEA had the second highest number of incident cases (74900); with 68% occurring in men and 32% in women. This was 10% of the global burden. SEA also had the second highest incidence rate (14.9/ht pyrs) (men: 21.4 /ht pyrs women: 9.0/ht pyrs). Of all new cancer cases 10.3% (men: 15%, women: 6.2%) were HCC.

Mortality

Altogether the two regions contributed almost half a million HCC deaths (~72% of global HCC deaths) [7]. The two regions together contributed 73% of the global male HCC deaths and 67% of the global female HCC deaths. Out of all cancer mortalities, 17% were from HCC in the two regions. HCC caused 20% of male cancer deaths and 12.5 of female cancer deaths [7]. The combined statistics for the two regions are dominated by the EA region statistics.

The EA region had the greatest number of HCC deaths, accounting for 61.8% of global HCC deaths. Sixty four percent of global male HCC deaths occurred in EA and almost 57% of all female HCC deaths were observed here. The male to female ratio for deaths was again 3:1. The mortality rate in the region was 31.7/ht pyrs in men and 11.7/ht pyrs in women, more than double the global rates for men and women. Of all deaths due to cancers in EA, HCC accounted for 17.6%. In men, 20% of cancer deaths were due to HCC, and in women this proportion was a little above 13%.

The SEA region contributed almost 10% of the global and 13.8% of combined EA and SEA HCC deaths. There was little difference between males and females in their respective contribution to the global HCC mortality (men: 9.8%; women: 10.2%). Within SEA 68% out of 69,200 HCC deaths occurred in men and 32% in women. The mortality rate in the region for men was 19.7/ht pyrs and for women 8.3/ht pyrs, only slightly better than Middle Africa. HCC in SEA resulted in 13.8% of all deaths due to any cancer. The proportion of deaths caused by HCC was 18.2% among men and 9.2% in women.

Summary

From the preceding discussion, it is clear that at present EA and SEA can justifiably be regarded as the HCC epicenter of the world. Not only are the absolute number of new cases being identified the largest, these two regions have the highest incidence rates for the disease.

Case fatality rate is very high so incidence rate does not differ much from the mortality rate. HCC causes a high proportion of cancer deaths in the region. These proportions are considerably higher for men than for women.

Table 1. Age adjusted incidence rates and proportion of incident cases out of all cancer cases in various regions and countries (GLOBOCAN 2008)

Region/ Country	Incidence rate (/100,000 person-yrs)			HCC cases (% of all Ca cases)		
	Overall	*Men*	*Women*	*Overall*	*Men*	*Women*
World	10.8	16.0	6.0	5.9	7.9	3.7
EA	24.0	35.5	12.6	12.7	16.0	8.3
SEA	14.9	21.4	9.0	10.3	15.1	6.2
China	25.7	37.4	13.7	14.3	18.1	9.1
Japan	11.2	17.6	5.8	6.3	7.1	5.2
Korea R	23.5	38.4	10.6	9.1	12.8	4.9
Taiwan	35.7	52.0	20.0	14.3	17.7	9.8
Korea DR	11.1	15.8	7.2	8.5	12.9	5.5
Mongolia	94.4	116.6	74.8	36.5	40.9	31.9
Vietnam	29.3	42.3	18.5	20.8	27.6	14.3
Thailand	29.7	40.6	19.9	19.6	28.3	12.6
Indonesia	6.7	10.3	3.5	4.5	7.0	2.4
Philippines	10.6	16.5	5.1	8.9	14.2	4.1
Myanmar	11.1	16.5	6.3	7.2	12.2	3.7
Cambodia	15.2	25.8	7.8	10.9	16.9	5.9
Laos	33.8	48.7	20.6	21.2	30.0	13.2
Malaysia	5.7	8.4	3.0	3.8	5.9	1.9
Singapore	10.1	17.0	3.8	5.2	8.3	2.2
Brunei	5.2	6.0	3.8	2.9	3.1	2.7

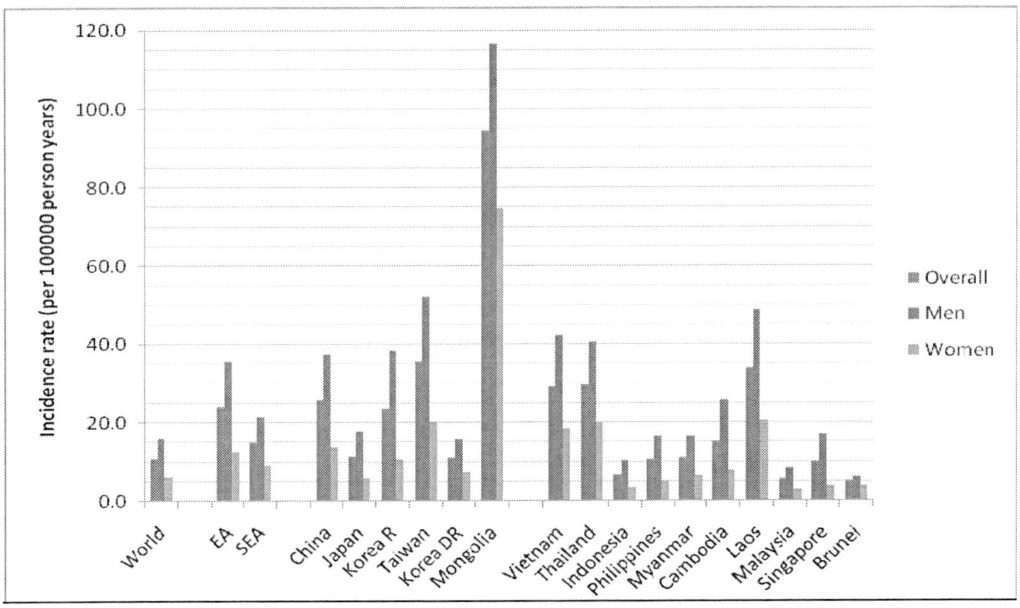

Figure 1. Age adjusted incidence rates for HCC – GLOBOCAN 2008.

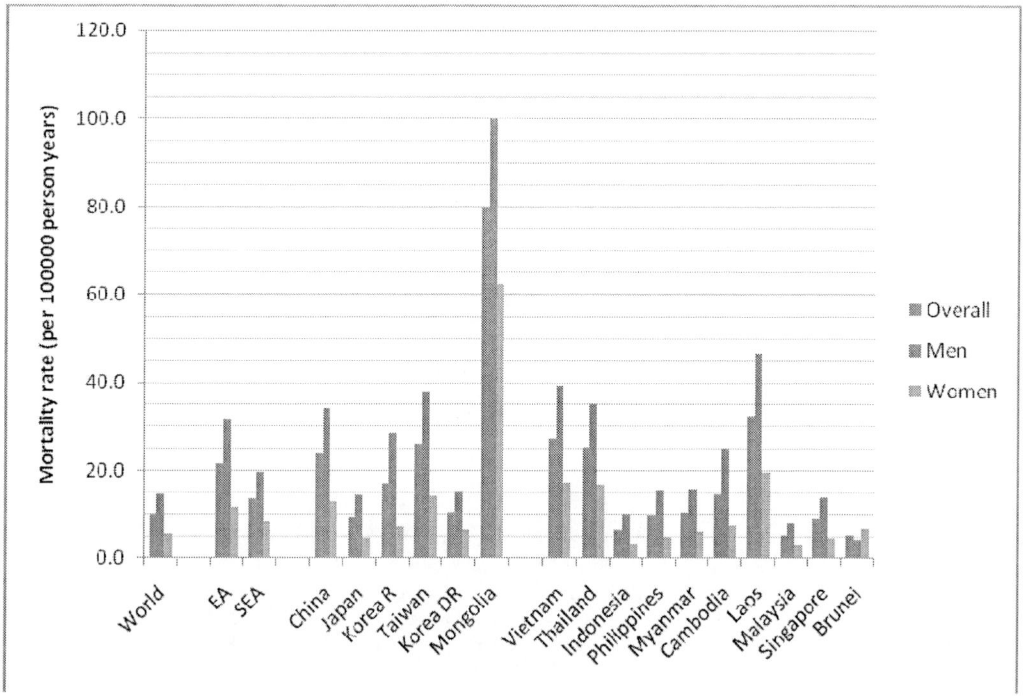

Figure 2. Age adjusted mortality rate for HCC – GLOBCAN 2008.

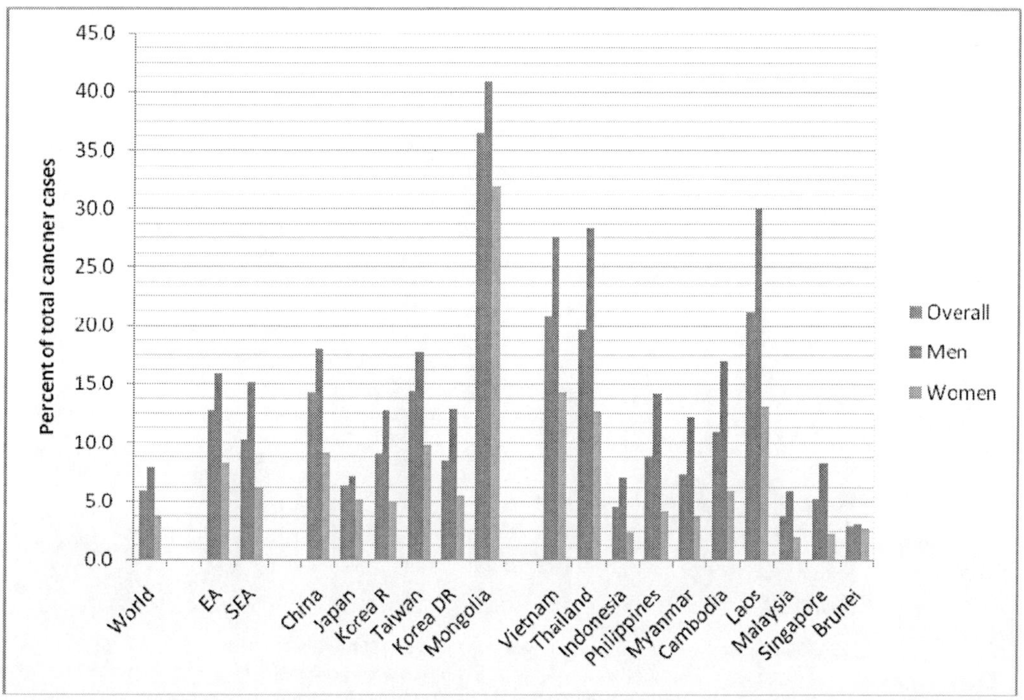

Figure 3. Proportion of HCC cases out of all cancer cases within geographical entity– GLOBOCAN 2008.

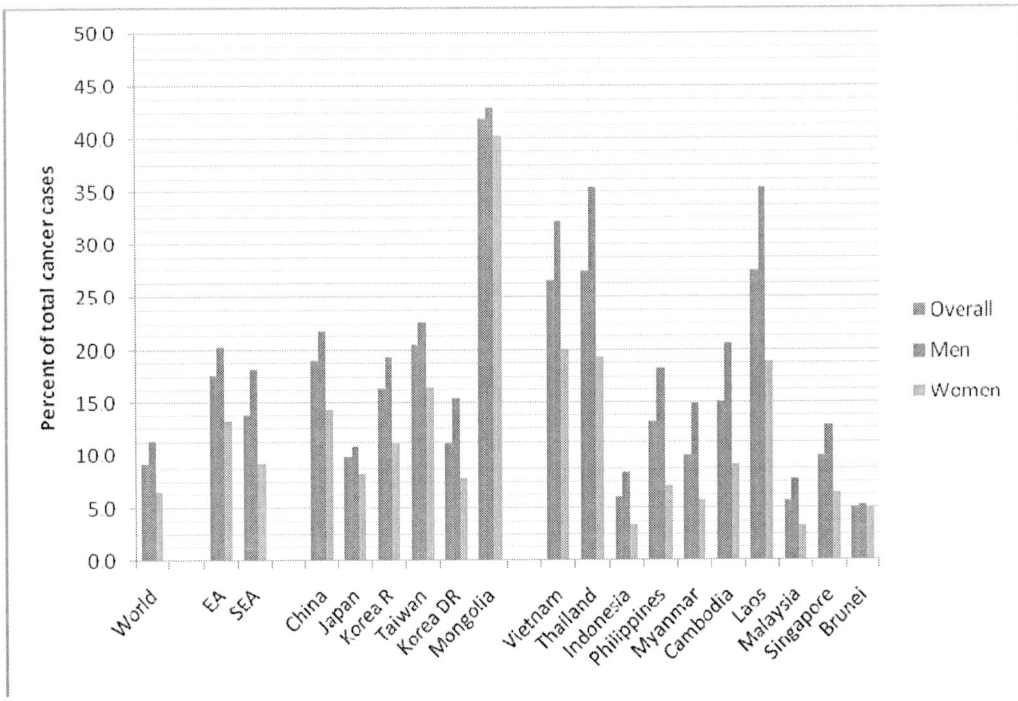

Figure 4. Proportion of HCC deaths out of all cancer deaths within geographical entity – GLOBOCAN 2008.

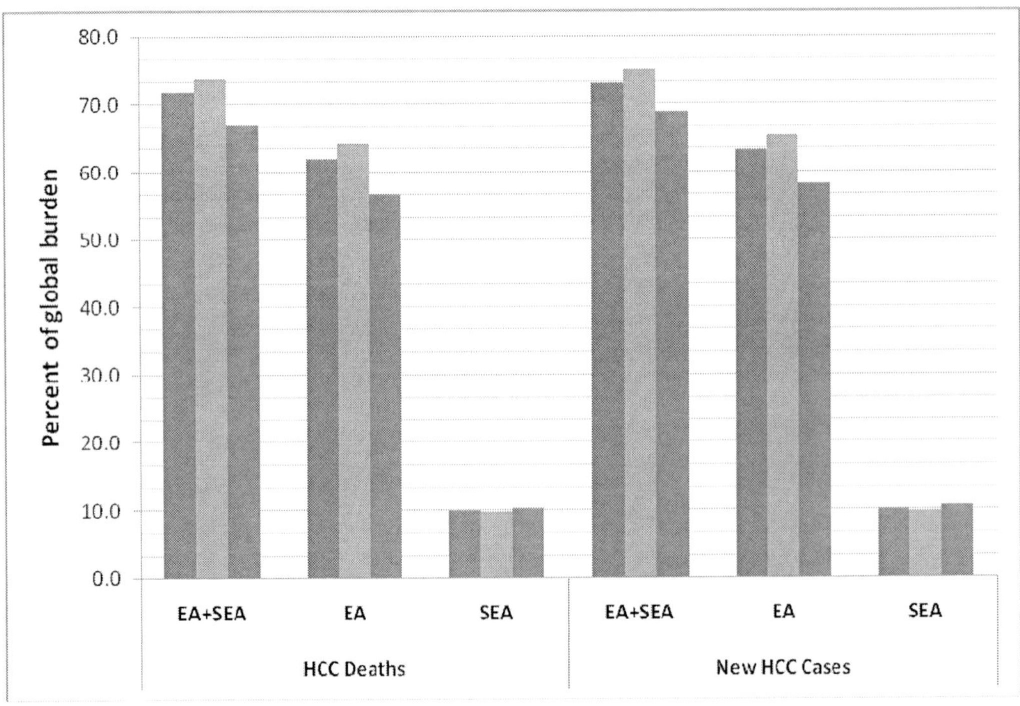

Figure 5. Share of East Asian and Southeast Asian Regions in Global HCC burden – GLOBOCAN 2008.

Country Commentaries

In this section, the countries are arranged in descending order of estimated number of HCC cases - EA countries will thus be presented first, followed by SEA countries. Estimated figures are for the year 2008 and show a high degree of heterogeneity in the morbidity and mortality of the disease. Unlike the GLOBOCAN report that ranks cancers according to incident numbers in 2008, we have chosen to report the ranking based on incidence rate as this will control for variation in the size of the population base.

China

The largest country in EA had the greatest number of cases (402,208) in 2008. This represents more than half (53.7%) of the global burden and 85% of the burden in EA. The disease ranked 3rd overall among men, and 4th among women with a male to female ratio of 2.7:1. The incidence rate was 25.7/ht pyrs; in men it was estimated to be 37.4/ht pyrs, and in women 13.7/ht pyrs. HCC caused 14.3% of all cancer cases. HCC in China in 2008, caused over half (53.4%) of the global HCC deaths (372,079) and over 86% of the EA deaths. This translated to a mortality rate of 23.7/ht pyrs (men: 34.1; women: 13.7) [7]. Out of all cancer deaths in China HCC contributed to 19.0%.

Hong Kong (SAR)

HCC was ranked the third most common cancer in men, although there was a slight decrease in the age-standardized incidence rate from the mid-1990s onward. According to 2005 statistics, the age-standardized rates for men and women are 30 and 8.3 per 100 000 persons, respectively [8].

Japan

The overall rank of HCC in Japan was 6th (38,901 cases) in 2008. In men it was ranked 5th and in women 7th, with a male to female ratio of 2:1. The incidence rate of HCC in Japan was 11.2/ht pyrs (men: 17.6; women: 5.8). Japan contributed to 8.2% of EA HCC cases. HCC cases made up 6.3% of all cancer cases within the country. Overall mortality rate was 9.2/ht pyrs (men: 14.5; women: 4.7). HCC was the cause of 9.8% of all deaths (proportionate mortality rate).

Republic of Korea (South Korea)

This country came third in the list of countries with most HCC cases in EA with 3.2% (15,277) of all EA cases. The overall rank of HCC in South Korea was 6th; 4th in men and 7th in women. The male to female ratio was 3:1. The overall incidence rate of HCC was 23.5/ht pyrs overall (men: 38.4; women; 10.6). HCC cases made up 9.1% of all cancer cases (men: 12.8%; women: 4.9%). S. Korea contributed 2.6% (11,231) of regional HCC deaths. Overall mortality rate was 17/ht pyrs (males: 28.4; women: 7.3) [7]. Of the total cancer deaths in S. Korea 16.3% were due to HCC [3].

Taiwan

HCC was ranked 2nd overall (11,179 cases), 1st in men and 3rd in women, with a male to female ratio of 2.4:1. It contributed 2.4% of the regional HCC burden. The incidence rate in

Taiwan was the second highest in EA region i.e. 35.7/ht pyrs (men: 52; women: 20). Two percent (8,412) of the annual regional HCC deaths occurred in Taiwan. The mortality rate was 25.9/ht pyrs (men: 38.2; women: 14.1) [7].

Democratic Republic of Korea (North Korea)

This country reported 3,148 cases and contributed almost 1% to the total regional HCC burden. The male to female ratio was 1.5:1. The cancer ranked 5th overall; in men it had the second highest incidence rate whereas in women it was 5th. The incidence rate was 11.1/ht pyrs (men: 15.8; women: 7.2). Of all cancer cases in the country 8.5% were from HCC (men: 12.9%: women: 8%). Overall mortality rate remained a little over 10/ht pyrs (men: 5.2; women: 6.6). HCC was the cause of 11.2% of all cancer deaths (men: 15.4%; women: 5.5%) [3].

Mongolia

This sparsely populated country had the highest reported incidence rates that far exceeded any other country in the world. HCC also was on the top of the list of cancer incidence for both men and women. In 2008 the incidence was 94.4/ht pyrs (men: 116.6; women: 74.8) with 1547 new cases identified. The male to female ratio was 1.4:1 one of smallest observed in the whole region especially on a background of high incidence. Among men 40% of all cancer cases were HCC and 30% among women. Overall, every 3rd cancer case was HCC. The country had a mortality rate for HCC of almost 80/ht pyrs (men: 100; women: 63). HCC was the cause of 40% of all cancer deaths.

Vietnam

Within the country HCC was the top ranking cancer both in men and women with overall incidence rate of 29/ht pyrs (men: 42.3; women: 18.5). The male to female ratio was 1.9:1. Overall every 5th case of cancer was HCC. Among all cancers in men 27% were HCC and in women it was 14%. Vietnam contributed almost third of the regional HCC morbidity and mortality burden in terms of number of cases and deaths. The country had the third highest HCC mortality rate among the countries within these two regions and the second highest in SEA. The mortality rate remained at over 27/ht pyrs overall (men: 39.2; women: 17.3). Almost one-third of all cancer deaths in men were due to HCC and one-fifth in women [3].

Thailand

The country ranked second in the region in regards to HCC incidence rate in 2008. The overall incidence of HCC was 29.7/ht pyrs (men: 40; women: 20). The male to female ratio was 1.8:1. Of all cancer cases almost 20% were due to HCC. Like Vietnam, Thailand also contributed a third to the regional HCC burden of morbidity and mortality. Over 14,000 deaths were observed in Thailand with a rate of 25.4/ht pyrs (men: 35.1; women: 16.6). Of all cancer deaths 27.5% were due to HCC [3].

Philippines

The incidence rate of HCC in this country of islands almost matched the global figure i.e. 10.6/ht pyrs (men: 16.5; women: 5.1). HCC ranked 2nd among male cancers, 6th among female ones and overall ranked 4th. The male to female ratio was a little over 3:1. Nine percent of all cancer cases were HCC. The country contributed almost 9% to the HCC morbidity and mortality of the region with a mortality rate of 9.9/ht pyrs (male: 15.4; women: 4.9) [3].

Myanmar

This is the second largest country in SEA, with an incidence rate of 11.1/ht pyrs with 6.5% of SEA HCC cases. Men were almost three times more likely to get HCC as compared to women with incidence rates of 16.5/ht pyrs and 6.3/ht pyrs respectively. Among male cancers it ranked 2nd in men and contributed over 12 percent of all cancer cases. The male to female ratio was 2.4:1. In terms of mortality the rate was 10.6/ht pyrs. One-tenth of all the cancer deaths were from HCC with the figure for men at almost 15% [3].

Cambodia

In Cambodia the overall incidence of HCC was 14.6/ht pyrs, (men: 25; women: 7.5). The cancer ranks 2nd among men and 4th in women. The male to female ratio was 2.4:1. HCC constitutes 10.9% of all cancer cases in the country. The mortality rate was more than double in men (20.6/ht pyrs) compared to that in women (9.1/ht pyrs) and the overall mortality rate in 2008 was 14.6/ht pyrs [3].

Laos

HCC ranks number 1 of all cancers as well as of cancers among men, and was 2nd in women with an overall incidence rate of 33.8/ht pyrs, (men: 48.7; women: 20.6), The incidence of HCC was higher than that of its neighbors China, Vietnam and Thailand. Although it contributes only 1.6% of the regional burden because of its small population, 21% of all cancers cases in Laos were HCC. The proportion was almost 30% in men and 13% for women. Mortality rates match closely with incidence rates and 27% (men: 46.8; women: 19.7) of all cancer deaths were due to HCC [3].

Malaysia

This was a country with incidence (5.7/ht pyrs) and mortality rates (5.4/ht pyrs) on the lower end of the spectrum both among men and women compared with that of its neighbors. HCC was ranked 11th among female cancers, the lowest in the region. The male to female ratio was among the highest i.e. 3.8:1. Only 3.8% of all cancer cases were HCC and 5.7% of all cancer deaths were due to HCC [3].

Singapore

The small multiethnic population living in this city state reported only 674 cases. The overall rank of this cancer was 7th among all cancers in Singapore with an incidence just above 10/ht pyrs (men: 17.0; women: 3.8). The male to female ratio was 3.8:1. Overall 5.2% of all cancer cases were HCC. In men this proportion was over 8% and in women the figure was 2.2%. Mortalities due to HCC were 612 with a mortality rate of 9/ht pyrs. In men the rate was 14/ht pyrs whereas in women it was only 4.5/ht pyrs. Of total cancer deaths 5.2% were from HCC with 8.3% and 2.2% for men and women respectively [3].

Table 2. Age adjusted mortality rates proportion of deaths out of all cancer deaths in various regions and countries (GLOBOCAN 2008)

Region/Country	Mortality rate (/100,000 person-yrs)			HCC deaths (%)		
	Overall	*Men*	*Women*	*Overall*	*Men*	*Women*
World	10.0	14.6	5.7	9.2	11.3	6.5
EA	21.6	31.7	11.7	17.6	20.3	13.3
SEA	13.6	19.7	8.3	13.8	18.2	9.2
China	23.7	34.1	13.1	19.0	21.8	14.3
Japan	9.2	14.5	4.7	9.8	10.8	8.3
Korea R	17.0	28.4	7.3	16.3	19.3	11.2
Taiwan	25.9	38.2	14.1	20.5	22.7	16.5
Korea DR	10.4	15.2	6.6	11.2	15.4	7.9
Mongolia	79.9	99.9	62.5	41.8	42.9	40.3
Vietnam	27.3	39.2	17.3	26.5	32.2	20.0
Thailand	25.4	35.1	16.6	27.5	35.4	19.4
Indonesia	6.6	10.0	3.5	6.0	8.4	3.4
Philippines	9.9	15.4	4.9	13.2	18.3	7.2
Myanmar	10.6	15.8	6	10.1	14.9	5.7
Cambodia	14.6	25.1	7.5	15.1	20.6	9.1
Laos	32.3	46.8	19.7	27.6	35.3	18.9
Malaysia	5.4	8.1	2.9	5.7	7.8	3.3
Singapore	9.0	14.0	4.5	10.0	12.8	6.4
Brunei	5.4	4.4	6.8	5.2	5.3	5.0

Brunei

The smallest country in the two regions had the lowest incidence and mortality rates. The cancer ranked 11th overall and 7th among male cancers [3]. Only 3% of all cancer cases were HCC and a little over 5% of all cancer deaths were due to HCC. However, as the total number of cases was 12 the estimates may not be robust.

Missing Data

There were a number of smaller countries for which GLOBOCAN has not yet published any estimates for example Timor-Leste [9]. This is also evident from the fact that the numbers from individual countries do not add up to the SEA figures. There is a difference of 91 HCC cases and 77 HCC deaths (see Table2).

Changing Etiology and Epidemiology

Etiology and Risk Factors

It is generally accepted that chronic liver disease and cirrhosis form the background of HCC in 70 – 90% of the cases. Several factors are thought to contribute to the above two conditions and these may be categorized as environmental and host factors. Environmental factors include infectious agents like Hepatitis B, C & D viruses, alimentary factors like alcohol and high calorie intake, and toxic agents like Aflatoxin 1B, steroids and some antibiotics [10, 11]. Host factors can be grouped as demographic characteristics such as gender and ethnicity. Metabolic conditions include non-alcoholic fatty liver disease (NAFLD) and obesity, and autoimmune disorders [12].

Whatever the case, liver cirrhosis remains the common pre-cancerous end-point and affects to a large extent the associated risks of HCC development [13]. It is also important to note that usually all factors that can lead to HCC development in the presence of liver cirrhosis, can also lead to HCC even in its absence, if the carcinogenic effect is strong enough to induce HCC before the development of liver cirrhosis [1, 14]. Figure 6 shows the pathways through which various factors cause HCC [15].

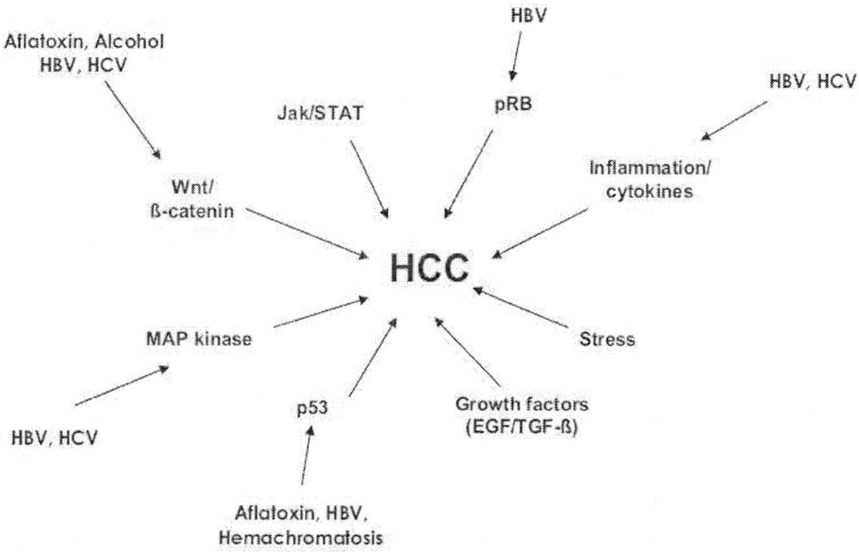

From: Aravalli RN, Steer CJ, Cressman EN. Molecular mechanisms of hepatocellular carcinoma. Hepatology. 2008 Dec;48(6):2047-63.

Figure 6. Cellular signalling pathways implicated in HCC. Several signaling pathways have been shown to be critical players in HCC. These pathways differ in different settings, because a variety of risk factors cause HCC, eath in their own unique manner.

Chronic Hepatitis B virus (HBV) infection is responsible for two thirds of all HCC cases [12]. Over half of the HCC in Asia and Africa have been attributed to HBV and here the infection is mainly transmitted vertically through mother to child [16]. However in Japan this proportion is only $1/5^{th}$ and in Japan, like many other developed countries, other modes of HBV transmission are more common than vertical transmission. It is evident that the variation in the prevalence of HCC reflects the variation in the prevalence of HBV [16].

The distribution of the eight HBV genotypes (A–H) differs regionally. Genotypes A and D prevail in Africa, Europe and India, while genotypes B and C are predominantly found in Asia [17]. A number of studies indicate an increased risk for HCC in the case of an infection with HBV genotype C in comparison to genotype B [18, 19]. However, it is not a uniform pattern as evidence contrary to this hypothesis also exists [20].

With chronic hepatitis C virus (HCV) infected patients the risk for the development of HCC increases by 17-fold, but the proportion of HCC patients with detectable HCV markers similarly vary with the regions [21]. This difference has been cited as contributing to the variation in incidence of HCC, although it may also be due to differences in the detection methods. In some regions of Asia as much as 9 out of 10 patients have been found to be positive for HCV markers [1, 22-24]. Because of the long latency period an accurate incidence is difficult to determine but the best available estimates show that of those patients who fail to clear HCV, two-third develops chronic hepatitis which eventually leads to cirrhosis. However, a review comprising of over 50 studies reports rate of progression to cirrhosis due to HCV of around 10% in 20 years time when community-based cohorts are studied [25].

A synergistic effect has been found between HBV and HCV and in the developing world, where almost 60% of HCC are attributed to HBV and 33% to HCV, this enhanced effect creates potentially alarming situations [26]. In Asia, the relative risk of developing HCC in cases infected with both HBV and HCV have been reported to be consistently higher than in cases with a single infection [27]. A meta-analysis of markers of HBV and HCV infection in patients with HCC suggests a synergism of the two infections in hepatocellular carcinogenesis with an OR of 22.5 (95% CI 19.5–26.0) for exposure to HBV, an OR of 17.3 (95% CI 13.9–21.6) for exposure to HCV and an OR of 165 (95% CI 81.2–374) where both HBV and HCV markers are present [28].

Chronic alcohol consumption leads to a fatty degeneration of hepatocytes and this in turn may lead to alcoholic liver fibrosis (30%) or to liver cirrhosis (10–20%). These conditions predispose to the development of HCC with an annual incidence of 1– 2% [29, 30]. An increase in the alcohol production and consumption corresponded to alcohol related disorders in China over the past three decades [31]. This is similar to findings from other countries like Taiwan, Japan, Korea and Vietnam [32-35]. Synergism among HBV, HCV and alcohol consumption have been reported from all over the globe in several studies [36-38].

It has been reported that in countries with high alcohol consumption and moderate burden of viral hepatitis, 85% of the HCC can be attributed to these three factors [39]. In the countries with the highest incidence of viral hepatitis infections and increasing alcohol consumption, this proportion can be anticipated to be even higher, making other risk factors less important.

Non-alcoholic steatohepatitis, diabetes mellitus, obesity and other metabolic factors are conditions that frequently co-exist and also have some common pathophysiological processes [40, 41]. The spectrum of non-alcoholic fatty liver disease (NAFLD) ranges from merely excessive fat accumulation in the liver (fatty liver) to inflammatory changes and fat deposition in hepatocytes (steatohepatitis) ultimately leading to cirrhosis. In the absence of a history of over consumption of alcohol it is known as non-alcoholic steatohepatitis (NASH). NASH is increasingly recognized to be an important causative factor of HCC in recent years. In several studies on patients with cryptogenic liver cirrhosis and HCC, there is suggestion that the prevalence of NASH was high in comparison to age- and sex- matched HCC patients with other well defined etiologies for their cancer [42-45].

The mycotoxin aflatoxin B1 has been classified as carcinogenic by the International Agency for Research on Cancer because of its strong hepatocarcinogenic potential. Aflatoxin

B1 is produced by the fungi of the *Aspergillus* species in regions where climate and food storage methods favor its development, such as in Asia and parts of Africa. In these regions it is a common contaminant of grain, nuts and vegetables. Among other biological effects, it leads to a characteristic mutation in the p53 tumor-suppressor gene that has been found in 30–60% of HCCs in aflatoxin-endemic areas [1]. The carcinogenic effect of aflatoxin is potentiated by simultaneous occurrence of viral hepatitis B. The synergistic effect of both has been shown by several studies [21, 46-48]. This is consistent with the observation that areas with a high prevalence of HCC have high aflatoxin intake and endemic HBV infection [49].

A few other factors and conditions have been positively and negatively associated with HCC. Iron overload, heamochromatosis and α_1-antitrypsin deficiency have been associated with a higher risk of HCC whilst a high intake of milk, yogurt, eggs, white meat, and consumption of coffee has been linked with a decreased the risk [50-57].

Global Trend

Since the year 2000, there have been three major reports on global cancer statistics [7, 58, 59]. In the 1st report, liver cancer was cited as the 3rd most deadly cancer causing around 9% of cancer deaths [58]. It also ranked 5th as the cause of new cancer cases with a total of 564,000 [58]. It mainly affected the populations in the less developed world, and was predominantly a male disease [58]. The case fatality rate reported was close to 100%.

The 2nd GLOBOCAN report (2002) ranked liver cancer as the 4th most common cancer causing around 626000 cases and a little less than 600000 deaths in that year [59]. For the first time region specific cancer incidence rates were reported. China had the highest incidence rate, Japan was third and rest of the South-East Asian region was 5th with incidence rates ranging 18 -37 for males and 5-14 for females per 100,000 person years.

The latest reported figures show an increasing number of new cancer cases occurring in the world and an unrelentingly high mortality rate (see above).

Trends in EA and SEA

Asia and particularly the EA and SEA regions have borne the brunt of HCC since the first reported statistics. The region comprises countries that are very heterogeneous in their socio-demographic characteristics and stage of economic development, with Japan, Singapore and South Korea classified as high income countries, Malaysia as being in the upper-middle income group, Mongolia, Vietnam, Philippines in the lower-middle income category and others like Myanmar, Laos & North Korea among countries having low incomes [60]. Consequently the high variability in the etiology and morbidity and mortality of HCC is not unexpected.

Observations are consistently made in EA and SEA countries with regards to high male to female incidence risk ratio and an increase in the incidence starting at the age of 35 – 40 years. Men have higher liver cancer rates than women – the male-to-female ratios usually ranges between 2:1 and 4:1 [61]. Men are more likely to be infected with HBV and HCV, consume alcohol, smoke cigarettes, and have increased iron stores. Non-environmental endogenous factors that may increase male risk include higher body mass index and higher levels of androgenic hormones. Several studies conducted in Taiwan reported a positive association between increased circulating testosterone levels and HCC in HBV-infected men [62, 63].

Trends in Asian Countries

The problems with ascertaining and comparing the trend are myriad ranging from the availability of the data to its comparability across various time points. The published data from selected countries presented below demonstrates how much the situation differs in various countries of the same region and even within a single country.

As an overview, HCC appears to be on the rise in Asia. It is generally a male dominated disease and has the greatest impact on the developing countries of Asia. Although this holds true for many countries in the region there have been signs of change in general trend for HCC or at least change in the magnitude of the background factors for HCC in some of the countries. The reasons for these exceptions are diverse, ranging from general healthcare improvement to targeted interventions against risk factors for HCC.

In general majority (80%) of HCC cases are related to chronic HBV infection, followed by HCV (15%) and other factors, such as alcoholic, metabolic liver disease, or aflatoxin exposure. Since HCC surveillance programs are still not widely available, most of the cases are diagnosed at an advanced stage [8].

China

The prevalence of HCC in China is 26–32 per 100 000 persons. However, in some areas the prevalence rate can be as high as 70–80 per 100 000. This high prevalence has been observed along the east coastal areas, whilst prevalence is lower i.e. <10 per 100 000 population in provinces located in the western regions of China. The major risk factor for HCC in China is clearly chronic HBV infection, followed by HCV infection. The odd ratios for different etiological agents are listed as follows: HBV: 12.45, HCV: 4.28, family history (may also be due to undiagnosed HBV): 3.45, aflatoxin B1: 2.82, alcohol intake: 1.88 [64]. If we track the figures available for almost four decades we will see a trend in the rising incidence of HCC. This increase is greater in men than in women. The Incidence in 1973 was around 20 in men and 10 in women which by 2006 was around 60 and 20 in men and women respectively [8]. One possible reason may just be improved detection. This, however, cannot be the entire explanation as the increase is higher in men than in women and against a background of continuously increasing vaccination again HBV [65, 66].

Hong Kong

Data from last decade showed no specific trends; with the age standardized incidence rate ranging from 35 – 40/100000 in men to a little above 10 in women [8]. With regards to etiology, several studies conducted in the period between 1981 and 2006 consistently showed that 75–80% of cases were related to chronic hepatitis B (CHB) infection [10–15]. Chronic HCV infection accounted for 3–6%, while co-infection with HBV and HCV accounted for 0.4–3%; chronic alcohol intake accounted for another 5% [8].

Japan

This country had observed a slow but steady increase in the incidence of HCC in the last 30 years though the increase has moderated in the past decade [67]. Viral hepatitis is the dominant cause of HCC in Japan, in contrast to most of the other EA and SEA countries [68]. Nationwide screening for HCV and HBV began in 2002 in Japan, and reduction of HCC is being anticipated in the years to come [68].

However, in Japan in contrast to China and Hong Kong, 79% of patients with HCC had chronic HCV infection and only 11% had chronic HBV infection. Sixty-three per cent of patients with HCC were older than 65 years. This may be related to the fact that the age of onset of HCC in patients with CHC is usually 10 years later than that of patients with CHB [69]. The incidence of HCV-related HCC seems to decline after the year 2000 [70]. This could be due to the decline in incidence of HCV infection after appropriate primary prevention has been initiated. A considerable proportion of HCC among patients negative for HBV and HCV had been found associated with steatohepatitis and diabetes [71].

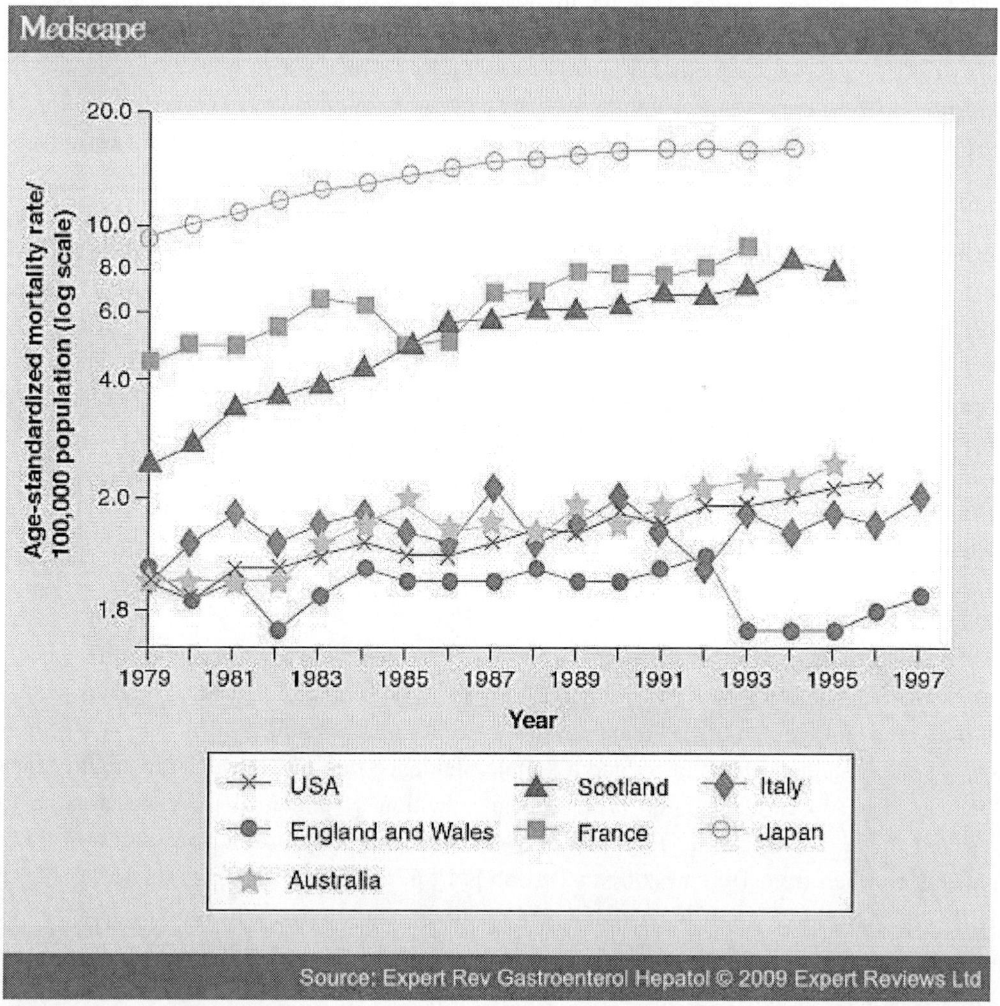

Korea

Data from 1995 to 2002 show that incidence rates have remained unchanged in women but have a downward trend in men. The rate fell from 50 to 40 in men during this period [8]. With regards to etiological agents, 72% of patients with HCC had chronic HBV infection, 20% had chronic HCV infection and less than 8% had other causes, including alcohol. Because of the implementation of a national HBV vaccination program in the late 1980s, the HBV carrier rates for males aged older than 20 years decreased from 8% in the 1980s to only 4.2% in 2005. With that, it is expected that the incidence of HCC will start to decrease in 2 to 3 decades time [8].

Singapore

From the late 1960s, the population-based Singapore Cancer Registry showed the HCC incidence to be four times higher in males than in females. Ethnic differences existed, with Singaporean Chinese experiencing the highest incidence followed by Malays and Indians. In that period a general declining trend in HCC incidence is observed [72]. More recently an almost 60% decrease in incidence among men and 47% in women have been documented when comparing the periods 1968-72 and 1998-02 with no change in ethnic distribution [8]. The reduction could be attributed to the drop in HBV infection especially after universal vaccination was introduced in 1985 and reduced Aflatoxin exposure [8].

Nevertheless if we compare 1988-92, when incidence among men was around 5 and women close to 1, with 1998-2002 the trend appeared to move in an upward direction with incidences 7 & 2 among males and females respectively [8]. Further investigations are required to explain this small but ominous increase.

In Singapore universal vaccination against hepatitis B commenced in 1985. The overall prevalence of chronic HBV infection in Singapore has fallen from 9–10% in 1980–81 to 4% in 1999. Data from to a cohort of 288 patients with HCC identified during 2002–2007 in the National University Hospital show that 74% were male and 76% were ethically Chinese; 35% have chronic HBV infection; 13% have chronic HCV infection and 31.4% were negative for HBV and HCV [8].

Taiwan

Published data from the country from 1979 to 2002 revealed that the difference in incidence rates between men and women is consistent with other countries. The rates increase in both men and women till 1998 and after that seem to have stabilized [8]. The latest figures show a male incidence rate of 53 and a female incidence rate of 21 which are slightly lower than the peak observed in 2000 [73]. The introduction of universal HBV vaccination has resulted in the reduction of HBV related HCC incidence. According to a study of 18423 patients enrolled from 1981 to 2001 in Taiwan [74], 67% of male HCC are related to chronic HBV infection, but 55% of female HCC are related to chronic HCV infection. The mean age of patients with HBV-related HCC is 53 ± 14 years, and for those with HCV-related HCC it is 65 ± 9.1 years ($P < 0.001$). The male-to-female ratio is 6.4 for HBV related HCC, while it is 1.7 for HCV-related HCC ($P < 0.001$). The percentage of HBV-related HCC has progressively decreased from 82 to 66% in men, and from 67 to 41% in women over the study period. In summary, the percentage of HBV-related HCC has declined progressively over the last 20 years. However, this is not due to a decrease in prevalence of chronic HBV infection but caused by an increase in HCV-related HCC [8].

Mongolia

In Mongolia the data of the last 10 years showed that number of cases and deaths due to HCC has increased steadily both in men and women. The number of deaths followed number of new cases until 2006 after which the difference increased consistently. It is unclear what the cause is but might be an indicator of the availability of better treatment facilities. The mortality rates have remained stable in Mongolia over time much more than incidence rates especially of men which showed big variations going as high as 120 to a low of 90. However, it seems less likely to be an artifact as women followed the trend without much variation (Personal Communication: Dr. Ariunaa Khasbazar, The Chemotherapy Department, National Cancer Center, Mongolia).

The reasons for this high incidence of HCC in Mongolia could largely be attributed to high prevalence of risk factors especially HBV, HCV and co-infection with delta virus and even triple infection that has been documented to exacerbate the progression of the liver damage [75, 76]. Triple infection was also reported from Mongolia and HCC patients had higher proportion of such infection as compared to those who only had chronic hepatitis (64% vs. 14%) [77]. Among children, 12.5% were found to be harboring the hepatitis virus with some harboring two or three types of viruses simultaneously. Despite vaccination 9.8% had active HBV infection and 2% had delta virus infection [78].

Reliability of Information

Obtaining reliable information from large populations is always a daunting task. It requires highly developed infrastructure to ensure representative coverage, minimize missing data and maintain data accuracy. Reporting epidemiological summaries in areas where such systems are either not in place or are very poor carry considerable risk of getting biased and imprecise estimates.

Although much of the variation in the burden of HCC can be accounted for the reasons discussed above, inadequate reporting of HCC cases cannot and should not be ignored as such inadequate data create artifacts in the overall picture. Even in countries as developed as the United States, under-reporting of such figures have been identified [79]. In the Asian region where a number of countries are under-developed and have poor infrastructure, the under-reporting of figures related to HCC should be expected.

The differences in the HCC incidence rates between North and South Korea illustrate this point. North Korea is relatively much less developed than its southern counterpart and the reported incidence of HCC in North Korea is almost half of that in South Korea [7].

If we examine the GLOBOCAN figures we find that the sources of data are highly varied. In some countries there are highly organized nationwide cancer registries with systems in place to ensure high quality data. In contrast there are countries where even birth and death registration are done in a very rudimentary manner, and the numbers are only estimates from where the incidence and mortality rates were calculated. For example, to get cancer incidence and mortality estimates for Cambodia, GLOBOCAN reports:

> Incidence rates for 'All sites but skin' estimated for males and females as the weighted average of Vietnamese and Thai cancer registries, were partitioned by site and age using proportions from Phnom Penh Cancer Registry (2001-2003) [80]
>
> Mortality was estimated from the 2008 national incidence estimate, using site-specific relative survival from Thai and Chinese cancer registries. The number of cancer deaths (all ages) was partitioned by sex and age using proportions from Chinese cancer registries mortality files. [80]

An even more extreme example is that of Indonesia for which data from Singapore, Malaysia and Papua New Guinea were used [81]. Unpublished data cannot attain a quality equivalent to that of the published data [82]. Several instances can be quoted where the numbers are obtained from just a single city or state level registry or at best a few of such registries [81, 82]. Therefore, although we base our findings on these numbers as these are the best available information, a lot needs to be done to overcome the data inadequacies and to arrive at an accurate picture of the real situation.

Future Directions

When considering the strategy for planning, research and public health action relating to HCC in East and Southeast Asia, a number of key issues must be taken into account. First, the HCC incidence burden has shown an increasing trend in the past decade, despite preventive strategies being adopted in some countries in the regions. Secondly, many countries in Asia have taken big strides and have achieved significant economic progress in the last 2 decades and the rest of the countries are catching up fast. In some countries, certain regions have developed economically far more than other regions. Thirdly, improving standards of living has resulted in an increased life expectancy at birth; as a result a greater number of people will be at-risk of HCC in the future. Fourthly, education and health awareness has increased the demand for better health care. An unabated increase in health consciousness is now a phenomenon independent of targeted campaigns as sources of information have diversified. In addition high impact disease specific public health campaigns will further augment this increasing demand for better health care. In this scenario of an increasing number of people at-risk, a growing number of people in need of care, more people attaining the capacity to afford better healthcare (be it diagnostic tests or high end treatment modalities for the disease), and rising health awareness, the demand for improved detection and treatment will increase tremendously. An anticipated increase in demand of diagnostic and treatment modalities must be preceded by an increased supply of these facilities and services. This in itself requires that considerable investments, both intellectual and financial, be committed today in order to meet expectations in the coming years.

An important weapon against the current main risk factor in HCC, i.e. HBV infection, is vaccination and hence it is possible to prevent HBV-related HCC. In contrast to this there is no immunological prevention for HCV. To reduce HCV infection requires increasing awareness among the population about HCV prevention and improved healthcare systems to avoid iatrogenic spread. Hence HCV will be expected to have a greater impact on the incidence of HCC in the future. Other risk factors that may become increasingly important could be those associated with metabolic syndrome, diabetes and obesity, in increasingly affluent societies.

Conclusion

HCC is one of the most common cancers in the world, and is particularly prevalent in Asia. There is a crucial need to focus our attention on improving our understanding of the disease - how best to treat it and the most appropriate means of controlling its etiological factors. Better information is required to provide the most appropriate care by choosing the most effective and efficient treatment strategies in the various sub-groups of HCC patients.

In the face of a high and increasing disease burden in Asia, it has become imperative to start planning large scale studies to search for definitive answers to address this important illness, in Asia in particular and the world in general.

Acknowledgments

We gratefully acknowledge the primary information on Mongolia provided by Dr Aruinaa Khasbazar from the National Cancer Center, Ulaan Baatar.

References

[1] El-Serag HB, Rudolph KL. Hepatocellular carcinoma: epidemiology and molecular carcinogenesis. *Gastroenterology.* 2007 Jun;132(7):2557-76.

[2] Ahmad OB, Boschi-Pinto C, Lopez AD, Murray CJL, Lozano R, M. I. *Age Standardization Of Rates: A New Who Standard;* 2001.

[3] Waterhouse JyC. *Cancer incidence in five continents.* Lyon 1976.

[4] IARC IAfRoC. HCC Incidence and Mortality Worldwide in 2008: Summary GLOBOCAN 2008 [cited 2010 01, Oct]; Available from: http://globocan.iarc.fr/factsheets/populations/factsheet.asp?uno=900

[5] IARC IAfRoC. The population dictionary. GLOBOCAN 2008 2010 [cited 2010 01 Oct]; Available from: http://globocan.iarc.fr/

[6] Wikipeida. East Asia. 2010 [cited 2010 Oct 01]; Available from: http://en.wikipedia.org/wiki/East_Asia.

[7] Wikipeida. Southeast Asia. 2010 [cited 2010 Oct 01]; Available from: http://en.wikipedia.org/wiki/Southeast_Asia.

[8] Ferlay J, Shin HR, Bray F, Forman D, Mathers C, Parkin DM. Estimates of worldwide burden of cancer in 2008: GLOBOCAN 2008. *International journal of cancer.* 2010 Jun 17.

[9] Yuen MF, Hou JL, Chutaputti A. Hepatocellular carcinoma in the Asia pacific region. *Journal of gastroenterology and hepatology.* 2009 Mar;24(3):346-53.

[10] IARC IAfRoC. Frequently asked questions. GLOBOCAN 2008 2010 [cited 2010 01 Oct]; Available from: http://globocan.iarc.fr/
[11] Arundel C, Lewis JH. Drug-induced liver disease in 2006. *Current opinion in gastroenterology*. 2007 May;23(3):244-54.
[12] Norris W, Paredes AH, Lewis JH. Drug-induced liver injury in 2007. *Current opinion in gastroenterology*. 2008 May;24(3):287-97.
[13] Schutte K, Bornschein J, Malfertheiner P. Hepatocellular carcinoma--epidemiological trends and risk factors. *Digestive diseases* (Basel, Switzerland). 2009;27(2):80-92.
[14] Fattovich G, Giustina G, Degos F, Tremolada F, Diodati G, Almasio P, et al. Morbidity and mortality in compensated cirrhosis type C: a retrospective follow-up study of 384 patients. *Gastroenterology*. 1997 Feb;112(2):463-72.
[15] Evert M, Dombrowski F. [Hepatocellular carcinoma in the non-cirrhotic liver]. *Der Pathologe*. 2008 Feb;29(1):47-52.
[16] Bosch FX, Ribes J, Diaz M, Cleries R. Primary liver cancer: worldwide incidence and trends. *Gastroenterology*. 2004 Nov;127(5 Suppl 1):S5-S16.
[17] Liu CJ, Kao JH, Chen DS. Therapeutic implications of hepatitis B virus genotypes. *Liver Int*. 2005 Dec;25(6):1097-107.
[18] Chan HL, Hui AY, Wong ML, Tse AM, Hung LC, Wong VW, et al. Genotype C hepatitis B virus infection is associated with an increased risk of hepatocellular carcinoma. *Gut*. 2004 Oct;53(10):1494-8.
[19] Chan HL, Tse CH, Mo F, Koh J, Wong VW, Wong GL, et al. High viral load and hepatitis B virus subgenotype ce are associated with increased risk of hepatocellular carcinoma. *J Clin Oncol*. 2008 Jan 10;26(2):177-82.
[20] Tseng TC, Liu CJ, Chen PJ, Lai MY, Lin CL, Kao JH, et al. Subgenotypes of hepatitis B virus genotype C do not correlate with disease progression of chronic hepatitis B in Taiwan. *Liver Int*. 2007 Sep;27(7):983-8.
[21] Donato F, Tagger A, Gelatti U, Parrinello G, Boffetta P, Albertini A, et al. Alcohol and hepatocellular carcinoma: the effect of lifetime intake and hepatitis virus infections in men and women. *American journal of epidemiology*. 2002 Feb 15;155(4):323-31.
[22] Yoshizawa H. Hepatocellular carcinoma associated with hepatitis C virus infection in Japan: projection to other countries in the foreseeable future. *Oncology*. 2002;62 Suppl 1:8-17.
[23] Ikeda K, Saitoh S, Arase Y, Chayama K, Suzuki Y, Kobayashi M, et al. Effect of interferon therapy on hepatocellular carcinogenesis in patients with chronic hepatitis type C: A long-term observation study of 1,643 patients using statistical bias correction with proportional hazard analysis. *Hepatology* (Baltimore, Md. 1999 Apr;29(4):1124-30.
[24] Bruno S, Battezzati PM, Bellati G, Manzin A, Maggioni M, Crosignani A, et al. Long-term beneficial effects in sustained responders to interferon-alfa therapy for chronic hepatitis C. *Journal of hepatology*. 2001 May;34(5):748-55.
[25] Freeman AJ, Dore GJ, Law MG, Thorpe M, Von Overbeck J, Lloyd AR, et al. Estimating progression to cirrhosis in chronic hepatitis C virus infection. *Hepatology* (Baltimore, Md. 2001 Oct;34(4 Pt 1):809-16.

[26] Nordenstedt H, White DL, El-Serag HB. The changing pattern of epidemiology in hepatocellular carcinoma. *Dig Liver Dis.* Jul;42 Suppl 3:S206-14.

[27] Chen CJ, Yu MW, Liaw YF. Epidemiological characteristics and risk factors of hepatocellular carcinoma. *Journal of gastroenterology and hepatology.* 1997 Oct;12(9-10):S294-308.

[28] Donato F, Boffetta P, Puoti M. A meta-analysis of epidemiological studies on the combined effect of hepatitis B and C virus infections in causing hepatocellular carcinoma. *International journal of cancer.* 1998 Jan 30;75(3):347-54.

[29] Morgan TR, Mandayam S, Jamal MM. Alcohol and hepatocellular carcinoma. *Gastroenterology.* 2004 Nov;127(5 Suppl 1):S87-96.

[30] Seitz HK, Stickel F. Risk factors and mechanisms of hepatocarcinogenesis with special emphasis on alcohol and oxidative stress. *Biological chemistry.* 2006 Apr;387(4):349-60.

[31] Zhou L, Conner KR, Phillips MR, Caine ED, Xiao S, Zhang R, et al. Epidemiology of alcohol abuse and dependence in rural chinese men. *Alcoholism, clinical and experimental research.* 2009 Oct;33(10):1770-6.

[32] Horie Y, Yamagishi Y, Kajihara M, Kato S, Ishii H. National survey of hepatocellular carcinoma in heavy drinkers in Japan. *Alcoholism, clinical and experimental research.* 2003 Aug;27(8 Suppl):32S-6S.

[33] Liu JD, Leung KW, Wang CK, Liao LY, Wang CS, Chen PH, et al. Alcohol-related problems in Taiwan with particular emphasis on alcoholic liver diseases. *Alcoholism, clinical and experimental research. 1998* May;22(3 Suppl):164S-9S.

[34] Yun EH, Lim MK, Oh JK, Park JH, Shin A, Sung J, et al. Combined effect of socioeconomic status, viral hepatitis, and lifestyles on hepatocelluar carcinoma risk in Korea. *British journal of cancer.* Aug 24;103(5):741-6.

[35] WHO. *WHO report on Global Status on Alcohol* 2004. 2004:1-3.

[36] Donato F, Tagger A, Chiesa R, Ribero ML, Tomasoni V, Fasola M, et al. Hepatitis B and C virus infection, alcohol drinking, and hepatocellular carcinoma: a case-control study in Italy. Brescia HCC Study. *Hepatology* (Baltimore, Md. 1997 Sep;26(3):579-84.

[37] Hassan MM, Hwang LY, Hatten CJ, Swaim M, Li D, Abbruzzese JL, et al. Risk factors for hepatocellular carcinoma: synergism of alcohol with viral hepatitis and diabetes mellitus. *Hepatology* (Baltimore, Md. 2002 Nov;36(5):1206-13.

[38] Kuper H, Tzonou A, Kaklamani E, Hsieh CC, Lagiou P, Adami HO, et al. Tobacco smoking, alcohol consumption and their interaction in the causation of hepatocellular carcinoma. *International journal of cancer.* 2000 Feb 15;85(4):498-502.

[39] Donato F, Gelatti U, Limina RM, Fattovich G. Southern Europe as an example of interaction between various environmental factors: a systematic review of the epidemiologic evidence. *Oncogene.* 2006 Jun 26;25(27):3756-70.

[40] Fan JG, Peng YD. Metabolic syndrome and non-alcoholic fatty liver disease: Asian definitions and Asian studies. *Hepatobiliary Pancreat Dis Int.* 2007 Dec;6(6):572-8.

[41] Qian Y, Fan JG. Obesity, fatty liver and liver cancer. *Hepatobiliary Pancreat Dis Int.* 2005 May;4(2):173-7.

[42] Marrero JA, Fontana RJ, Su GL, Conjeevaram HS, Emick DM, Lok AS. NAFLD may be a common underlying liver disease in patients with hepatocellular carcinoma in the United States. *Hepatology* (Baltimore, Md. 2002 Dec;36(6):1349-54.

[43] Bugianesi E, Leone N, Vanni E, Marchesini G, Brunello F, Carucci P, et al. Expanding the natural history of nonalcoholic steatohepatitis: from cryptogenic cirrhosis to hepatocellular carcinoma. *Gastroenterology.* 2002 Jul;123(1):134-40.

[44] Takamatsu S, Noguchi N, Kudoh A, Nakamura N, Kawamura T, Teramoto K, et al. Influence of risk factors for metabolic syndrome and non-alcoholic fatty liver disease on the progression and prognosis of hepatocellular carcinoma. *Hepato-gastroenterology.* 2008 Mar-Apr;55(82-83):609-14.

[45] Regimbeau JM, Colombat M, Mognol P, Durand F, Abdalla E, Degott C, et al. Obesity and diabetes as a risk factor for hepatocellular carcinoma. *Liver Transpl.* 2004 Feb;10(2 Suppl 1):S69-73.

[46] Hsia CC, Kleiner DE, Jr., Axiotis CA, Di Bisceglie A, Nomura AM, Stemmermann GN, et al. Mutations of p53 gene in hepatocellular carcinoma: roles of hepatitis B virus and aflatoxin contamination in the diet. *Journal of the National Cancer Institute.* 1992 Nov 4;84(21):1638-41.

[47] Wang LY, Hatch M, Chen CJ, Levin B, You SL, Lu SN, et al. Aflatoxin exposure and risk of hepatocellular carcinoma in Taiwan. *International journal of cancer.* 1996 Sep 4;67(5):620-5.

[48] Wu HC, Wang Q, Yang HI, Ahsan H, Tsai WY, Wang LY, et al. Aflatoxin B1 exposure, hepatitis B virus infection, and hepatocellular carcinoma in Taiwan. *Cancer Epidemiol Biomarkers Prev.* 2009 Mar;18(3):846-53.

[49] Gomaa AI, Khan SA, Toledano MB, Waked I, Taylor-Robinson SD. Hepatocellular carcinoma: epidemiology, risk factors and pathogenesis. *World J Gastroenterol.* 2008 Jul 21;14(27):4300-8.

[50] Bravi F, Bosetti C, Tavani A, Bagnardi V, Gallus S, Negri E, et al. Coffee drinking and hepatocellular carcinoma risk: a meta-analysis. *Hepatology* (Baltimore, Md. 2007 Aug;46(2):430-5.

[51] Bravi F, Bosetti C, Tavani A, La Vecchia C. Coffee drinking and hepatocellular carcinoma: an update. *Hepatology* (Baltimore, Md. 2009 Oct;50(4):1317-8.

[52] Fairbanks KD, Tavill AS. Liver disease in alpha 1-antitrypsin deficiency: a review. The American journal of gastroenterology. 2008 Aug;103(8):2136-41; quiz 42.

[53] Kew MC. Hepatic iron overload and hepatocellular carcinoma. *Cancer letters.* 2009 Dec 1;286(1):38-43.

[54] Klatsky AL, Morton C, Udaltsova N, Friedman GD. Coffee, cirrhosis, and transaminase enzymes. Archives of internal medicine. 2006 Jun 12;166(11):1190-5.

[55] Kowdley KV. Iron, hemochromatosis, and hepatocellular carcinoma. *Gastroenterology.* 2004 Nov;127(5 Suppl 1):S79-86.

[56] Rosen HR. Liver disease associated with alpha1-antitrypsin deficiency. *Clinics in liver disease.* 1998 Feb;2(1):175-85.

[57] Talamini R, Polesel J, Montella M, Dal Maso L, Crispo A, Tommasi LG, et al. Food groups and risk of hepatocellular carcinoma: A multicenter case-control study in Italy. *International journal of cancer.* 2006 Dec 15;119(12):2916-21.

[58] Parkin DM. Global cancer statistics in the year 2000. *The lancet oncology.* 2001 Sep;2(9):533-43.

[59] Parkin DM, Bray F, Ferlay J, Pisani P. Global cancer statistics, 2002. CA: *a cancer journal for clinicians.* 2005 Mar-Apr;55(2):74-108.

[60] World Bank. World Bank List of Econmomies. 2010 [cited 2010 Oct 18]; Available from: http://data.worldbank.org/about/country-classifications/country-and-lending-groups

[61] McGlynn KA, Tsao L, Hsing AW, Devesa SS, Fraumeni JF, Jr. International trends and patterns of primary liver cancer. *International journal of cancer.* 2001 Oct 15;94(2):290-6.

[62] Yu MW, Chen CJ. Elevated serum testosterone levels and risk of hepatocellular carcinoma. *Cancer research.* 1993 Feb 15;53(4):790-4.

[63] Yu MW, Yang YC, Yang SY, Cheng SW, Liaw YF, Lin SM, et al. Hormonal markers and hepatitis B virus-related hepatocellular carcinoma risk: a nested case-control study among men. *Journal of the National Cancer Institute.* 2001 Nov 7;93(21):1644-51.

[64] Luo RH, Zhao ZX, Zhou XY, Gao ZL, Yao JL. Risk factors for primary liver carcinoma in Chinese population. World J Gastroenterol. 2005 Jul 28;11(28):4431-4.

[65] Sun Z, Ming L, Zhu X, Lu J. Prevention and control of hepatitis B in China. *Journal of medical virology.* 2002 Jul;67(3):447-50.

[66] Zhou YH, Wu C, Zhuang H. Vaccination against hepatitis B: the Chinese experience. *Chinese medical journal.* 2009 Jan 5;122(1):98-102.

[67] Shariff MI, Cox IJ, Gomaa AI, Khan SA, Gedroyc W, Taylor-Robinson SD. Hepatocellular carcinoma: current trends in worldwide epidemiology, risk factors, diagnosis and therapeutics. *Expert review of gastroenterology & hepatology.* 2009 Aug;3(4):353-67.

[68] Kiyosawa K, Umemura T, Ichijo T, Matsumoto A, Yoshizawa K, Gad A, et al. Hepatocellular carcinoma: recent trends in Japan. *Gastroenterology.* 2004 Nov;127(5 Suppl 1):S17-26.

[69] But DY, Lai CL, Yuen MF. Natural history of hepatitis-related hepatocellular carcinoma. *World J Gastroenterol.* 2008 Mar 21;14(11):1652-6.

[70] Tanaka H, Imai Y, Hiramatsu N, Ito Y, Imanaka K, Oshita M, et al. Declining incidence of hepatocellular carcinoma in Osaka, Japan, from 1990 to 2003. *Annals of internal medicine. 2008* Jun 3;148(11):820-6.

[71] Umemura T, Ichijo T, Yoshizawa K, Tanaka E, Kiyosawa K. Epidemiology of hepatocellular carcinoma in Japan. *Journal of gastroenterology.* 2009;44 Suppl 19:102-7.

[72] Chia KS, Lee HP, Lee J. Incidence of primary liver cancer in Singapore, 1968-1982. *Annals of the Academy of Medicine, Singapore.* 1989 May;18(3):313-6.

[73] Taiwan Cancer Registry. *Cancer incidence in Taiwan* 1998 -2002. 2010.

[74] Lu SN, Su WW, Yang SS, Chang TT, Cheng KS, Wu JC, et al. Secular trends and geographic variations of hepatitis B virus and hepatitis C virus-associated hepatocellular carcinoma in Taiwan. *International journal of cancer.* 2006 Oct 15;119(8):1946-52.

[75] Kurbanov F, Tanaka Y, Elkady A, Oyunsuren T, Mizokami M. Tracing hepatitis C and Delta viruses to estimate their contribution in HCC rates in Mongolia. *Journal of viral hepatitis.* 2007 Sep;14(9):667-74.

[76] Oyunsuren T, Kurbanov F, Tanaka Y, Elkady A, Sanduijav R, Khajidsuren O, et al. High frequency of hepatocellular carcinoma in Mongolia; association with mono-, or co-infection with hepatitis C, B, and delta viruses. *Journal of medical virology.* 2006 Dec;78(12):1688-95.

[77] Tsatsralt-Od B, Takahashi M, Nishizawa T, Endo K, Inoue J, Okamoto H. High prevalence of dual or triple infection of hepatitis B, C, and delta viruses among patients with chronic liver disease in Mongolia. *Journal of medical virology.* 2005 Dec;77(4):491-9.

[78] Tsatsralt-Od B, Takahashi M, Endo K, Agiimaa D, Buyankhuu O, Ninomiya M, et al. Prevalence of hepatitis B, C, and delta virus infections among children in Mongolia: progress in childhood immunization. *Journal of medical virology.* 2007 Aug; 79(8):1064-74.

[79] Altekruse SF, McGlynn KA, Reichman ME. Hepatocellular carcinoma incidence, mortality, and survival trends in the United States from 1975 to 2005. *J Clin Oncol.* 2009 Mar 20;27(9):1485-91.

[80] IARC IAfRoC. Data sources and methods: Cambodia. GLOBOCAN 2008 2010 [cited 2010 Oct 19]; Available from: http://globocan.iarc.fr/method/method.asp?country=116.

[81] IARC IAfRoC. Data sources and methods: Inodnesia. GLOBOCAN 2008 2010 [cited 2010 Oct 19]; Available from: http://globocan.iarc.fr/method/method.asp?country=360

[82] IARC IAfRoC. Data sources and methods: Phlippines. GLOBOCAN 2008 2010 [cited 2010 Oct 19]; Available from: http://globocan.iarc.fr/method/method.asp?country=608.

In: Hepatocellular Carcionoma: A Global Challenge
Editor: Isabelle Chemin

ISBN: 978-1-61470-644-1

Chapter III

Hepatocellular Carcinoma in Latin America

Flor Helene Pujol[1,*], Sonia Roman[2], Arturo Panduro[2], Maria Cristina Navas[3] and Elizabeth Lampe[4]

[1]Laboratorio de Virología Molecular, CMBC, IVIC, Apdo 20632, Caracas, Venezuela

[2]Servicio de Biología Molecular en Medicina, Antiguo Hospital Civil de Guadalajara, Fray Antonio Alcalde y Centro Universitario de Ciencias de la Salud, Universidad de Guadalajara. Calle Hospital #278, Col. Retiro, Guadalajara, Jalisco, Mexico

[3]Laboratório de Hepatites Virais, Instituto Oswaldo Cruz - FIOCRUZ, Rio de Janeiro, Brazil

[4]Grupo de Gastrohepatología, Facultad de medicina, Universidad de Antioquia, Medellìn, Colombia

Abstract

Latin America (LA) represents a heterogeneous region in terms of ethnic admixtures and exhibits an intermediate incidence of Hepatocellular carcinoma (HCC). The mains factors associated to HCC development in LA are alcohol consumption, HBV and HCV infection. HCV infection is more frequently found in HCC cases in countries like Argentine, Brazil and Mexico, while in Colombia and Peru, HBV infection seems to be more prevalent. HCV genotype 1 is the most frequent genotype in LA, followed by either genotype 2 or 3. This last genotype has been more frequently found among HCC cases in Brazil. Among the eight HBV genotypes (A–H), the ones most commonly found in LA are the worldwide distributed A and D, and the American F and H The American HBV genotype F has been associated to a rapid development of HCC in Alaska. More studies are needed to analyze if this situation is also frequent in the LA countries where this genotype is frequent. In order to reduce its incidence, more efforts are needed to improve the strategies for prevention and treatment of HCC in the region.

1. Hepatocellular Carcinoma Incidence in Latin America

Information on Hepatocellular carcinoma (HCC) in Latin America (LA) is scarce. While around 750,000 persons develop liver cancer each year in the world, this incidence is ranked as intermediate in LA (5.2 per 100.000) (Figure 1). This pathology is the fifth and ninth cause of cancer among men and women respectively in LA, a situation similar to the world average [1]. However, this information is based frequently on incomplete data for some countries, and regional variations might be significant. For example, a tendency towards higher incidences of liver cancer seems to occur in Central America, compared to South America. Generally, as observed worldwide, the frequency of liver cancer is higher in men than women in the region (Figure 1). A large frequency of underreporting is also expected in rural populations and groups getting lower sanitary assistance, which might have high prevalence of hepatitis B virus infection (HBV).

Regional variations have also been described in HCC incidence worldwide, according to age. These differences are probably due to:

- The differential contribution of the most frequent HCC etiological factors: hepatitis B and C viruses (HBV, HCV), alcohol and others,
- The age of acquisition of the viral infections,
- The type and variant of infecting viruses,
- Regional differences in host and ambient factors that might influence the rate of evolution of HCC [2].

HCC was reported as rarely present in Mexico, with a low incidence rate of 0.22 per 100.000 per year [3]. Furthermore, since Mexico is considered a low endemic region for HBV infection, estimations based on HBsAg prevalence rate indicate that only 0.2% of HBsAg-positive patients will develop liver cirrhosis and 0.01% HCC [4]. However, from 1953 to 2007, approximately 1000 HCC cases were reported with an incidence rate from 0.21 to 1.87% (Roman S and Panduro A, manuscript in preparation). Differences in incidence with the Database from the International Agency of Research in Cancer (Figure 1) might be due to for example, to the fact that in Mexico a relatively high frequency of non primary liver cancer are observed and may contribute to increase the frequency of liver cancer reported by the database. In Brazil, clinical and epidemiological data regarding HCC has shown that the incidence of such a tumor is rather low (< 5/100,000). However, there are great regional differences in the frequencies of HCC in different States of Brazil, as it is a country with a large geographical area with great cultural, ethnic and socioeconomic diversity (Figure 2). HCC is more frequent in the States of the South and of the Southeast of the country, as well as in some States of the Amazon region [5]. Despite its relatively low prevalence in Brazil, HCC has a very considerable morbidity and mortality, and thus brings high costs to the whole health system. Lifetime after diagnosis of a patient with HCC clinically detectable is extremely short. Therefore, the incidence rate becomes equivalent to that of mortality [6].

* Correspondance: Dr. Flor H. Pujol. E-mail: fhpujol@gmail.com.

Colombia is a country relatively low incidence of liver cancer with incidences of primary liver and bile duct cancers of 3.1 in males and 2.7 in females, [1]. Each year nearly 1,300 deaths are reported from malignant liver neoplasmas and intrahepatic bile ducts that correspond to a mortality rate of 3.23 and 3.09/100 000 in men and women respectively [7]. However it should be considered that these data are underestimated.

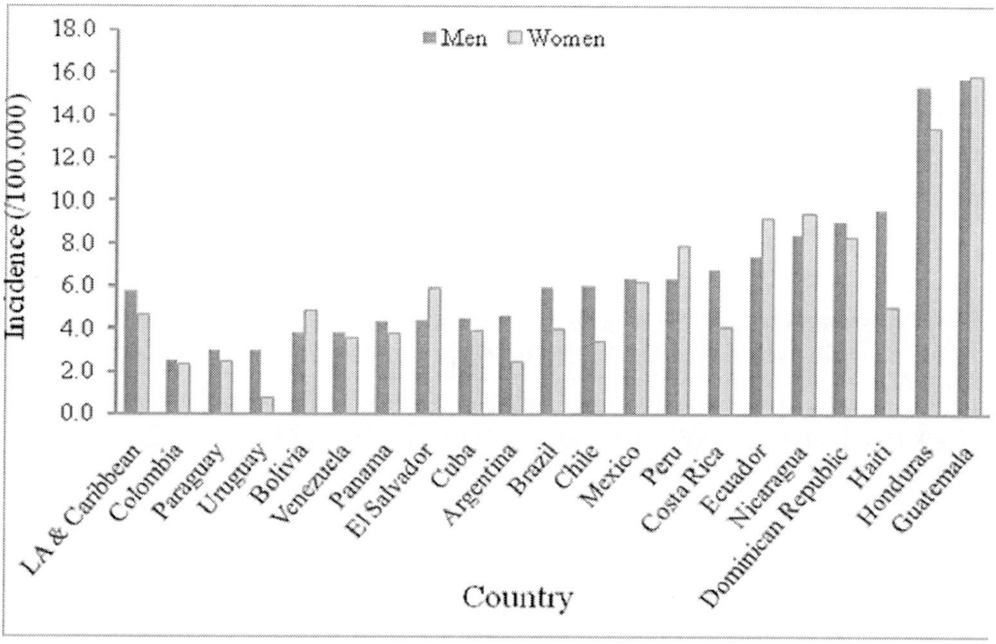

Figure 1. Liver cancer incidence in different LA countries. Incidence is reported as per 100.000 habitants. Data from the IARC Cancerbase [1].

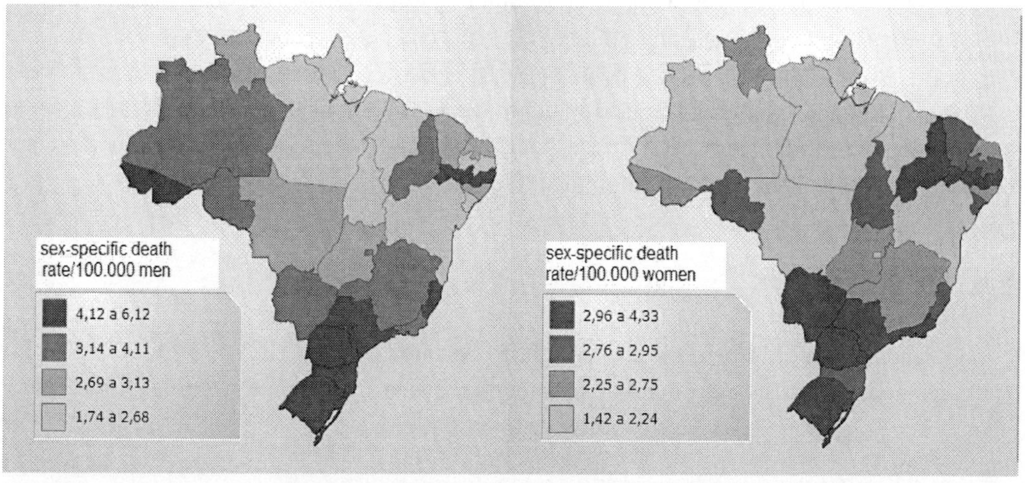

Figure 2. Geographic distribution of estimated crude mortality rates of hepatocellular carcinoma per 100,000 men (left figure) and per 100,000 women (right figure) by State, between the years of 2001 to 2007. Data from the Mortality Information System (SIM) of the Ministry of Health (MOH/SVS/DASIS/CGIAE/SIM).

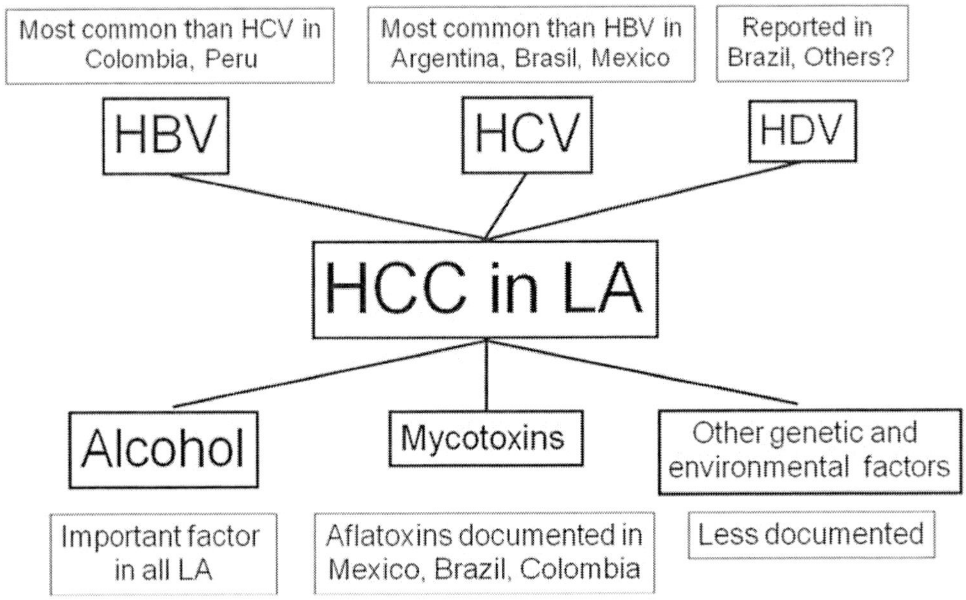

Figure 3. HCC etiological factors in LA. The differential contribution of viral hepatitis viruses is shown for some countries.

2. HCC Etiology in LA

Different etiological factors have been found linked to the development of HCC:

- Viral infection, mainly HBV and HCV infections.
- Non-viral factors, as alcohol consumption, iron overload, tobacco and oral uses, exposure to aflatoxins and other mycotoxins and betel quid chewing [8,9].

LA represents a heterogeneous region in terms of ethnical admixture, and in some aspects socio-cultural practices. These factors among others influence the extent the contribution to the different HCC etiological factors in each country (Figure 3).

2.1. HCV

Around 170 million persons are thought to be infected with HCV worldwide [10]. Six HCV genotypes, and a large number of subtypes inside them, have been described. HCV genotypes 1, 2, and 3 have a worldwide distribution. HCV subtype 3a is frequent in intravenous drug abusers in Europe and the United States. HCV genotype 4 appears to be prevalent in Africa and the Middle East, and genotypes 5 and 6 seem to be more restricted to South Africa and Asia, respectively [11]. HCV genotype 1b has also been frequently associated with a more severe liver disease, although this association might be due to the fact that individuals infected with this genotype have a longer mean duration of infection [12]. A recent meta-analysis showed however HCV subtype 1b associated to a higher risk factor for

HCC development [13]. Hepatic steatosis is a common consequence of HCV infection, has been recently associated with the development of HCC, and is more frequently found among HCV genotype 3 infected patients [14]. More studies are needed to confirm and understand the correlation between HCV genotype 3, the presence of steatosis and progression to HCC [15].

Around 7 million persons are estimated to be infected with HCV in LA, the prevalence ranging from 1 to 2% [10,16]. HCV genotype 1 is the most frequent genotype in LA, followed by either genotype 2 or 3 [17]. For example, in Brazil, Chile, and Mexico, HCV genotype 3 is more common than genotype 2, while in Argentine and Venezuela, the latest is more frequent than genotype 3 [18-20]. The other genotypes are rarely found in the region. HCV is with alcohol the most frequent cause of HCC and transplantation all around LA. A prospective study analyzing cases from 9 countries from LA showed that HCV was the most frequent cause of HCC, with a male:female ratio of 2.6 [21].

In a study carried out at four hospitals in Colombia during the period 2001 to 2007, the prevalence of molecular markers of HCV infection in 46 HCC cases was about 20% (Navas MC, personal communication). A national survey conducted in 1997 including 287 cases of HCC from 19 medical centers showed that hepatitis B virus (HBV) and hepatitis C virus (HCV) are the main responsible agents in Brazil, but with regional differences. The association with HCV infection was more frequent in Southern States and in great urban concentrations [5,22-24]. Studies on hepatitis C virus in Brazil indicate a moderate prevalence in the country as a whole. In the Amazon, among blood donors the prevalence rate varies from 0.8 to 5.9% (Lampe E, personal communication). In all regions, genotype 1 is the most frequent. Genotype 2 is more prevalent in the Center-West region, while genotype 3 was more common in the South [19]. There is only one study relating the frequency of HCV genotypes in Brazilian HCC patients, carried out in São Paulo State. HCV genotype 3 was more frequent among HCC cases, compared to HCV infected patients with liver cirrhosis without HCC. More studies involving a large number of cases should be carried out to confirm these data and to further characterize Brazilian HCV genotype 3 isolates, to elucidate genetic features that might be related to its carcinogenic potential [25].

2.2. HBV

Around 350-400 millions persons are chronic carriers of HBV in the world [26], and 11 million persons are estimated infected with HBV in LA [27], a region exhibiting an intermediate prevalence of infection, varying from 2 to 7% [28]. Great differences in HBV prevalence and genotype distribution can be found in those countries [2,29]. Vertical and low age acquisition of HBV is less frequent than in Asia or Africa [30,31]. The Southern regions of South America (Chile, Uruguay, Paraguay and Argentine) and Central America exhibit lower prevalence of HBV infection, compared to the higher prevalence found in the Amazonian region. A very high prevalence of infection (up to 30%) is found among Amerindians [29].

Among the eight HBV genotypes (A–H), the ones most commonly found in LA are the worldwide distributed A and D, and the American F and H [29]. Although HBV genotypes F and H are indigenous to America, the relative frequency of HBV genotype F in Latin America is in close correlation with the degree of admixture of the general population with Amerindians [29]. The most prevalent HBV genotypes in LA have been found in different studies associated to a relatively high frequency of HCC development [32,33]. These associations might depend however also on the infecting subgenotypes, and on host genetic and environmental factors. Although HBV genotype F have been associated in Alaska to HCC development at younger age [34], these HCC were not associated with the presence of viruses harboring basal core promoter mutation, suggesting that at least in some of the HBV genotype F subgenotypes, HCC development might undergo through different mechanisms that whose observed in the Old World genotypes [32].

In Colombia and Peru, HBV seems to be even more important than HCV in the etiology of HCC [35] (Navas MC, personal communication). HBV DNA was detectable in 60-70% of HCC cases in the series of 46 patients from different hospital location in Colombia (Navas MC, personal communication). In both countries, the predominant HBV genotype, as in Venezuela, is genotype F [29]. In Venezuela, the most common HBV subgenotype is F3, and this subgenotype seems to be less prone to be associated to HCC development, when compared to more frequently associated ones, as genotype C (Pujol FH, personal communication).

In contrast, low HBV prevalence rate (HBsAg marker) has been reported among the Mexican urban population, with the exception of the native Mexicans of the rural areas [4,36]. The predominant HBV genotype in Mexico is genotype H followed by genotypes D and A [36,37]. The association between HBV genotype H and the development of HCC has not been as thoroughly analyzed. Additionally, the highest number of genotype G cases has been reported from Mexico [37]. In Brazil, the Amazon basin is considered a region of high endemicity for HBV. But even in the low prevalence areas of the South or Southeast, there are regional pockets where the prevalence of HBV infections is very high. This prevalence is higher among males than females and is two times more frequent in low socio-economic level populations [38]. HBV genotype A (subgenotype A1) is the most prevalent in the North, Northeast and Southeast and genotype D is the most common genotype in the South of Brazil. In general, genotype F has shown a low prevalence in the whole country, except in some Amerindian Communities of Amazonia [39]. The association of HBV infection with HCC development is particularly significant in the regions of high prevalence of HBV infection [40,41]. In Argentine, HBV genotype F was found more frequently among acute cases, compared to chronic ones, although the clinical presentation of HBV genotype F in chronic cases showed a tendency to adverse effects [42].

Occult HBV infection (OBI) refers to the presence of HBV DNA detectable by PCR in liver and/or serum, in the absence of a detectable circulating HBV surface antigen [43]. There is growing evidence that OBI might be also associated to HCC development [43-45]. OBI has been documented in LA, although its frequency might be more associated with some specific genotypes [25,36,46]. In addition to HBV, HDV co-infection is frequent in some native groups from LA and has been associated to severe episodes of fulminant hepatitis in the region [17]. Hepatitis D virus infection has been shown to be an independent risk factor for HCC development [47]. However, HDV co-infection has been shown to be associated with a higher frequency of HCC in Brazil [48].

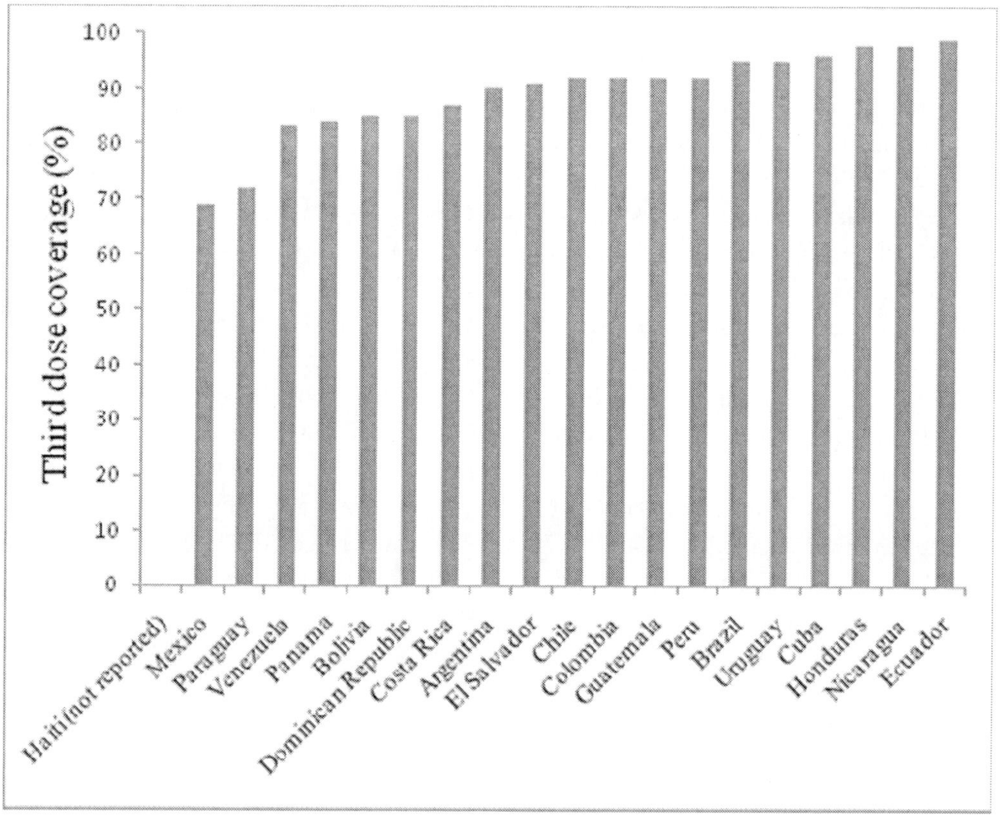

Figure 4. HBV vaccination coverage in LA. Data from the Immunization surveillance, assessment and monitoring, WHO.

2.3. Other Factors

Several factors have been shown to contribute significantly to the development of HCC. One of the first and more significant factors associated to HCC in LA is alcohol consumption, ranking first to second after HCV infection in different countries [21]. Cirrhosis mainly due to alcohol consumption is one of the ten leading causes of mortality in Mexico [49]. Despite the high prevalence of alcoholic liver cirrhosis, case-control studies regarding the association between alcohol consumption and HCC are limited in Mexico by the fact that death occurs earlier in the cirrhotic patient due to long term complications, while the average age of death for HCC occurs at least one or two decades later.

Aflatoxins (AFB) and fumonisins are mycotoxins contaminating several foodstuffs, including maize, cereals, groundnuts and tree nuts, particularly in developing countries. Among the aflatoxins, the most common and potent aflatoxin B1 (AFB1), is metabolized predominantly in the liver in AFB1-epxide, which is able to form a promutagenic DNA adduct. In some areas, up to 50% of HCC exhibits the R249S mutation in the TP53 tumour suppressor gene [50,51]. In addition, epidemiological studies have shown a synergism in HCC development between aflatoxin exposure and HBV infection. The mechanisms involved in this situation are not known yet [50,52]. Mexicans have the highest per capita consumption of corn (300 g/person/day) in the world and an aflatoxin exposure that ranges from 14-85 ng/kg/body weight/day [53,54]. However, in the preparation of mexican tortillas, the process of "nixtamalization" - adding of alkaline lime, either CaO or Ca(OH)2 to the corn grains and then washing them- has been practiced ever since pre-Hispanic times. This action can reduce the amount of aflatoxins and appears to exert a protective effect against the development of HCC [55]. Aflatoxins have also been described to be present in the urine of Cuban children [56]. R249S mutation has been found in HCC samples from Brazilian patients, which may suggest aflatoxin (AFB1) exposure and indicates that this mutation is an important factor of HCC carcinogenesis in Brazil [57]. Although AFB1 contamination has been controlled in Brazil, there are still cases of food samples presenting AFB1 levels above the tolerated level. A survey of aflatoxin contamination in selected Colombian foods was conducted on samples collected in supermarkets and stock centers [58]. Aflatoxins were detected in 22 samples, including 14 of 109 samples of corn and corn products. Given that corn is part of the common diet in Colombia, it is likely that AFB1 may represent a significant exposure at least in a fraction of the population. In 46 HCC cases, the prevalence of TP53 mutations was about 1/3 and occurred at the common aflatoxin mutation hotspot, codon 249 (Navas MC, personal communication).

3. HCC Prevention and Treatment in LA

The HBV vaccination benefits in reducing HCC incidence have been shown in several Asian countries [59]. HBV vaccine coverage in LA has significantly been increasing in this last decade (Figure 4). Many of the LA countries report vaccine coverage over 90%. In Mexico, vaccine coverage was relatively low in these last two years, but similar to the other countries in previous ones [60]. In Brazil, HBV vaccine is offered by the public health system since the 1990s. A few commitments to reduce viral hepatitis prevalence in the country are being implemented by the Ministry of Health, like increasing the vaccine supply to extend vaccination to older groups. For the reduction of vertical transmission of hepatitis B virus the offer of serological screening test for all pregnant women will be intensified and all newborns of mothers with the HBV infection will receive vaccine and immunoglobulin. In Colombia, the benefit of HBV vaccination in reducing HBV prevalence has already been reported [61].

Other prevention strategies in LA include the reduction of HBV and HCV transmission, where the safety of blood donation has been increased. However, many issues still need to be addressed to reduce the residual risk of transmission of HBV and HCV, like increasing the number of voluntary donations, and better donor selection and screening [62]. In Mexico and other LA countries, HBV infection is significantly transmitted by sexual activity [4]. Current prevalence trends derived from age-adjusted population-based estimations indicate that HBV infection is higher in elderly subjects than in childhood, consequence of the time gap between the implementation of the mandatory detection of HBsAg in blood donors and universal vaccination policies [4]. Similarly, chronic HCV infection in Mexico is mostly common among adult women in a ratio of 3:1 compared to men and was mainly transmitted by blood transfusion during the 1980's [63-65]. Consequently, it is not unfamiliar that HCV chronic infection be detected in a higher proportion (up to 40%) than HBV chronic infection in HCC cases [3,66]. In order to prevent severe complications of chronic hepatitis C and HCC development, the Brazilian Ministry of Health will also intensify the offer of tests to detect HCV infection in order to encourage early diagnosis, thereby increasing the possibility of curative treatment.

Therapeutic options and guidelines are available for both HBV and HCV in LA [67,68], although these options may not be available for all infected patients. In Brazil, in 2009, a new Clinical Therapeutic Protocol and Guidelines for the treatment of chronic hepatitis B and co-infections was released by the Ministry of Health, including drugs as tenofovir, entecavir and adefovir in addition to interferon and ribavirin.

Orthotopic liver transplantation (OLT) has been improved in LA over years to provide a therapeutic option for early HCC. Due to the scarcity of liver donors compared to the demand, strict criteria must be used to be eligible for OLT [69]. The "Milan criteria" are widely accepted in many countries [70,71]. The major criteria include the presence of a single small tumor or up to 3 with smaller dimensions and no macrovascular invasion. Limitations for OLT include risk before and after this kind of intervention and the difficulty in finding an adequate donor [58,69,72,73]. HCV is the most frequent cause of hepatic disease in patients who underwent orthotopic liver transplantation (OLT) in many LA countries [70,74,75]. In Venezuela, OLT has been increasingly performed recently, following the "Milan criteria". In Colombia, in particular in Medellin, an average survival of 5 years in 80% of the patients has been obtained with OLT when using cadaveric donors (Restrepo JC, personal communication). Treatment modalities for HCC in Mexico are mainly surgical resection with an overall survival of 8 months to due to late diagnosis and advance liver disease [76].

Conclusion

HCC occurs with an intermediate incidence in LA. The most frequent etiologies are alcohol consumption and/or HCV infection in many countries, although HBV infection is the leading cause in others. The complex ethnic admixture and socio-cultural practices existing in LA is also associated to differences in incidence and etiology of HCC in the region. More studies are needed to elucidate if specific viral strains, indigenous to the region, may lead to a more severe progression to HCC. In particular, the association with HCC development of the American HBV genotypes and subgenotypes warrants further studies. Efforts should focus on improving the strategies for prevention and treatment of HCC in the region.

References

[1] Ferlay J, Shin HR, Bray F, Forman D, Mathers C and Parkin DM. GLOBOCAN 2008, Cancer Incidence and Mortality Worldwide: IARC CancerBase No. 10 [Internet]. Lyon, France: *International Agency for Research on Cancer;* 2010. Available from: http://globocan.iarc.fr.

[2] Yang JD, Roberts LR 2010, Hepatocellular carcinoma: a global view. *Nat Rev Gastroenterol Hepatol.* 2010;7:448-458.

[3] Vivas Arceo C, Bastidas Ramirez BE, Panduro A. Hepatocellular carcinoma is rarely present in Western Mexico. *Hepatology Research* 1999; 44:1401-1403.

[4] Roman S, Panduro A, Aguilar-Gutierrez Y, Maldonado M, Vazquez-VanDyck, Martinez-Lopez E, Ruiz-Madrigal B, Hernandez-Nazara Z. A low steady HBsAg seroprevalence is associated with a low incidence of HBV-related liver cirrhosis and hepatocellular carcinoma in Mexico: a systemic review. *Hepatology International* 2009;3:343-335.

[5] Goncalves CS, Pereira FE, Gayotto LCC. Hepatocellular carcinoma in Brazil: report of a national survey (Florianopolis, SC, 1995). *Rev Inst. Med Trop S. Paulo*, 1997; 39: 165-170.

[6] Pimenta JR, Massabki PS. Hepatocellular carcinoma: a clinical outlook. *Rev Bras Clin Med,* 2010; 8:59-67.

[7] Ochoa LF, Montoya LP. Mortalidad por cáncer en Colombia en el año 2000: cuando aumentar no es mejorar. *CES Medicina.* 2003; 17: 7-22.

[8] Blonski W, Kotlyar DS, Forde KA. Non-viral causes of hepatocellular carcinoma. *World J Gastroenterol.* 2010; 16: 3603-3615.

[9] Wang LY, You SL, Lu SN, Ho HC, Wu MH, Sun CA, Yang HI, Chien-Jen C. Risk of hepatocellular carcinoma and habits of alcohol drinking, betel quid chewing and cigarette smoking: a cohort of 2416 HBsAg-seropositive and 9421 HBsAg-seronegative male residents in Taiwan. *Cancer Causes Control.* 2003; 14: 241-250.

[10] Shepard CW, Finelli L, Alter MJ. Global epidemiology of hepatitis C virus infection. *Lancet Infect Dis.* 2005; 5: 558-567.

[11] Simmonds P. The origin and evolution of hepatitis viruses in humans. *J Gen Virol* 2001; 82: 693-712.

[12] Zein NN. Clinical significance of hepatitis C virus genotypes. *Clin Microbiol Rev. 2000;* 13: 223-235.

[13] Raimondi S, Bruno S, Mondelli MU, Maisonneuve P. Hepatitis C virus genotype 1b as a risk factor for hepatocellular carcinoma development: a meta-analysis. *J Hepatol.* 2009; 50: 1142-1154.

[14] Monto A. Hepatitis C and steatosis. *Semin Gastrointest Dis.* 2002; 13: 40-46.

[15] Zhu AX, Chung RT. Hepatic steatosis in patients with chronic hepatitis C virus infection. Another risk factor for hepatocellular carcinoma? *Cancer.* 2003; 97: 2948-2950.

[16] Méndez-Sánchez N, Gutiérrez-Grobe Y, Kobashi-Margáin RA. Epidemiology of HCV infection in Latin America. *Ann Hepatol.* 2010;9: S2-S27.

[17] Pujol FH. Molecular epidemiology of hepatitis viruses in Latin America and Amerindians. *Virus Rev Res.* 2009; 14: 7-15.

[18] Cristina J. Genetic diversity and evolution of hepatitis C virus in the Latin American region. *J Clin Virol.* 2005; 34(Suppl 2): S1-S7.

[19] Campiotto S, Pinho JR, Carrilho FJ, Da Silva LC, Souto FJ, Spinelli V, Pereira LM, Coelho HS, Silva AO, Fonseca JC, et al. Geographic distribution of hepatitis C virus genotypes in Brazil. *Braz J Med Biol Res.* 2005; 38: 41–49.

[20] Panduro A, Roman S, Khan S, Tanaka Y, Kurbanov F, Martinez-Lopez E, Campollo O, Hernandez-Nazara Z, Mizokami M. Molecular epidemiology of hepatitis C virus genotypes in West Mexico. *Virus Research* 2010; 151: 19-25.

[21] Fassio E, Díaz S, Santa C, Reig ME, Martínez Artola Y, Alves de Mattos A, Míguez C, Galizzi J, Zapata R, Ridruejo E, de Souza FC, Hernández N, Pinchuk L; Multicenter Group for Study of Hepatocarcinoma in Latin America; Asociación Latinoamericana para el Estudio del Hígado (ALEH). Etiology of hepatocellular carcinoma in Latin America: a prospective, multicenter, international study. *Ann Hepatol.* 2010; 9: 63-69.

[22] Leão-Filho GC, Lopes EPA, Ferraz AAB, Moura I, Pernambuco JR, Reis C, Silva AEB, Ferraz MCG. Hepatitis G Virus Infection in Patients with Hepatocellular Carcinoma in Recife, Brazil. *Jpn J Clin Oncol* 2007; 37: 632–636.

[23] Narciso GR, Nader LA, Maggione LS, Kupsi C. Profile of the hepatocellular carcinoma in patients with diagnosis of chronic C hepatitis. *Sciencia Medica, Porto Alegre:PUCRS,* 2006; 9: 157-161.

[24] Pannain VLN; Bottino AC; Santos RTM; Coelho HSM; Ribeiro-Filho J; Alves VAF. Detecção imunoistoquímica das oncoproteínas p21ras, c-myc e p53 no carcinoma hepatocelular e no tecido hepático não-neoplásico. *Arq Gastroenterol.* 2004; 41: 225-228.

[25] Alencar RS, Gomes MM, Sitnik R, Pinho JR, Malta FM, Mello IM, Mello ES, Bacchella T, Machado MC, Alves VA, Carrilho FJ. Low occurrence of occult hepatitis B virus infection and high frequency of hepatitis C virus genotype 3 in hepatocellular carcinoma in Brazil. *Braz J Med Biol Res.* 2008; 41: 235-240.

[26] McMahon BJ. Epidemiology and natural history of hepatitis B. *Semin Liver Dis.* 2005;25: S3-S8.

[27] Custer B, Sullivan SD, Hazlet TK, Iloeje U, Veenstra DL, Kowdley KV. Global epidemiology of hepatitis B virus. *J Clin Gastroenterol.* 2004;38: S158-S168.

[28] Tanaka J. Hepatitis B epidemiology in Latin America. *Vaccine.* 2000;18: S17-S9.

[29] Devesa M, Pujol FH. Hepatitis B virus genetic diversity in Latin America. *Virus Res.* 2007;127: 177-184.

[30] Duarte MC, Cardona N, Poblete F, González K, García M, Pacheco M, Botto C, Pujol FH, Williams JR. A comparative epidemiological study of hepatitis B and hepatitis D virus infections in Yanomami and Piaroa Amerindians of Amazonas State, Venezuela. *Trop Med Int Health.* 2010;15: 924-933.

[31] Parana R, Almeida D. HBV epidemiology in Latin America. *J Clin Virol.* 2005;34: S130-S133.

[32] McMahon BJ. The influence of hepatitis B virus genotype and subgenotype on the natural history of chronic hepatitis B. *Hepatol Int.* 2009;3: 334-342.

[33] Pujol FH, Navas MC, Hainaut P, Chemin I. Worldwide genetic diversity of HBV genotypes and risk of hepatocellular carcinoma. *Cancer Lett.* 2009;286: 80-88

[34] Livingston SE, Simonetti J, McMahon B, Bulkow L, Hurlburt KJ, Homan CE, Snowball MM, Cagle HH, Williams JL, Chulanov VP. Hepatitis B virus genotypes in Alaska Native People with hepatocellular carcinoma: preponderance of genotype F. *J Infect Dis* 2007;195: 5–11.

[35] Bustíos Sánchez C, Díaz Ferrer J, Román Vargas R, Dávalos Moscol M, Zumaeta Villena E. Clinical - Epidemiological characteristics of the Hepatocellular Carcinoma and treatment in the department of digestive system diseases of the National Hospital "Eduardo Rebagliatti Martins" (HNERM) – ESSALUD Rev Gastroenterol Peru. 2009;29: 17-23.

[36] Roman S, Tanaka Y, Khan A, Kurbanov, Hideaki K, Mizokami M, Panduro A. Occult hepatitis B in the genotype H-infected Nahuas and Huichol native Mexican population. *J Med Virol.* 2010;82: 1527-1536.

[37] Sanchez LV, Tanaka Y, Maldonado M, Mizokami M, Panduro A. Difference of hepatitis B virus genotype distribution in two groups of Mexican patients with different risk factors. High prevalence of genotype H and G. *Intervirology.* 2007;50: 9-15.

[38] Pereira LM, Martelli CM, Merchán-Hamann E, Montarroyos UR, Braga MC, de Lima ML, Cardoso MR, Turchi MD, Costa MA, de Alencar LC, Moreira RC, Figueiredo GM, Ximenes RA; Hepatitis Study Group. Population-based multicentric survey of hepatitis B infection and risk factor differences among three regions in Brazil. *Am J Trop Med Hyg.* 2009;81: 240-247.

[39] Mello FC, Souto FJ, Nabuco LC, Villela-Nogueira CA, Coelho HS, Franz HC, Saraiva JC, Virgolino HA, Motta-Castro AR, Melo MM, Martins RM, Gomes SA. Hepatitis B virus genotypes circulating in Brazil: molecular characterization of genotype F isolates. *BMC Microbiol.* 2007;7: 103.

[40] Cotrim H, Mota E, Leite L, Silva L, Lyra L. A case-control study on the association of hepatitis B virus infection and hepatocellular carcinoma in northeast Brazil. *Rev Saude Publica.* 1992;26: 301-305.

[41] Miranda EC, Moia LJ, Amaral IS, Barbosa MS, Conde SR, Araújo MT, Cruz ER, Demachki S, Bensabath G, Soares MC. Hepatitis B and C virus infection and the hepatocellular carcinoma in the East Amazon, Brazil. *Rev Soc Bras Med Trop.* 2004;37: S47-S51.

[42] Pezzano SC, Torres C, Fainboim HA, Bouzas MB, Schroder T, Giuliano SF, Paz S, Alvarez E, Campos RH, Mbayed VA. Hepatitis B virus in Buenos Aires, Argentina: genotypes, virological characteristics and clinical outcomes. *Clin Microbiol Infect.* 2010: in press.

[43] Hollinger FB, Sood G. Occult hepatitis B virus infection: a covert operation. *J Viral Hepat.* 2010; 17: 1-15.

[44] Chemin I, Zoulim F. Hepatitis B virus induced hepatocellular carcinoma. *Cancer Lett.* 2009;286: 52-59.

[45] De Mitri MS, Cassini R, Bernardi M. Hepatitis B virus-related hepatocarcinogenesis: molecular oncogenic potential of clear or occult infections. *Eur J Cancer.* 2010;46: 2178-2186.

[46] Gutiérrez C, Devesa M, Loureiro CL, León G, Liprandi F, Pujol FH. Molecular and serological evaluation of surface antigen negative hepatitis B virus infection in blood donors from Venezuela. *J Med Virol.* 2004;73: 200-207.

[47] Romeo R, Del Ninno E, Rumi M, Russo A, Sangiovanni A, de Franchis R, Ronchi G, Colombo M. A 28-year study of the course of hepatitis Delta infection: a risk factor for cirrhosis and hepatocellular carcinoma. *Gastroenterology.* 2009;136: 1629-1638.

[48] Kiesslich D, Crispim MA, Santos C, Ferreira Fde L, Fraiji NA, Komninakis SV, Diaz RS. Influence of hepatitis B virus (HBV) genotype on the clinical course of disease in patients coinfected with HBV and hepatitis delta virus. *J Infect Dis.* 2009;199: 1608-1611.

[49] Anuario Estadístico de Mortalidad, series 2001-2008. Secretaria de Salud de Mexico. Cited July 2010. http://www.sinais.salud.gob.mx/mortalidad/index.html.

[50] Wild CP, Montesano R. A model of interaction: aflatoxins and hepatitis viruses in liver cancer aetiology and prevention. *Cancer Lett.* 2009;286: 22-28.

[51] Wild CP, Gong YY. Mycotoxins and human disease: a largely ignored global health issue. *Carcinogenesis.* 2010;31: 71-82.

[52] Gouas D, Shi H, Hainaut P. The aflatoxin-induced TP53 mutation at codon 249 (R249S): biomarker of exposure, early detection and target for therapy. *Cancer Lett.* 2009;286: 29-37.

[53] Liu Y & Wu F. Global burden of aflatoxin-induced hepatocellular carcinoma: A risk assessment. *Environmental Health Perspectives* 2010;118: 818-824.

[54] Guzman-de-Peña D & Peña-Cabriales JJ. Regulatory considerations of aflatoxin contamination of food in Mexico. *Rev Latinoamer Microbiol.* 2005;47: 160-164.

[55] Anguiano-Ruvalcaba GL, Verver & Vargas-Cortina A, Guzman-de-Peña D. Inactivation of aflatoxin B1 and aflatoxicol through "nixtamalizacion" of corn and their regeneration by acidication of corn dough. *Salud Publica Mex* 2005;47: 369-375.

[56] Alvarez MT, Castañeda C, Escobar A, Fragoso T. Aflatoxin detection in urine in liver diseases in childhood. *G E N.* 1991;45: 205-219.

[57] Nogueira JA, Ono-Nita SK, Nita ME, de Souza MM, do Carmo EP, Mello ES, Scapulatempo C, Paranaguá-Vezozzo DC, Carrilho FJ, Alves VA. TP53 mutation has high prevalence and is correlated with larger and poorly differentiated HCC in Brazilian patients. *BMC Cancer.* 2009;9: 204-249.

[58] Diaz GJ, Espitia E. Occurrence of aflatoxin M1 in retail milk samples from Bogotá, Colombia. *Food Addit Contam.* 2006;23: 811-815.

[59] Williams R 2006, Global challenges in liver disease. *Hepatology.* 2006 Sep;44: 521-526.

[60] WHO. *Immunization surveillance, assessment and monitoring.* 2010.

[61] De la Hoz F, Perez L, de Neira M, Hall AJ. Eight years of hepatitis B vaccination in Colombia with a recombinant vaccine: factors influencing hepatitis B virus infection and effectiveness. *Int J Infect Dis.* 2008;12: 183-189.

[62] Schmunis GA, Cruz JR. Safety of the blood supply in Latin America. *Clin Microbiol Rev.* 2005;18: 12-29.

[63] Chiquete E and Panduro A. Low prevalence of anti-hepatitis C virus antibodies in Mexico: A systematic review. *Intervirology.* 2007;50: 1-8.

[64] Chiquete E, Sanchez LV, Panduro A. Routes of infection and clinical outcome of Mexican women reactive to anti-hepatitis C virus antibodies. *Hepatol Res.* 2006;36: 1001-106.

[65] Vazquez-Vandyck, Roman S, Vazquez JL, Huacuja L, Khalsa G, Troyo-SanRoman R, Panduro A. Effect of Breathwalk on body composition, metabolic and mood state in

chronic hepatitis C patients with insulin resistance sydrome. *World J Gastroenterol.* 2007;13: 6213-6218.

[66] Mondragon-Sanchez R, Gurduño-Lopez AL, Hernandez-Castillo E, Gomez-Gomez E, Ruiz-Molina JM. Hepatocellular carcinoma and hepatitis C in Mexico. *Hepatogastroenterology.* 2005;52: 1159-1162.

[67] Daruich J, Gadano A, Fainboim H, Pessoa M, Cheinquer H. Latin American guideline for the treatment of chronic hepatitis B. *Acta Gastroenterol Latinoam.* 2007;37: 168-177.

[68] Latin American Association for the Study of the Liver. Latin American Association for the Study of the Liver Practice Guidelines. Diagnosis, management, and treatment of hepatitis C. *Ann Hepatol.* 2010;9: S8-S26.

[69] Alsina AE. Liver transplantation for hepatocellular carcinoma. *Cancer Control.* 2010 17: 83-86.

[70] Coelho GR, Vasconcelos KF, Vasconcelos JB, Barros MA, Costa PE, Borges GC, Júnior JT, Brasil IR, Filho DH, Viana CF, Rocha TD, Mesquita DF, Garcia JH. Orthotopic liver transplantation for hepatocellular carcinoma: one center's experience in the Northeast of Brazil. *Transplant Proc.* 2009;41: 1740-1742.

[71] Gabrielli M, Vivanco M, Hepp J, Martínez J, Pérez R, Guerra J, Arrese M, Figueroa E, Soza A, Yáñes R, Humeres R, Rios H, Palacios JM, Zapata R, Sanhueza E, Contreras J, Rencoret G, Rossi R, Jarufe N. Liver transplantation results for hepatocellular carcinoma in Chile. *Transplant Proc.* 2010;42: 299-301.

[72] Hepp J, Innocenti FA. Liver transplantation in Latin America: current status. *Transplant Proc.* 2004;36: 1667-1668.

[73] Tanwar S, Khan SA, Grover VP, Gwilt C, Smith B, Brown A. Liver transplantation for hepatocellular carcinoma. *World J Gastroenterol.* 2009 15: 5511-5516.

[74] González I, Abdo AA, López O, Hernández JC, Samada M, Cepero M, Ramos L, Ysla R, Madrigal G, Collera SA, Dominguez J, Diaz J, Benitez PP, Castellanos R. First 100 liver transplants at the medico-surgical research center (CIMEQ). *Transplant Proc.* 2006;38: 2473-2474.

[75] González-Rapado L, Abdo A, Hernández H, Cepero M, Samada M, Ramos L, Ysla R, Gómez F, Delgado D, Melián K, González C, Pérez J, Bernardos A. Results of liver transplantation at the Cuban Center for Medical and Surgical Research. *Transplant Proc.* 2008;40: 2983-2984.

[76] Meza-Junco J, Montaño-Lopez A, Candelaria M. Modalidades de tratamiento para pacientes con carcinoma hepatocelular: una serie retrospectiva de una sola institución en Mexico. *Gastroenterologia y Hepatologia* 2004;27: 11-17.

In: Hepatocellular Carcionoma: A Global Challenge
Editor: Isabelle Chemin
ISBN: 978-1-61470-644-1

Chapter IV

Epidemiology of Hepatocellular Carcinoma in Europe

Nathalie Ganne-Carrie * ***and Jean-Claude Trinchet***
Service d'Hépato-gastroentérologie, Hôpital Jean Verdier, AP-HP, UFR SMBH, Université Paris, Bondy, France

Abstract

Hepatocellular carcinoma(HCC), the main form of primary liver cancer, occurs mostly in the setting of cirrhosis. Chronic HCV infection, alcohol consumption, and obesity/diabetes are the main risk factors in Europe. The overall annual incidence of liver cancer in Europe was estimated around 60 000 cases in 2008 (two-third in men) but with a wide spectrum according to different countries. There is an increasing gradient from Northern to Southern Europe, reflecting geographical differences in exposure to risk factors for HCC. Mortality is very close to incidence, reflecting the poor prognosis of patients. Upward trends in incidence and mortality from liver cancer have been reported in several European countries, but with a large pattern of outcomes. In France, in contrast with persistently increasing incidence, a slight decrease in mortality from late-1990s has been recently reported after several decades of continuous increase. Significant improvement in HCC incidence and mortality in the future will require effective control of exposure to the main causes of cirrhosis, promotion of periodic ultrasonographic surveillance and effective antiviral control of HCV and HBV infections in patients with cirrhosis, and further improvements in curative treatments for HCC.

Keywords: Hepatocellular carcinoma, cirrhosis, epidemiology, prevention, screening, diagnosis

* Correspondance: Dr Nathalie GANNE, MD PhD. Hôpital Jean Verdier, Service d'Hépato-gastroentérologie, Avenue du 14 Juillet, 93143 Bondy Cedex – France, Tél : +33 1 48 02 62 80, Fax : +33 1 48 02 62 02, Email : nathalie.ganne@jvr.aphp.fr.

Introduction

HCC is the most frequent primary liver cancer. Liver cancer is the fifth most common malignancy worldwide in men and the seventh in women [1]. It is also the third leading cause of cancer-related mortality worldwide with almost 700 000 related deaths recorded in 2008, exceeded only by cancer of lung and stomach [1]. In more than 90% of cases, HCC occurs in patients with a chronic liver disease, mostly cirrhosis. Accordingly the epidemiology of HCC is closely linked to the geographical distribution of the causes of chronic liver diseases [2]. On a worldwide scale, chronic infections by hepatitis B virus (HBV) and hepatitis C virus (HCV) are predominant, with about 350 millions and 170 millions of chronic carriers respectively, mostly in Africa and Asia [3]. In Europe, the prevalence of HBV and HCV chronic carriers is markedly lower than in Africa and Asia, and both excessive alcohol consumption and obesity/diabetes represent important factors of chronic liver diseases [4, 5]. Moreover an important increase in HCC incidence during the three past decades has been reported in several countries in Europe, as in North America and Japan [6, 7].

This chapter is aimed at reviewing the main data and trends about epidemiology and risk factors for HCC in Europe, with focus for the situation in France.

Risk (Predictive) Factors

As previously indicated, HCC occurs almost always in patients with chronic liver diseases. Consequently epidemiological characteristics of HCC in one given area depend on regional prevalences of the different causes of chronic liver diseases, on time and duration of exposure, and possibly on some cofactors specific to the area. In Africa and Asia, HBV infection is highly prevalent and occurs mostly at birth from maternal contamination or during the first years of childhood. In those areas, exposure to aflatoxin B1, a potent carcinogen produced by contamination of food grains with *Aspergillus fumigatus*, is common and results in a major increase in HCC risk [8]. Consequently many cases of HCC occur at young age, often during third or fourth decade. Moreover HCC can occur before cirrhosis in chronic HBV infection explaining that up to 40% of patients are not cirrhotic at time of diagnosis in those areas [2].

By contrast in Europe HCC is rarely associated with HBV infection. The main causes of chronic liver diseases are chronic alcohol consumption and chronic HCV infection [4], but also non alcoholic steatohepatitis (NASH) [9]. This latter disease is caused by obesity and diabetes, whose prevalences are increasing markedly in many European countries as in North America [10-12]. Exposure to those three factors begins usually in adolescents or young adults, 15-20 years later than HBV infection in highly endemic areas. Consequently HCC occurs during the fifth and sixth decades in most of the European patients. However HCC can occur early in patients with more than one cause of liver disease (most often alcohol and HCV, or alcohol and NASH) or with other cofactors such as human immunodeficiency virus (HIV) infection [13]. Almost all the patients with alcohol and HCV-related HCC have cirrhosis at the time of cancer diagnosis. The situation seems to be different for NASH-related HCC with a significantly higher percentage (but still imprecise) of patients without cirrhosis at HCC diagnosis [14]. HCC can also occur in the setting of rare causes of chronic liver diseases such as hereditary hemochromatosis [15] or primary biliary cirrhosis [16] but on the whole the number of patients is low.

Besides etiologies of chronic liver diseases, a large number of factors may modify the individual risk for HCC [17]. Most of epidemiological studies have shown a markedly higher prevalence of HCC in males than in females with a ratio above 2 [1]. However this difference is usually less important for HCV infection than for alcohol consumption. The reasons for this difference are not well known. It could result either on sex-related factors, such as sex hormones, or on epidemiological differences about exposure to etiological factors such as alcohol consumption in males [18]. A lot of other clinical and biological factors (related to liver function, portal hypertension, molecular carcinogenetic pathways, etc.) have been linked to HCC risk [17, 19]. Some studies have demonstrated that individual risk can be estimated using predictive scores combining simple clinical factors [11, 20, 21]. Moreover smoking has been recently recognized as another risk factor for HCC, which has been added to the list of tobacco-related malignancies by the International Agency for Research on Cancer in 2004 [22, 23].

In France chronic alcohol consumption remains the first cause (about 60-70%) of cirrhosis associated with HCC [24, 25]. HCV is the second cause (30%) [26] due to high rate of chronic infection, concerning about 280 000 patients in a recent survey from the French Institut National de Veille Sanitaire (INVs) (http://www.invs.sante.fr/publications/2006/prevalence _b_c/index. html). Chronic HBV infection has been estimated to affect about 230 000 subjects in the same survey but it is likely that the rate of inactive carriers is high in this population, resulting in a lower influence of HBV in HCC epidemiology in France. Association between alcohol and virus, mainly HCV, accounts for about 5% of cases [25]. Moreover, obesity and diabetes are increasing in French population (for instance obesity prevalence was 14.5% in 2009 in ObEpi survey *versus* 8.5% in 1997) [27], resulting probably in a growing prevalence (even if still imprecise) of NASH.

Among HCC patients, only a very small percentage (likely less than 5%) has no chronic liver disease ("normal" liver) [28, 29]. Some tumours correspond histologically to fibrolamellar HCC [30]. Epidemiology and risk factors seem to be different from usual HCC and remain largely unknown. Some cases result from malignant transformation of hepatocellular adenoma in the context of exogenous anabolic steroid administration [18] or hereditary metabolic disorders such as glycogenosis [31]. Exposure to environmental factors such as vinyl chloride monomer or other chemical carcinogens has been suggested but is still controversial [32].

Incidence and Mortality

Most of the data concerning HCC incidence and mortality in this chapter have been extracted from GLOBOCAN (http://www.iarc.fr/en/media-centre/iarcnews/2010/globocan 2008.php) and European Cancer Observatory (ECO) (http://eu-cancer.iarc.fr/cancer-7-liver.html,en) websites which are two large databases managed by the International Agency for Research on Cancer. Two recent publications have summarized estimates about worldwide [1] and European [26] cancer burden in 2008 including liver cancer. The rates of incidence and mortality have been age-standardized (Age Standardized Rate (ASR) per 100 000 person-years)) using World or European standard populations. Concerning incidence and mortality ASRs in Europe, there are frequent discrepancies between studies due to various selection criteria for calendar periods and included countries [4, 6, 26]. Moreover precise knowledge of HCC epidemiology is hampered by difficulty to separate HCC from other primary liver tumors, mainly due to frequent lack of histological data. Overall morphological verification rates range from 40% in Eastern Europe to 65% in Western Europe resulting in high rates of unknown types of tumor in some countries (for instance 56% in Russian Federation) [4]. Accordingly most of epidemiological studies concern only "primary liver cancer" (codes 155 and C22 in International Classification of Diseases (ICD)-9 and ICD-10 respectively) and not specifically HCC (codes 155.0 and C22.0 in ICD-9 and ICD-10 respectively). It is well established that 80-90% of all primary liver tumors correspond to HCC. Other primary liver tumors correspond almost exclusively to intrahepatic cholangiocarcinoma (codes 155.1 and C22.1 in ICD-9 and ICD-10 respectively), a biliary cancer also frequently encountered in the setting of cirrhosis particularly from viral origin [33, 34]. Even if global statistics about primary liver cancer reflect mainly HCC epidemiology, modifications may also be related to intrahepatic cholangiocarcinoma. An important increase in primary liver cancer incidence in England and Wales has been linked (at least partially) to a dramatic increase in intrahepatic cholangiocarcinoma incidence over the last three decades of the 20th century [35].

Incidence

The annual incidence of liver cancer was estimated to 748 000 cases in 2008 worldwide (ASR 10.8 per 100 000) with about 70% of cases in males (ASR 16.0 *versus* 6.0 per 100 000 in females) [1]. However, there are important differences according to geographical areas, mainly due to different exposure to risk factors for HCC as indicated above [1]. The areas of high incidence are mostly concentrated in developing countries (ASR 18.9 and 7.6 per 100 000 in males and females respectively in 2008) [1]. Almost 85% of cases of liver cancer in the World occur in sub-Saharan Africa and Eastern and South-Eastern Asia (55% in China) (Figure 1) [1]. By contrast, the incidence is usually lower in developed areas (ASR 8.1 and 2.7 per 100 000 in males and females respectively in 2008) [1]. In Europe, the overall annual incidence was estimated around 60 000 cases in 2008 (two-third in men) [26] but with a wide spectrum according to different areas (Figure 2). Overall there is an increasing gradient of incidence from Northern Europe (ASR 5.6 and 2.4 per 100 000 in males and females respectively) to Southern Europe (ASR 14.5 and 4.9 per 100 000 in males and females respectively) and, to a lesser extent, from Central and Eastern Europe (ASR 7.3 and 3.4 per 100 000 in males and females respectively) to Western Europe (ASR 10.6 and 3.1 per 100 000 in males and females respectively) [26]. Countries in Southern Europe such as Italy and Spain have medium-high incidence (ASR 12.8 and 8.5 per 100 000 respectively) while Scandinavian countries have the lowest incidence (ASR below 5 per 100 000) (Figure 2) (http://eu-cancer.iarc.fr/cancer-7-liver.html,en). The higher incidence was observed among males in Moldavia (ASR 20.3 per 100 000) [26]. As stated above, those differences reflect likely the geographical differences between exposure to risk factors for HCC. Chronic viral infections, mostly HCV, are highly prevalent in Southern Europe (Spain, Italy, Greece) but lower in Scandinavian countries [4, 36]. Europe has also the highest level of alcohol consumption in the World but with large variations between countries [4, 37].

Some evidence suggests that global pattern of liver cancer has changed markedly over the three or four last decades [2, 7]. In broad outline, some developing countries (mainly in Asia) have experienced decrease in liver cancer incidence (likely due to decline in HBV and environmental factors exposure) [7] whereas several developed countries have experienced marked increases [7, 38, 39]. In Europe important increases in incidence have been reported over the 15-year time period 1978-1992 in France, Switzerland, United Kingdom, Italy and Spain [7]. Those increases relate primarily to men (who represent the vast majority of patients with HCC) but also to women to a lesser extent [7]. By contrast, rates remained stable at low levels or even decreased over time in Scandinavian countries, both in males and females [7].

The underlying explanations for increase in incidence rates in Europe are still imprecise. Possible explanations include changes in coding for primary liver tumors, in diagnostic procedures, in management of cirrhosis, and in prevalences of major risk factors for HCC. Since the introduction of ICD-9 in 1978, coding of HCC and intrahepatic cholangio-carcinoma are clearly separated. However the precise type of liver tumors remains often unknown in databases, particularly in most of the Eastern European countries [4]. Consequently most of epidemiological studies do not distinguish between HCC and intrahepatic cholangiocarcinoma. Recent increase in global incidence of liver cancer in United Kingdom has been linked to rises in both HCC and cholangiocarcinoma incidences [35]. Concerning diagnosis of liver tumors, the rapid development of new imaging methods (ultrasonography, CT-scan, MRI) during the past 30-year period has led to a marked improvement in tumor identification and to the development of non invasive (without biopsy) diagnosis of HCC [40]. Obviously this may result in artefactual increases in incidence of liver cancer even if extent is unknown. Furthermore many progresses have been done for two decades in the management of the main complications of cirrhosis. Dramatic improvements in treatment and prevention for both variceal bleeding [41] and severe bacterial infections [42] have resulted in improved survival of cirrhotic patients and consequently increased opportunity for the occurrence of HCC. Increases in liver cancer incidence in Europe may also be explained by changes in prevalences of major risk factors for cirrhosis. Many patients infected by HCV in the 1970s have currently reached the cirrhotic stage and are therefore at risk for HCC [43]. Immigration from HCV and HBV endemic areas is considerable in several European countries resulting in rises in prevalence of patients with chronic liver diseases. Alcohol consumption has decreased markedly but remains at a high level in many European countries [37]. Moreover, obesity and diabetes prevalences are increasing in most of the developed countries [44]. They represent major comorbidities for liver diseases and HCC occurrence [45]. However the respective influences of all those factors are still indeterminate.

The epidemiological situation in France is characterized by high rates of alcohol consumption and HCV infection [4] and by increasing prevalences of obesity and diabetes [44]. The number of new cases of liver cancer has been estimated to 7100 in 2008 (5550 in males, 1550 in females) [26] corresponding to a medium-high incidence rate (ASR 8.7 per 100 000 both sexes; 15.4 and 3.2 per 100 000 in males and females respectively) close to Spain and Italy (Figure 2). Between 1980 and 2005, a regular increase in number of cases (1768 to 6433, both sexes) and incidence rate (ASR 4.1 to 10.4 and 0.8 to 2.0 per 100 000 in males and females respectively) has been reported in the Network of the French Cancer Registries (FRANCIM) database (Figure 3) [46]. As in several other developed countries, this important increase is likely attributable to persistent high level of alcohol consumption, high number of patients contaminated with HCV several decades ago becoming cirrhotic, improvement in management of cirrhosis, and rising level of metabolic syndrome. However some recent data from FRANCIM suggest that incidence rate of liver cancer has slowed down slightly in men for the more recent period (annual rate of change: +3.8% over 1980-2005, +1.9% over 2000-2005) [46]. Nevertheless this trend remains to be confirmed.

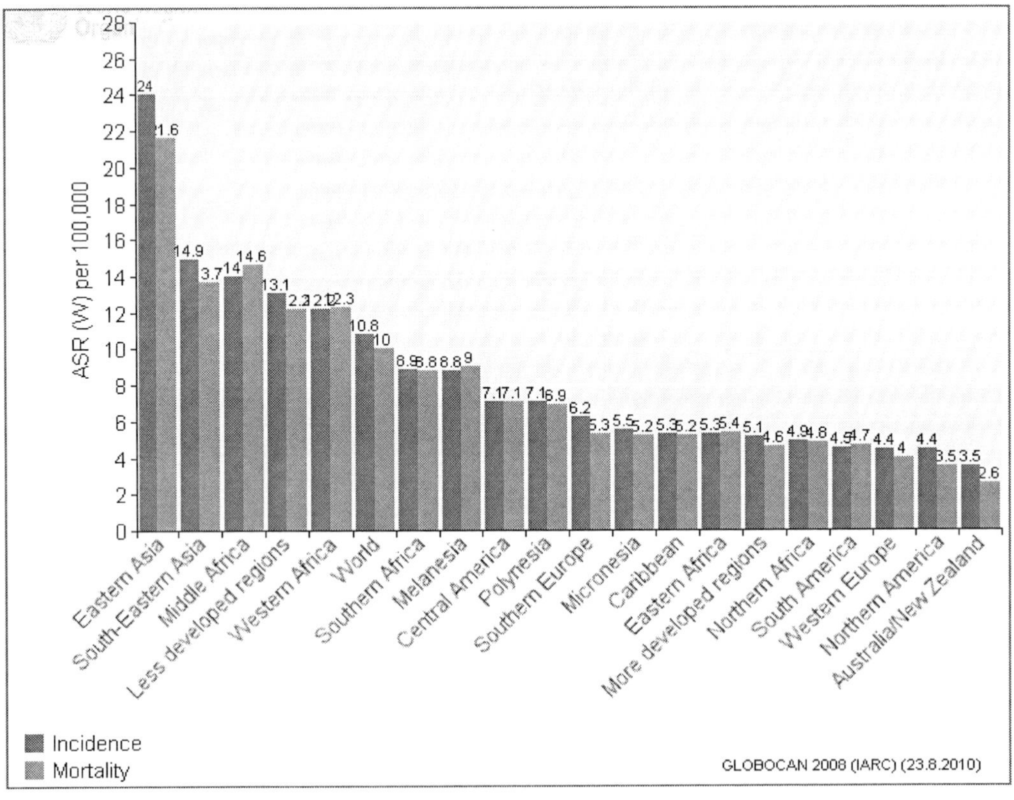

Figure 1. Estimated incidence and mortality rates for liver cancer in the different parts of the World in 2008 (Age Standardized Rate per 100 000, both sexes). Arrows: data from Southern and Western Europe *(from GLOBOCAN 2008, http://www.iarc.fr/en/media-centre/iarcnews/2010/globocan2008.php, accessed on 23 august 2010).*

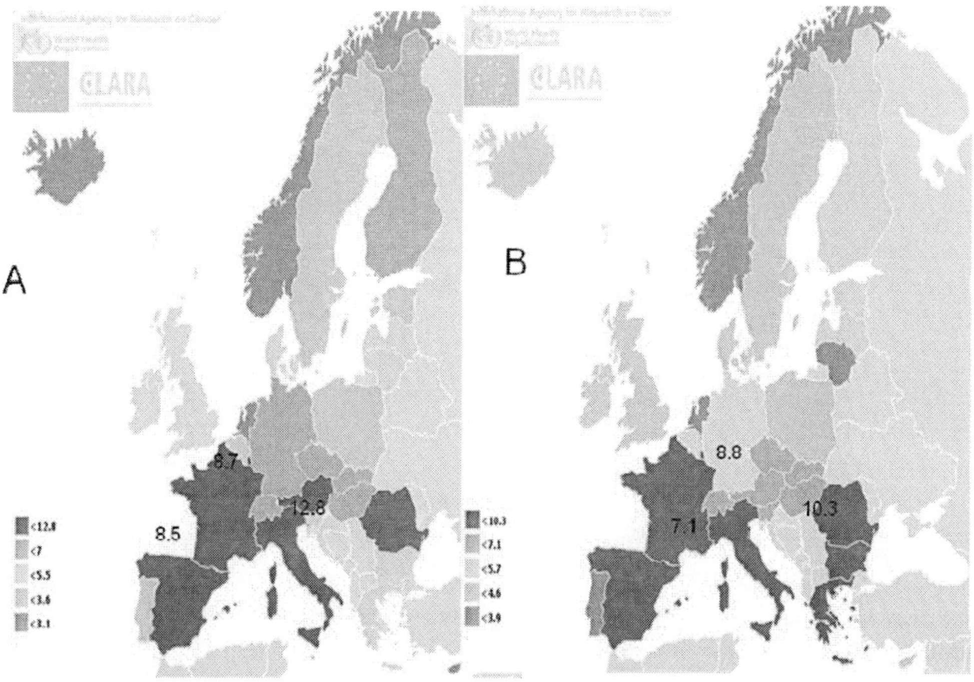

Figure 2. Estimated incidence (A) and mortality (B) from liver cancer in Europe in 2008 (Age Standardized Rate per 100 000, both sexes) *(from European Cancer Observatory, International Agency for Research on Cancer, Lyon, France. http://eu-cancer.iarc.fr, accessed on 24 august 2010).*

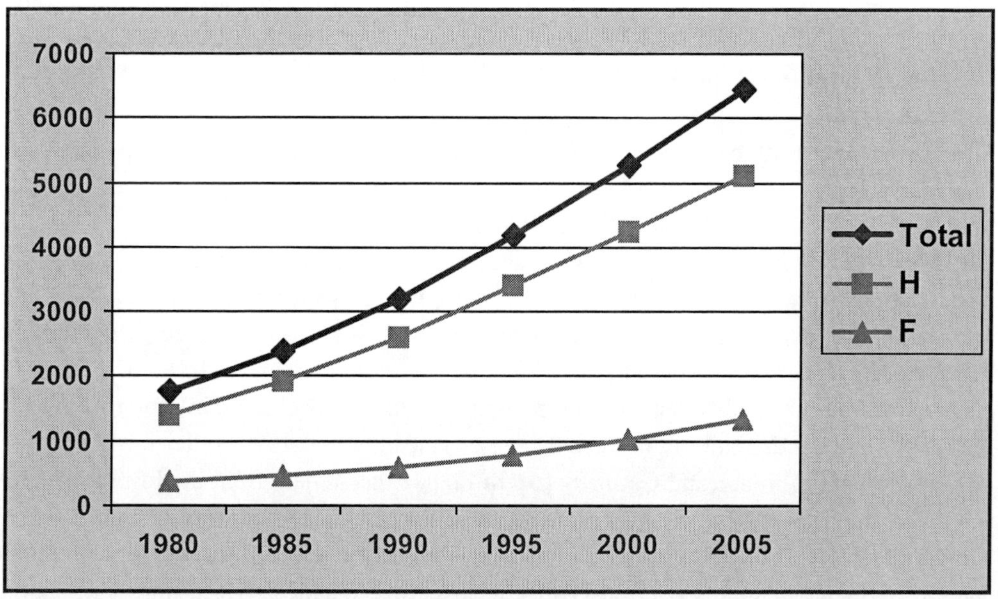

Figure 3. Annual incidence of liver cancer between 1980 and 2005 in France (numbers of cases). H: men, F: women *(established from Belot et al. Rev Epidemiol Sante Publique 2008;56:159-75).*

Mortality

The mortality from liver cancer was estimated to 696 000 cases in 2008 worldwide (ASR 10.0 per 100 000) with about 70% of males (ASR 14.6 versus 5.7 per 100 000 in females) [1]. Mortality statistics are very close to incidence statistics reflecting the very poor prognosis of patients with liver cancer (median of survival largely below one year and ratio of mortality to incidence of 0.93) [1]. This trend is similar in all geographic areas worldwide. In Europe, the number of death from liver cancer was estimated to 60 000 in 2008 (ASR 9.5 and 3.5 per 100 000 in males and females respectively), practically equal to the number of new cases. This very poor prognosis is mainly related to too late diagnosis of primary liver cancer worldwide [40]. Even in developed countries, most of the patients have advanced tumor at diagnosis, often associated with vascular invasion or metastasis, precluding to perform curative treatment [40].

In France, the number of deaths from liver cancer was estimated to 7700 in 2008 (ASR 15.4 and 3.25 per 100 000 in males and females respectively). The CépiDC (database on mortality provided by the Institut National de la Santé et de la Recherche Médicale (INSERM)) bring more precise data about histological type of liver cancer (http://www.cepidc.vesinet.inserm.fr/). In 2008, the numbers of patients dying from HCC and intrahepatic cholangiocarcinoma were 4038 and 1610 respectively (53% and 21% of total respectively). However, tumor type was not reported in 1871 cases (25% of total, ICD-10 code C22.9) even if most of them corresponded likely to HCC. Rare primary liver cancers (hepatoblastoma and sarcomas, ICD-10 codes C22.1 to C22.7) represented only 23 cases (0.3% of total). HCC is currently the leading cause of death in patients with viral cirrhosis [47]. In a random sample of 999 French patients who died with hepatitis viral infection in 2001, HCC was found in 33% and 35% of patients with HCV and HBV infections respectively [48].

In accordance with close relationship to incidence, upward trends in mortality from liver cancer have been reported in developed areas such as United States, Japan and several major European countries [2, 7]. However some studies suggest that the situation is more complex. In a recent study covering 23 European countries over the period 1980-2004 [6], diverging trends were observed in Europe. For instance, mortality rates increased continuously in men over the entire period in Austria, Germany, Greece, Spain, and United Kingdom, but decreased since the mid-1990s, after increases in the previous period, in France and Italy. Results were markedly different in women with continuous decreases in mortality rates in Austria and Italy and, similarly to men, decreases since the mid-1990s, after increases in the previous period, in France and Germany [6]. In France recent data from the Institut National de Veille sanitaire (http://www.invs.sante.fr/ surveillance/cancers) confirm a slight decrease in mortality rates from liver cancer from late-1990s after several decades of continuous increase. Artefactual increase in survival due to earlier diagnosis (lead-time bias) and/or improvement in management and curative treatments [49] are potential explanations for this favourable trend, which must be confirmed.

Conclusion

HCC, the main form of primary liver cancer which occurs mostly in the setting of cirrhosis, represents an important burden in term of public health in Europe. Epidemiological characteristics vary largely among countries, depending on respective prevalences and outcomes of chronic liver disease etiologies. Chronic HCV infection, alcohol consumption, and also obesity/diabetes (to an increasing extent), are the main risk factors for HCC. Moreover, frequent advanced stage at diagnosis results in poor survival, with a ratio of mortality to incidence close to 1.

Even if epidemiological data are still incomplete and heterogeneous, they bring enough informations to suggest how to decrease the incidence and mortality from HCC. To obtain an effective control of exposure to the main causes of cirrhosis is obviously a major topic (decrease in alcohol consumption, fight against overweight, treatment of diabetes and insulin resistance, control of risk of contamination by HCV, large promotion of HBV vaccine, effective treatment of HCV and HBV chronic hepatitis before severe lesions). In patients with cirrhosis, periodic surveillance using ultrasonography is likely a cost-effective procedure to detect HCC at curable stage [50]. However it is likely that many patients with compensated cirrhosis are not submitted to adequate surveillance in developed countries, such as suggested by a recent study from the United States [51], and some important efforts must be done to promote this official recommandation [40]. Moreover several studies suggest that effective antiviral control of HCV and HBV infections may decrease markedly the incidence of HCC even in patients with cirrhosis [52, 53]. Finally significant improvements in curative treatment for HCC (transplantation, resection and percutaneous radiofrequency) have been performed over the last two decades [40] which may explain (at least partially) the slight decrease in mortality observed recently in some European countries such as in France [49].

References

[1] Ferlay J, Shin HR, Bray F, Forman D, Mathers C, Parkin DM. Estimates of worldwide burden of cancer in 2008: GLOBOCAN 2008. *Int J Cancer* 2010;127:2893-2917.

[2] McGlynn KA, London WT. Epidemiology and natural history of hepatocellular carcinoma. *Best Pract Res Clin Gastroenterol* 2005;19:3-23.

[3] Marcellin P. Hepatitis B and hepatitis C in 2009. *Liver Int* 2009;29 Suppl 1:1-8.

[4] Ribes J, Cleries R, Esteban L, Moreno V, Bosch FX. The influence of alcohol consumption and hepatitis B and C infections on the risk of liver cancer in Europe. *J Hepatol* 2008;49:233-42.

[5] El-Serag HB, Hampel H, Javadi F. The association between diabetes and hepatocellular carcinoma: a systematic review of epidemiologic evidence. *Clin Gastroenterol Hepatol* 2006;4:369-80.

[6] Bosetti C, Levi F, Boffetta P, Lucchini F, Negri E, La Vecchia C. Trends in mortality from hepatocellular carcinoma in Europe, 1980-2004. *Hepatology* 2008;48:137-45.

[7] McGlynn KA, Tsao L, Hsing AW, Devesa SS, Fraumeni JF, Jr. International trends and patterns of primary liver cancer. *Int J Cancer* 2001;94:290-6.

[8] Gomaa AI, Khan SA, Toledano MB, Waked I, Taylor-Robinson SD. Hepatocellular carcinoma: Epidemiology, risk factors and pathogenesis. *World J Gastroenterol* 2008;14:4300-8.

[9] Saunders D, Seidel D, Allison M, Lyratzopoulos G. Systematic review: the association between obesity and hepatocellular carcinoma - epidemiological evidence. *Aliment Pharmacol Ther* 2010;31:1051-63.

[10] Calle E, Rodriguez C, Walker-Thurmond K, Thun M. Overweight, obesity, and mortality from cancer in a prospectively studied cohort of U.S. adults. *N Engl J Med* 2003;24:1625-38.

[11] N'Kontchou G, Paries J, Htar MT, Ganne-Carrie N, Costentin L, Grando-Lemaire V, Trinchet JC, Beaugrand M. Risk factors for hepatocellular carcinoma in patients with alcoholic or viral C cirrhosis. *Clin Gastroenterol Hepatol* 2006;4:1062-8.

[12] Veldt BJ, Chen W, Heathcote EJ, Wedemeyer H, Reichen J, Hofmann WP, de Knegt RJ, Zeuzem S, Manns MP, Hansen BE, Schalm SW, Janssen HL. Increased risk of hepatocellular carcinoma among patients with hepatitis C cirrhosis and diabetes mellitus. *Hepatology* 2008;47:1856-62.

[13] Degos F, Tural C. Hepatocellular carcinoma in human immunodeficiency virus (HIV)-infected patients: is it really different, and if so, why? *J Hepatol* 2007;47:447-50.

[14] Paradis V, Zalinski S, Chelbi E, Guedj N, Degos F, Vilgrain V, Bedossa P, Belghiti J. Hepatocellular carcinomas in patients with metabolic syndrome often develop without significant liver fibrosis: a pathological analysis. *Hepatology* 2009;49:851-9.

[15] Harrison SA, Bacon BR. Relation of hemochromatosis with hepatocellular carcinoma: epidemiology, natural history, pathophysiology, screening, treatment, and prevention. *Med Clin North Am* 2005;89:391-409.

[16] Cavazza A, Caballeria L, Floreani A, Farinati F, Bruguera M, Caroli D, Pares A. Incidence, risk factors, and survival of hepatocellular carcinoma in primary biliary cirrhosis: comparative analysis from two centers. *Hepatology* 2009;50:1162-8.

[17] Fattovich G, Stroffolini T, Zagni I, Donato F. Hepatocellular carcinoma in cirrhosis: incidence and risk factors. *Gastroenterology* 2004;127:S35-50.

[18] Giannitrapani L, Soresi M, La Spada E, Cervello M, D'Alessandro N, Montalto G. Sex hormones and risk of liver tumor. *Ann N Y Acad Sci* 2006;1089:228-36.

[19] Ioannou GN, Morrow OB, Connole ML, Lee SP. Association between dietary nutrient composition and the incidence of cirrhosis or liver cancer in the United States population. *Hepatology* 2009;50:175-84.

[20] Ganne-Carrie N, Chastang C, Chapel F, Munz C, Pateron D, Sibony M, Deny P, Trinchet JC, Callard P, Guettier C, Beaugrand M. Predictive score for the development of hepatocellular carcinoma and additional value of liver large cell dysplasia in Western patients with cirrhosis. *Hepatology* 1996;23:1112-8.

[21] Velazquez RF, Rodriguez M, Navascues CA, Linares A, Perez R, Sotorrios NG, Martinez I, Rodrigo L. Prospective analysis of risk factors for hepatocellular carcinoma in patients with liver cirrhosis. *Hepatology* 2003;37:520-7.

[22] Hassan MM, Spitz MR, Thomas MB, El-Deeb AS, Glover KY, Nguyen NT, Chan W, Kaseb A, Curley SA, Vauthey JN, Ellis LM, Abdalla E, Lozano RD, Patt YZ, Brown TD, Abbruzzese JL, Li D. Effect of different types of smoking and synergism with

hepatitis C virus on risk of hepatocellular carcinoma in American men and women: case-control study. *Int J Cancer* 2008;123:1883-91.

[23] Imaizumi T, Higaki Y, Hara M, Sakamoto T, Horita M, Mizuta T, Eguchi Y, Yasutake T, Ozaki I, Yamamoto K, Onohara S, Kawazoe S, Shigematsu H, Koizumi S, Kudo S, Tanaka K. Interaction between cytochrome P450 1A2 genetic polymorphism and cigarette smoking on the risk of hepatocellular carcinoma in a Japanese population. *Carcinogenesis* 2009;30:1729-34.

[24] Chevret S, Trinchet JC, Mathieu D, Abou Rached A, Beaugrand M, Chastang C, Groupe d'Etude et de Traitement du Carcinome Hépatocellulaire. A new prognostic classification for predicting survival in patients with hepatocellular carcinoma. *J Hepatol* 1999;31:133-141.

[25] Borie F, Tretarre B, Bouvier AM, Faivre J, Binder F, Launoy G, Delafosse P, Tissot J, Peng J, Grosclaude P, Guizard AV, Gras-Aygon C. Primitive liver cancers: epidemiology and geographical study in France. *Eur J Gastroenterol Hepatol* 2009;21:984-9.

[26] Ferlay J, Parkin DM, Steliarova-Foucher E. Estimates of cancer incidence and mortality in Europe in 2008. *Eur J Cancer* 2010;46:765-81.

[27] Charles MA, Basdevant A, Eschwege E. OBEPI Roche 2009 - Enquête épidémiologique nationale sur le surpoids et l'obésité. http://www.roche.fr/gear/newcontents/servlet/staticfilesServlet?type=data&communityId=re719001&id=static/attachedfile/re7300002/re72700003/AttachedFile_10101.pdf 2009.

[28] Grando-Lemaire V, Guettier C, Chevret S, Beaugrand M, Trinchet JC. Hepatocellular carcinoma without cirrhosis in the West: epidemiological factors and histopathology of the non-tumorous liver. Groupe d'Etude et de Traitement du Carcinome Hepatocellulaire. *J Hepatol* 1999;31:508-13.

[29] Bralet MP, Regimbeau JM, Pineau P, Dubois S, Loas G, Degos F, Valla D, Belghiti J, Degott C, Terris B. Hepatocellular carcinoma occurring in nonfibrotic liver: epidemiologic and histopathologic analysis of 80 French cases. *Hepatology* 2000;32:200-4.

[30] El-Serag HB, Davila JA. Is fibrolamellar carcinoma different from hepatocellular carcinoma? A US population-based study. *Hepatology* 2004;39:798-803.

[31] Franco LM, Krishnamurthy V, Bali D, Weinstein DA, Arn P, Clary B, Boney A, Sullivan J, Frush DP, Chen YT, Kishnani PS. Hepatocellular carcinoma in glycogen storage disease type Ia: a case series. *J Inherit Metab Dis* 2005;28:153-62.

[32] Sherman M. Vinyl chloride and the liver. *J Hepatol* 2009;51:1074-81.

[33] Kalaitzakis E, Gunnarsdottir SA, Josefsson A, Bjornsson E. Increased risk for malignant neoplasms among patients with cirrhosis. *Clin Gastroenterol Hepatol* 2010;(in press).

[34] Tao LY, He XD, Qu Q, Cai L, Liu W, Zhou L, Zhang SM. Risk factors for intrahepatic and extrahepatic cholangiocarcinoma: a case-control study in China. *Liver Int* 2010;30:215-21.

[35] West J, Wood H, Logan RF, Quinn M, Aithal GP. Trends in the incidence of primary liver and biliary tract cancers in England and Wales 1971-2001. *Br J Cancer* 2006;94:1751-8.

[36] Rantala M, van de Laar MJ. Surveillance and epidemiology of hepatitis B and C in Europe. A review. *Euro Surveill* 2008;13:pii=18880.

[37] Popova S, Rehm J, Patra J, Zatonski W. Comparing alcohol consumption in central and eastern Europe to other European countries. *Alcohol Alcohol* 2007;42:465-73.

[38] Taylor-Robinson SD, Foster GR, Arora S, Hargreaves S, Thomas HC. Increase in primary liver cancer in the UK, 1979-94. *Lancet* 1997;350:1142-3.

[39] Deuffic S, Poynard T, Buffat L, Valleron AJ. Trends in primary liver cancer. *Lancet* 1998;351:214-5.

[40] Bruix J, Sherman M. Management of hepatocellular carcinoma. *Hepatology* 2005;42:1208-36.

[41] Triantos CK, Burroughs AK. Prevention of the development of varices and first portal hypertensive bleeding episode. *Best Pract Res Clin Gastroenterol* 2007;21:31-42.

[42] Ghassemi S, Garcia-Tsao G. Prevention and treatment of infections in patients with cirrhosis. *Best Pract Res Clin Gastroenterol* 2007;21:77-93.

[43] Deuffic S, Poynard T, Valleron AJ. Correlation between hepatitis C virus prevalence and hepatocellular carcinoma mortality in Europe. *J Viral Hepat* 1999;6:411-3.

[44] Charles MA, Eschwege E, Basdevant A. Monitoring the obesity epidemic in France: the Obepi surveys 1997-2006. *Obesity (Silver Spring)* 2008;16:2182-6.

[45] Stickel F, Hellerbrand C. Non-alcoholic fatty liver disease as a risk factor for hepatocellular carcinoma: mechanisms and implications. *Gut* 2010;59:1303-7.

[46] Belot A, Grosclaude P, Bossard N, Jougla E, Benhamou E, Delafosse P, Guizard AV, Molinie F, Danzon A, Bara S, Bouvier AM, Tretarre B, Binder-Foucard F, Colonna M, Daubisse L, Hedelin G, Launoy G, Le Stang N, Maynadie M, Monnereau A, Troussard X, Faivre J, Collignon A, Janoray I, Arveux P, Buemi A, Raverdy N, Schvartz C, Bovet M, Cherie-Challine L, Esteve J, Remontet L, Velten M. Cancer incidence and mortality in France over the period 1980-2005. *Rev Epidemiol Sante Publique* 2008;56:159-75.

[47] Benvegnu L, Gios M, Boccato S, Alberti A. Natural history of compensated viral cirrhosis: a prospective study on the incidence and hierarchy of major complications. *Gut* 2004;53:744-9.

[48] Marcellin P, Pequignot F, Delarocque-Astagneau E, Zarski JP, Ganne N, Hillon P, Antona D, Bovet M, Mechain M, Asselah T, Desenclos JC, Jougla E. Mortality related to chronic hepatitis B and chronic hepatitis C in France: evidence for the role of HIV coinfection and alcohol consumption. *J Hepatol* 2008;48:200-7.

[49] Guiu B, Minello A, Cottet V, Lepage C, Hillon P, Faivre J, Bouvier AM. A 30-year, population-based study shows improved management and prognosis of hepatocellular carcinoma. *Clin Gastroenterol Hepatol* 2010;8:986-91.

[50] Thompson Coon J, Rogers G, Hewson P, Wright D, Anderson R, Jackson S, Ryder S, Cramp M, Stein K. Surveillance of cirrhosis for hepatocellular carcinoma: a cost-utility analysis. *Br J Cancer* 2008;98:1166-75.

[51] Davila JA, Morgan RO, Richardson PA, Du XL, McGlynn KA, El-Serag HB. Use of surveillance for hepatocellular carcinoma among patients with cirrhosis in the United States. *Hepatology* 2010;52:132-41.

[52] Singal AK, Singh A, Jaganmohan S, Guturu P, Mummadi R, Kuo YF, Sood GK. Antiviral therapy reduces risk of hepatocellular carcinoma in patients with hepatitis C virus-related cirrhosis. *Clin Gastroenterol Hepatol* 2010;8:192-199.

[53] Liaw YF, Sung JJ, Chow WC, Farrell G, Lee CZ, Yuen H, Tanwandee T, Tao QM, Shue K, Keene ON, Dixon JS, Gray DF, Sabbat J. Lamivudine for patients with chronic hepatitis B and advanced liver disease. *N Engl J Med* 2004;351:1521-31.

In: Hepatocellular Carcionoma: A Global Challenge
Editor: Isabelle Chemin ISBN: 978-1-61470-644-1

Chapter V

Challenges in Risk Assessment for Hepatocellular Carcinoma: Example of Hepatitis B Virus Infection

Myriam Lereau[1,2], *Doriane Gouas*[2], *Nora Martel*[1], *Tatiana Dupinay*[1] *and Isabelle Chemin*[1]
[1]Université Lyon 1, France, Centre de Recherche en Cancérologie de Lyon, Lyon, France
[2] International Agency for Research on Cancer, Lyon, France

Abstract

A number of risk factors appear to play a role in hepatocellular carcinoma (HCC), hepatitis B infection being one of the most important. Hepatitis B surface antigen (HBsAg) is the hallmark of hepatitis B virus (HBV) since it is the best and most reliable diagnostic marker. However, since most studies do not rely on longitudinal observations but mostly on cross-sectional studies little is known on time changes in those markers and their incidence. Chronic inflammation and cytokines are key determinants in the development of fibrosis and liver cell proliferation. Integration of HBV DNA into host cellular DNA is crucial during HBV chronic infection by disrupting or promoting expression of cellular genes that are important in cell growth and differentiation. In addition, expression of HBV proteins may have a direct effect on cellular functions, and some of these gene products can promote malignant transformation. Several HBV genes have been found in infected tumoral tissues more frequently than others, including truncated pre-S2/S and hepatitis B X genes. The proteins expressed from these integrated genes have been shown to have intracellular activities that may account for their association with HCC, including effects on cellular growth and apoptosis. A major player involved in this form of viral transactivation is the X protein (HBx) that displays pleiotropic functions and has been implicated in the malignant transformation of chronically-infected liver cells. Occult hepatitis B virus infection is characterized by persistence of HBV DNA in HBsAg-negative individuals. There are evidences that occult HBV constitutes a risk factor for the development of HCC and that the mechanisms whereby overt HBV might induce tumor formation are maintained in those atypical HBV infections.

Introduction

Chronic hepatitis B virus (HBV) infection is a primary risk factor for the development of cirrhosis and hepatocellular carcinoma (HCC) worldwide. HBV carriers are identified by detection of the hepatitis B virus surface antigen (HBsAg) in their blood and persistence of HBsAg over a time interval of 6 months defines chronic hepatitis B. If HBsAg detection means ongoing HBV infection its disappearance may have different meanings either true clearance of the virus or just its decline to low grade persisting occult HBV infection. Moreover, co-infection of HBV with HIV or HCV could lead to down-regulation of HBsAg production or interference with its detection. It has indeed become evident through a large number of studies that HBV may persist in the form of serologically silent infections, leading to the concept of seronegative or occult infection. In a recent expert guideline, occult HBV infection (OBI) has been defined as the presence of HBV DNA in the liver, in the absence of HBsAg and with low titers or even absence of HBV DNA in serum. Such infection may significantly contribute to the population burden of HBV-related diseases since occult HBV infections are spread worldwide. Many studies have been carried out on OBI in different parts of the world since the early 1980s. Some of these studies have suggested that OBI may play a role in chronic liver damage and in the development of HCC, particularly in patients with chronic hepatitis C. It is to note that both integrated viral DNA and covalently closed circular HBV genomes (HBV cccDNA) are present in the liver of patients with OBI, and the persistence of free viral genomes is associated with continuance of viral transcription and replication. Thus, the direct and indirect mechanisms whereby overt HBV may induce tumor formation appear to be mostly maintained by OBI.

HBV Presentation

Structure of the Genome

Human hepatitis B virus (HBV) is a small enveloped DNA virus belonging to the *Hepadnavidiae* family. One unique feature is that the viral genome is a non-covalently closed circular DNA of about 3.2kb with a partially double-stranded region over 50% to 80% of its length, giving rise to a relaxed circular DNA (RC DNA) (Figure 1A). The (-) strand is complete and contains the entire genetic inheritance of the virus; a viral polymerase is covalently linked to its 5' end. The (+) strand is incomplete, with a fixed 5' end and a variable 3' end; it overlaps the 5' and 3' of the (-) strand, thus ensuring the genomic circularity.

Four overlapping open reading frames (ORF) encode the 7 viral proteins:

- The C gene encodes the pre-core protein or HBe antigen (HBeAg) and the capsid/core protein or HBcAg;
- The S gene encodes the 3 surface proteins: L (large), M (medium) and S (small, HBsAg);
- The P gene encodes the viral polymerase;
- And the X gene is the smallest ORF and encodes HBxAg.

Besides the splicing events of mRNAs, HBV increases its genetic complexity by using different initiation sites of transcription. Moreover, alternative codons for initiation of the protein synthesis allow generating several proteins from one single ORF, as for HBeAg/ HBcAg and the three surface proteins.

Replication Cycle

HBV is also qualified as a DNA para-retrovirus as its replication cycle contains a retro-transcription step. The cycle starts with the entry of the infectious particle, also called virion, into the hepatocyte by endocytose (Figure 1B). The mechanism of entry has not been completely elucidated so far. However several studies suggest that it would be mediated by interactions between viral envelope proteins and two types of cellular receptors at the surface [1]: the first type would be of high affinity and the second type of low affinity would belong to heparan sulfate proteoglycans. Moreover Leistner et al. proposed a model: *in vivo* HBV would be initially trapped in the liver in the space of Dissé by heparan sulfate proteoglycans, then bind to a high affinity receptor through the pre-S1 attachment site and the N-terminal myristic acid [2].

After the fusion of the viral envelop with the cell membrane, the nucleocapsid is released into the cytoplasm. Then a model has been set up from *in vitro* studies: the capsid would be directed *via* the microtubules to the center of microtubule organization which is located in the periphery of the nucleus; the capsid contains a NLS sequence which would allow its interaction with importin α and β and facilitate its translocation into the nuclear pore; finally the capsid would be dismantled into HBcAg dimers inside the pore, allowing the release of the genomic RC DNA into the nucleus [3].

Once inside the nucleus, the RC DNA undergoes several modifications before being converted into a very stable double-stranded covalently-closed circular DNA (cccDNA). This cccDNA forms a "mini-chromosome" which serves as a viral "tank" inside the infected cells: it is transcribed by the cellular RNA polymerase into different mRNAs and pre-genomic RNA (pgRNA), the latter being the mRNA of the entire genome. mRNAs are translated in the endoplasmic reticulum into different viral proteins which are able to assemble into new viral particles. The pgRNA is then encapsided with the viral polymerase and cellular heat shock proteins [4]. Inside the capsid the polymerase has several enzymatic activities to convert the pgRNA into RC DNA: it serves as primer for the (-) strand synthesis, retro-transcriptase, RNase H and DNA-dependent DNA polymerase [5].

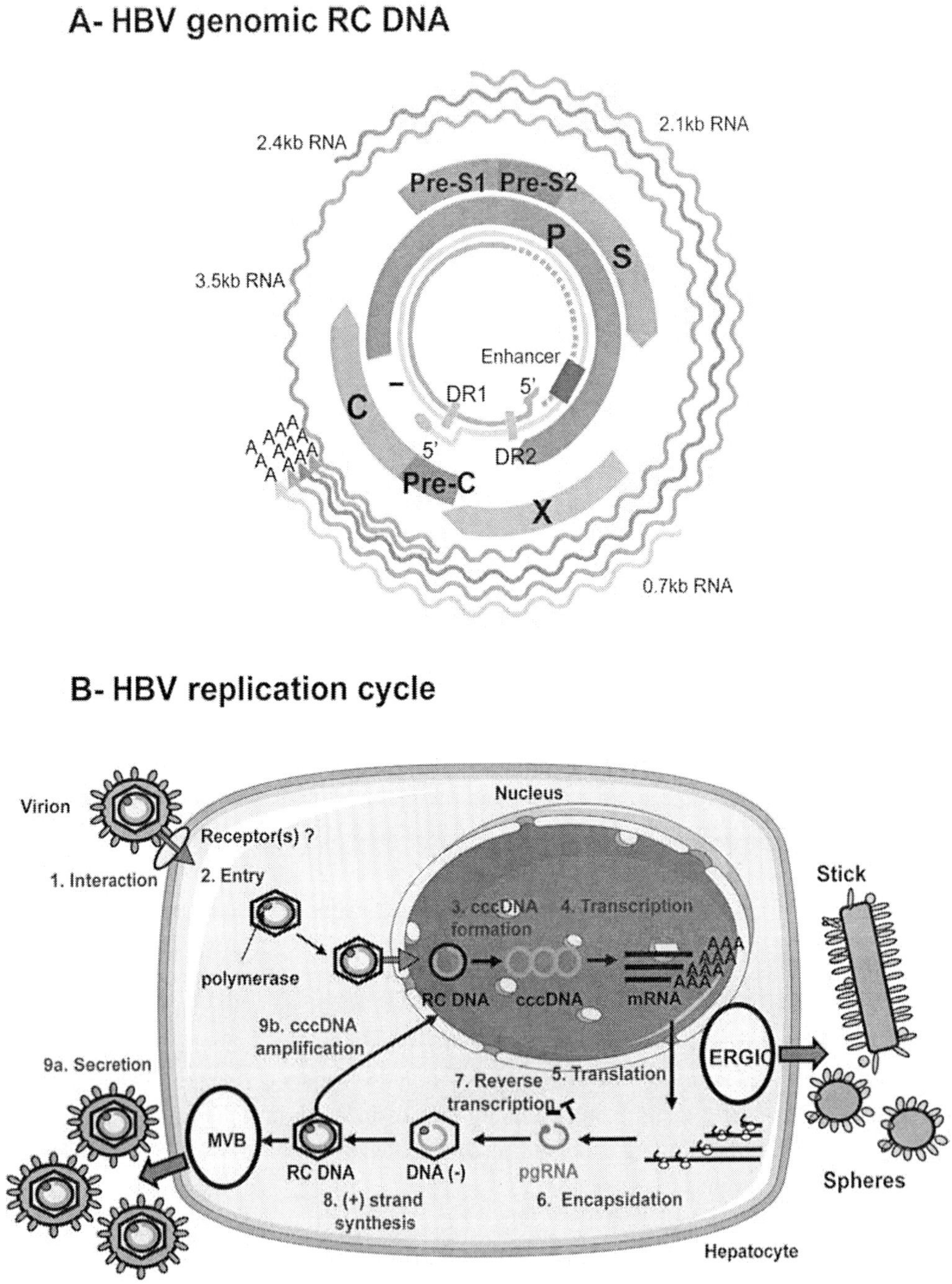

Figure 1. HBV characteristics. (A) Structure of HBV genomic DNA. HBV genome contains the four ORF S, P, C and X. The corresponding mRNAs and lengths are indicated in the same colors as genes. Adapted from Jay H. Hoofnagle, 2002. (B) HBV replication cycle. Nine steps describe the life cycle of the virus, which ends in secretion of infectious particles through MVB or secretion of non-infectious particles (spheres and sticks) through ERGIC. MVB: Multi-Vesicular Bodies; ERGIC: Endoplasmic Reticulum-Golgi Intermediate Compartment. The cell was drawn thanks to Servier Medical Art (http://www.servier.fr/smart/home_smart.asp).

Finally the nucleocapsid containing the neo-synthesized RC DNA can be directed either to multi-vesicular bodies to be matured and secreted after association with envelop proteins and insertion into the cell membrane in order to form new infection particles [6], or to the nucleus in order to amplify the cccDNA pool.

In parallel, the viral DNA can also integrate into the host genome in a relatively random way as fragments of variable length.

Viral Proteins: Role in HCC

Hepatocarcinogenesis mediated by HBV is associated with the chronicity of infection. The evolution of HBV infection towards chronicity depends on the age and the immune system of the individual at the time of infection: 5 to 10% of immune-competent individuals and 90% of newborns or children develop a chronic infection [7]. The mechanisms responsible for the malignant transformation during a chronic infection by HBV involve host and viral factors. HBV is not cytophatic by itself but liver injuries caused by chronic HBV infection are considered to be immune-mediated. Moreover a direct role of the virus in hepatocarcinogenesis is well established. However, it is not known whether the viral infection causes the initiation of the tumor or the subsequent inflammation leading to liver regeneration and to cirrhosis acts as a tumorous promoter in hepatocarcinogenesis. Several studies suggest that some viral proteins, especially surface proteins and HBxAg, may contribute to HBV-induced carcinogenesis by interacting with host factors leading to an alteration of cellular gene expression. Nevertheless, the role of these proteins through direct or indirect mechanisms is still not clear.

Surface Proteins: Endoplasmic Reticulum Stress

Expression of the various types of surface proteins depends on the replicative status of the HBV genome. During the acute phase of HBV infection, HBsAg is predominant. On the contrary, during the chronic phase, the HBV genome integrates into the host genome and the L protein becomes predominant. A number of truncated surface genes with a partially deleted pre-S1 or pre-S2 region have already been identified and may contribute to HCC development by accumulating in the endoplasmic reticulum (ER) and inducing ER stress [8].

ΔS-L mutants from L protein are frequently detected in the serum of chronically infected patients [9]. Studies have shown that the weaker the viral replication is, the more these mutants appear and this evolution could be a consequence of the host immune pressure [10]. Moreover, ΔS-L mutants have been shown to accumulate in the ER and induce genomic instability by generating an oxidative stress, DNA damage and mutations [8].

HBx Protein: The Super-HBV Gangster in HCC

HBx is a regulatory protein of 154 amino acids known to exhibit a transcriptional transactivation function. Previous observations suggest that HBx has two independent cell proliferative (pro-oncogenic domain) and death-promoting (pro-apoptotic domain) activities (Figure 2).

Since HBx has no DNA-binding activity, it exerts these functions through interaction with cellular factor(s). Nevertheless, how HBx operates in cellular transformation remains unclear. As a multifunctional protein exhibiting numerous activities, HBx may be referred as "*the super-HBV gangster in HCC*". Indeed, it affects gene transcription, intracellular signal transduction, cell proliferation, apoptotic cell death and DNA repair (Figure 2) and any or all of these activities could contribute to HCC.

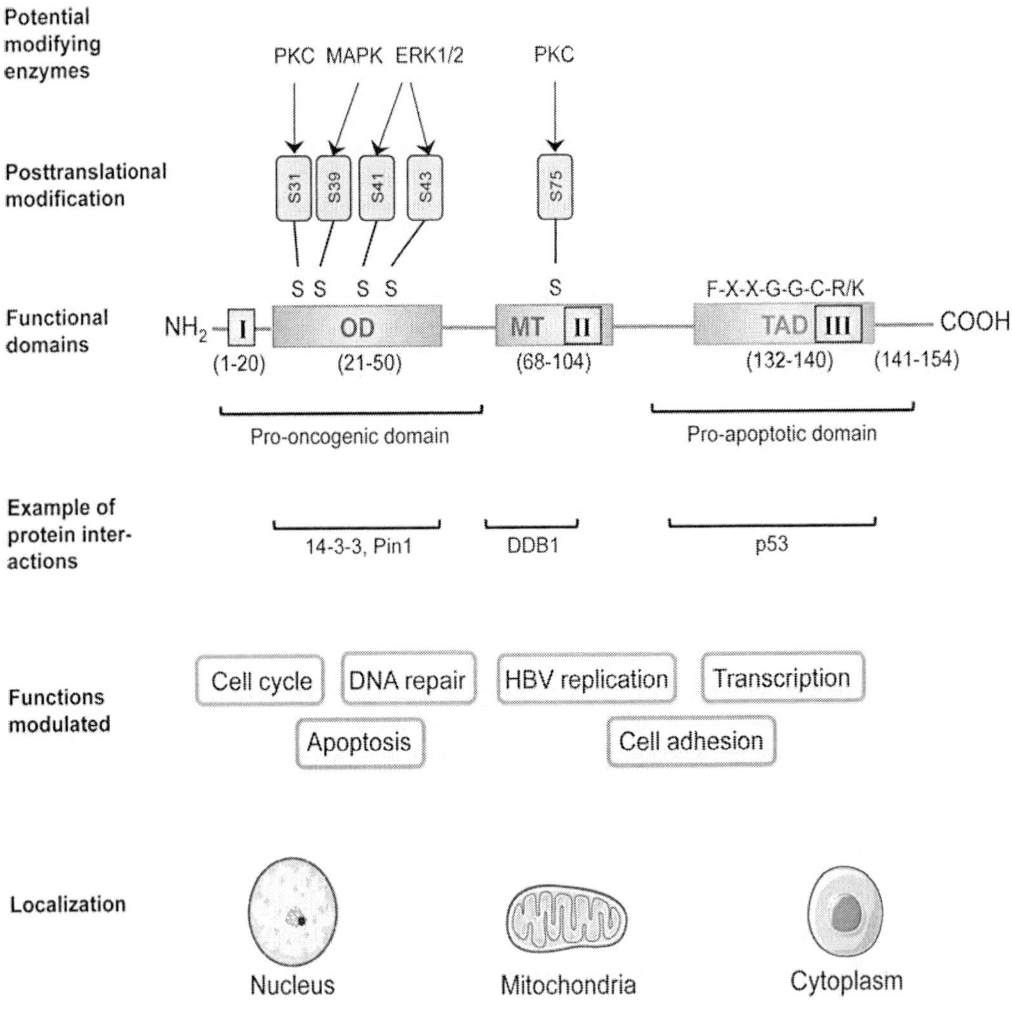

Figure 2. Structure, posttranslational modification and role of HBx. The protein contains three domains from N- to C-terminal region: an oligomerization domain (OD; aa 21-50); a mitochondria association domain (MT; aa 68-104), which is essential for cell death but not for transactivation function; and a transactivation domain (TAD; aa 132-140). Five posttranslational modifications have been described so far (Serines 31, 39, 41, 43 and 75) involving PKC and MAPK pathways. Moreover, HBx displays two independent pro-oncogenic and pro-apoptotic domains that allow it to modulate cell cycle, DNA repair, HBV replication, transcription, apoptosis and cell adhesion. HBx has been shown to interact with several cellular proteins like p53 in its C-terminal region. Even if its localization is still a matter of debate, HBx may be found in the mitochondria or in the nucleus and/or in the cytoplasm depending to its concentration.

The localization of HBx remains a matter of debate. Some studies demonstrated its localization in the cytoplasm or in the mitochondria, whereas others found the protein preferentially in the nucleus, or present in both the cytoplasm and the nucleus [11-14]. As a possible explanation to these contradictory findings, other studies from different laboratories have shown that HBx expressed at very low level is predominantly nuclear, whereas high levels of expression lead to a cytoplasmic accumulation [15, 16]. Overall, it seems that there is a dual localization of HBx: during virus replication, HBx could fluctuate depending on its concentration, but also on the accessibility of cellular partners involved in its nuclear import and export. Its cellular partners will be developed in the next part of this chapter.

Influence of Genotypes

Eight genotypes (A through H) of HBV have been identified that differ from each other in whole-genome sequencing by at least 8% [17-21]. In addition, the major HBV genotypes apart from E and H have been divided into subgenotypes (1, 2, 3, etc.) based on phylogenetic analyses and genetic divergence of complete genomes. Genotype A is common in North-Western Europe, North America, and Africa. Genotypes B and C are predominant in East and South-East Asia, Oceania and among aboriginal populations in Australia. Genotype D is found worldwide and is predominant in the Mediterranean, Middle East, and India, whereas genotype E has been so far confined to populations in western parts of sub-Saharan Africa apart from one report from India [22, 23]. Genotype G has been identified in samples from several countries, and is found in patients co-infected with another HBV genotype. Genotypes F and H are found mainly in Central and South America, and are the indigenous genotypes of Amerindian populations [17, 22, 24, 25].

Several studies analyzed the outcomes of HBV infection in relation to specific infecting HBV genotypes. Genotype A1 is associated with HCC in young men who are usually HBeAg-negative and anti-HBe–positive, have low levels of HBV DNA, and rarely display cirrhosis, while genotype A2 is associated with HCC in older persons. Compared to genotype D, genotype A2 is associated with a lower risk of HCC and has a greater resolution of active hepatitis [26]. A study from India reported that genotype D was associated with more severe liver disease and HCC in younger patients than genotype A [27]. Most of the current knowledge is based on studies of Asian patients which are infected principally by genotypes B and C. Genotype B causes a shorter duration of high levels of HBV replication with spontaneous HBeAg seroconversion and therefore results in less active liver disease. Genotype B-associated HCC was found primarily in persons older than 60 years. In most of the studies, genotype C has been associated with an increased risk of HCC and HBeAg seroconversion occurs 10-30 years later than genotypes A, B, D, and F1. Genotype C-associated HCC occurred in significantly younger persons ($\leq$50 years) [26, 28-31]. Genotype F1 is associated with HCC in Alaskan natives. Certain HBV genotypes and subgenotypes, including genotypes C, B2-5, and F1, appear to be associated with a higher risk of developing HCC, and others, including genotypes B1, B6, and A2, appear to be associated with a lower risk of complications of HBV (Table 1) [26].

Finally, treatment responses to interferon-α apparently vary according to the viral genotype, infections with strains A and B responding better than those due to genotype C or D.

Table 1. Association between HBV genotypes and disease outcomes

Genotype	Geographic Region	Disease Association
A1	Sub-Saharan Africa	HCC in young males often without cirrhosis
A2	Northern Europe	HCC and cirrhosis in older persons
B1	Japan	HCC and cirrhosis in older persons
B2-6	East Asia	HCC and cirrhosis occur at younger age than B1
C	China, Korea, South-East Asia, Japan, South Pacific Islands	Higher risk of HCC and cirrhosis compared with genotypes B, A, D and F1
D1-4	Russia, Middle East, Mediterranean, North Africa, Eastern Europe, Indian Subcontinent	Anti-HBe chronic hepatitis B, HCC, and cirrhosis in older individuals
F1	Alaska, Central America, South America	HCC in children and young adults in Alaska only

Genetic Mechanisms of HCC

Genetic mechanisms are involved in the development of HCC: HBV integration into the host genome induces genetic instability and viral proteins encoded by integrated sequences act as trans-activating factors of cellular pathways.

HBV Integration

During the course of HBV chronic infection, viral DNA integration can occur into the host genome. This event is not essential for the viral replication but would allow the persistence of the viral genome in the liver. Integration of HBV DNA into the host genome is found in 85–90% of HBV-related HCCs [32]. Moreover this would occur early before HCC appearance as some integration events were observed in the liver of patients suffering from acute and active chronic hepatitis [33, 34]. Whether the integration occurs randomly into the host genome is still a matter of debate. Several significant sites have been described, like *hTERT* [35-38], the chromosome 17 containing *TP53* [39-41], and the chromosome 3 [33]. However, no specific genes have been identified so far to be a preferential target for HBV insertion, unlike for the woodchuck hepatitis B virus (WHV), which preferentially inserts its DNA genome into *c-Myc* or *N-Myc* genes in the woodchuck genome. Viral genome insertions are shown to be facilitated by cellular conditions that disrupt host genomic stability or increase cellular DNA replication, such as exposure to oxidative stress or DNA-damaging agents, deficiency of the DNA repair machinery, co-infection with other viruses and chronic liver injuries that increase hepatocyte turnover [32].

Genetic Instability

The insertion itself can induce general genetic instability in host cells: integrated viral sequences are often characterized by rearrangements and/or partial deletions and HBV integration can also induce deletions in the host genome at the integration site. For example, a deletion of 2285 base pairs (bp) in the promoter region of *hTERT* and a deletion of 863 bp in HBV integrated sequence have been reported in one HCC case [35].

HBV Integration Exerts a *cis* Effect

Most of HCC cases contain one or several copies of integrated viral DNA [38]. Numerous studies analyzing the integration profile of HBV DNA in human tumors have shown a clonal proliferation of cells with the same integration site. Many of integration sites are located in or near genes involved in cellular signal pathways or playing key cellular functions (Table 2).

Table 2. HBV integration sites and signaling pathways

Pathways	Genes	References
Ras	*IRAK2, MAPK1*	[38]
Calcium	*SERCA1*	[36]
	NTRK2, IP3R1, IP3R2	[38]
Transcription	*TRAP150*a	[36]
	TRUP, EMX2-like	[38]
	RARb	[42]
Cell cycle	*cyclin A*	[43, 44]
	NMP84p	[36]
DNA replication	*MCM8*	[36]
	hTERT	[35-38]

Thus integration itself could exert a *cis* effect by deregulating important cellular components. In one study, HBV integration was observed in the intron 2 of the gene encoding Cyclin A, leading to the synthesis of a chimeric protein Cyclin A – HBV by using the viral promoter PreS2/S [44]. This protein was stabilized as the N-terminus of Cyclin A was truncated and replaced by PreS2/S sequences. In the cell line Huh4 which is derived from a HCC, a viral integration was observed in the promoter region of *hTERT* [37]: transcription occurred through viral and endogen promoters; moreover HBV enhancer sequence was located at about 1.6kb upstream the initiation site of transcription leading to a *cis* activation.

Taken together, though the insertion of HBV DNA into the host genome might be a random event, it contributes to the formation of an unstable environment, and occasionally induces genomic alterations that may facilitate hepatocyte transformation. Therefore, HBV integration may contribute, at least in part, to the development of most of HBV-induced HCCs.

HBV Integration Exerts a *Trans*-Activation Effect

In most integrated subviral HBV genomes, the ORF for HBx or Pre-S2 regulatory protein is conserved and can be transcribed [45]. These proteins are transcriptional transactivators and are known to be involved in liver cell proliferation and hepatocarcinogenesis.

A category of pre-S2 activators has been described and corresponds to pre-S/S 3'-truncated sequences [45, 46]. These sequences encode C-terminally truncated M (M^t) surface proteins that display a regulatory protein function. This truncation induces modification in the conformation of this M^t protein and allows the pre-S2 region to interact with cytosolic proteins and to activate signaling pathways in the host cell. L proteins can play a role in *trans*-activation as well. Indeed, they display a topology where their pre-S region is entirely directed into the cytoplasm. Truncated L mutants have also been described. These pre-S2 activators activate and interact directly with PKC-α, which results in the phosphorylation of the pre-S2 domain. This activation induces the c-Raf-1/MEK/ERK cascade that favors tumor progression [47, 48]. Transgenic mice for M^t protein developed liver tumors after 10 months. In addition, transgenic mice for L protein developed liver tumors as well [49]. In that case, the overexpression of L protein induces a permanent inflammation that would lead to tumorigenesis. Thus, the regulatory function of L protein would be a supplemental factor favoring the tumor development in mice: protein accumulation due to the stress and inflammation result in critical mutations, and the permanent activation of the c-Raf-1/MEK/ERK pathway in parallel favors tumorigenesis. Moreover, ΔS2-L mutants can positively regulate cyclin A expression and induce cell cycle progression [50].

HBx is also a *trans*-activator of several genes *in vitro*, among which oncogenes like *MYC* [51], *JUN* [52] and *FOS* [53], which would favor the development of HCC [54], and *FAK* that could favor migration and cellular invasion [55]. Furthermore, HBx could inhibit apoptosis induced by p53, TNF, Fas or TGF-beta, while it was shown to promote cell death by inducing mitochondrial aggregation and cytochrome c release (Figure 2) or by sensitizing cells to TNF. Moreover, HBx interacts with DDB1 (UV-damaged DNA-binding protein 1), which plays a role in DNA repair and in cell cycle regulation. Through this interaction, HBx interferes with cell cycle progression into S-phase and induces lagging chromosomes during mitosis [56]. This effect may cause cell proliferation to slow down, and at the same time may create a form of genetic instability contributing to cancer. Studies on the role of HBx have shown that HBx is often accompanied by the loss of C-terminus domain, the full-length protein being detectable in only about 20% of HCC cases with integrated HBx. They have shown that truncated HBx protein can be produced and many 3'-truncated *HBX* gene products retain the transactivation function. In a recent study, Ma and collaborators have shown that transfection of a truncated form of HBx (lacking the p53 interaction domain) increased cell proliferation, whereas transfection of full length HBx had an anti-proliferative, pro-apoptotic effect [57]. While some studies concluded that COOH-truncated HBx proteins retain transcriptional transactivation ability, others found that they have lost most of the activities associated with wild-type HBx, in particular that they can enhance (instead of inhibit) the transforming activity of Ras and Myc [58]. It is possible that the *HBX* gene used in these experiments as well as the lifelong expression of HBx could impact on the development of HCC. However, even if further studies are needed to confirm that HBx can directly induce transformation in mice, its role as a cofactor of carcinogenesis is well accepted.

Occult HBV Infections

Prevalence of Occult HBV and HCC

Chronic HBV infection is one of the main factors for the development of fibrosis, cirrhosis and HCC worldwide. This infection is characterized by the presence for more than 6 months of HBsAg and HBV DNA. Thanks to the improvement of detection tools for HBV since the 80's, occult HBV infections (OBI) were described. OBI is defined by the presence of HBV DNA in the liver tissue and/or in the serum of HBsAg-negative patients associated usually with a low HBV viremia (10^1 to 10^4 copies/ml). Two types of OBI can be distinguished: (i) seropositive OBI with the presence of HBV DNA in the liver and/or in the serum with anti-HBs and/or anti-HBc seroconversion, and (ii) seronegative OBI characterized by the presence of HBV DNA in the liver and/or in the serum in the absence of anti-HBs and HBc seroconversion [59]. The prevalence of OBI worldwide is not clear due to the different sensitivity and specificity of the methods used for detection [60]. An Italian study concerning people without liver disease revealed OBI in 16.3% of the population and in association with anti-HBc positive status [61]. However, in a Korean study concerning healthy adults, OBI was found in 0.7% of the population [62]. OBI was also investigated among chronic hepatitis patients with unknown etiology. In a cohort of 50 HBsAg-negative patients with non-A non-C non-E hepatitis, OBI was present in 30% of the cases and responsible for liver lesions [63]. In an HBsAg-negative hemophilia Japanese cohort in which a high prevalence of infection with transfusion-transmissible agents occurred, 51.2% of patients were positive for OBI [64]. OBI is usually characterized by a low level HBV replication leading to low viremia. However, in particular context OBI can reactivate and a high HBV viremia can be observed. Such cases of reactivations occur mostly with an immune-depressive status induced by therapies and/or related to diseases that involve the immune system [65].

OBI is the consequence of the persistence of cccDNA in the nucleus of hepatocytes [66]. Most of patients with OBI are infected with replication competent virus showing a suppression of replication and gene expression. OBI may be explained by the appearance of mutations in the immunodominant loop of HBV surface antigen, thus altering HBsAg antigenicity, or the suppression of viral replication due to (i) mutations in the viral polymerase or (ii) virus-host interactions and epigenetic factors [67].

Occult strains usually persist as free episomal forms which are transcriptionnally active, thus maintaining (i) a chronic liver inflammation, (ii) the tumorigenic properties of the virus *via* HBx protein, and (iii) a potential viral integration in the host genome, leading to hepatoma transformation [68]. To understand the implication of OBI in HCC development, an Italian team analyzed in HCC patients with OBI the molecular and functional aspects of the HBV strains involved. It appeared clearly that HBV strains are *in vitro* replication competent without harboring any mutation that could be responsible for an *in vivo* inhibition of HBV replication [69]. This study underlines the fact that HBV strains in OBI are replication competent and by this way can exert also, with a low level of HBV replication, the oncogenic potential of the virus. Experiments in animal models demonstrated that woodchucks, once infected with WHV, are at risk of developing HCC even after the 'apparent' clearance of the virus [70]. In this context, a retrospective cohort of cirrhotic patients without overt HCV or HBV infection were screened for the presence of HBV DNA (C and X genes) by sensitive PCR. The carcinogenesis rates related to OBI were investigated in two groups, HBV DNA-positive group and HBV DNA-negative group: the rates were 27.0% and 11.8% after 5 year, and 100% and 17.6% after 10 years, respectively. Therefore the presence of HBV DNA in the cirrhotic liver increased the risk of HCC development by 8, demonstrating a clear correlation between OBI and HCC in cirrhotic patients [71].

HBV and HCV Co-infection

Hepatitis C virus (HCV) is a member of the *flaviviridae* family, which affects 130 million people worldwide and is responsible for cirrhosis, fibrosis and HCC. This virus is mainly transmitted by blood products and drug injection. It is estimated that 7 to 20 million people are co-infected by HBV/HCV worldwide with a higher prevalence in HBV endemic regions (Asia, South America and Sub-Saharian Africa). In areas with a low prevalence for HBsAg (< 1% for example in Europe), HBV/HCV co-infection is considered as very rare.

HBV and HCV have little in common during their life cycle except their preferential replication in the same target organ: the liver. HBV/HCV co-infection is associated with a more severe liver disease, a faster development of HCC and a higher mortality rate compared with HBV or HCV mono-infection [72].

Several studies have shown that HBV/HCV co-infected patients have lower levels of HBV DNA, associated with a decreased activity of HBV polymerase and a diminution of HBsAg and HBcAg in the liver. During co-infection HCV seems to have a dominant effect leading to the suppression of HBV replication. Little is known about the molecular mechanism of inhibition of HBV during co-infection with HCV: *in vitro* studies suggest a suppression of HBV DNA transcription by the hepatitis C core protein [73, 74]. However another study observed an inhibition of HCV by active HBV replication in chronic carriers [75]. Nothing indicates a direct interaction between both viruses and it was proposed that molecular indirect effects of host-viral interactions may be responsible for a dual inhibition [76-78].

It is to notice that HCV infected patients are a population with a high rate of OBI. HBV DNA is detectable in one third of HBsAg-negative HCV carriers in the Mediterranean basin [79] and the prevalence seems to be higher in East Asian countries. Studies made in the Japanese population reported a prevalence between 37% and 95 % [80]. Another study reported a prevalence of 43.6% in HCV-positive patients for whom the degree of inflammatory cell infiltration and irregular regeneration of hepatocytes was significantly greater than for HBV DNA-negative patients [81]. Furthermore the probability for developing HCC was significantly higher in HBV DNA-positive patients (76.3%) than in HBV DNA-negative patients (23.7%). Finally OBI in co-infection with HCV is responsible for advanced liver fibrosis and HCC development [81, 82].

HBV and HIV Co-infection

Human immunodeficiency virus (HIV) is a member of the lentivirus family affecting 40 million people worldwide and responsible for the Acquired Immune Deficiency Syndrome. It shares the same routes of transmission as HBV (sexual, blood transfusion, mother-to-child), leading to a high frequency of co-infections: it is estimated that 2-4 million HIV-positive individuals are chronically infected with HBV [83]. With the introduction of highly active anti-retroviral treatment (HAART) to cure HIV, HIV infection is considered as a chronic disease and hepatic disease due to HBV or HCV is one of the first causes of morbidity and mortality in HIV-positive patients [84]. Furthermore drugs used to treat HIV, principally lamivudine, are also active against HBV and may increase the risk of drug-related hepato-toxicity and impact on the selection of drug-resistant HBV mutants and escape mutants.

During HBV/HIV co-infection HBV does not seem to affect HIV disease but the opposite is not true. Some studies reported a higher rate of HBV chronicity than during HBV mono-infection [85], a higher level of HBV replication, a lower rate of spontaneous loss of HBeAg and/or HBsAg, and a lower anti-HBs and anti-HBe seroconversion. Importantly, progression to fibrosis, cirrhosis and HCC is faster than during HBV mono-infection [86].

In HIV-positive patients, OBI is correlated with anti-HBc seroconversion status and HCV triple co-infection. In a HIV(+), HBsAg(-), anti-HBc(+) cohort, 15% of patients were positive for HBV DNA with a clear correlation between OBI and HCV positivity: 21% *versus* 8% for HCV(-) individuals [87]. In a HIV(+) Brazilian cohort, OBI was found in 14% (6/43) of patients in association with a HCV(+) status, a low HBV viral load but not with alanine aminotransferase (ALT) elevated levels. HBV strains were isolated by a molecular analysis from HIV-positive patients treated by HAART and HBV strains harboring modifications were identified: one modification in the S gene that can affect antigenicity, and another in the P gene conferring drug resistance [88]. Interestingly, the strain harboring drug resistance mutations displayed a low viremia. This underlines the multi-factorial mechanism of OBI. Actually, it is clear that in HIV-positive patients, one of the first risks associated with OBI is the selection and reactivation of HBV resistant strains or escape mutants due to a cessation of HAART treatment or an immunosuppressive status [88, 89], thus complicating clinical treatment and increasing liver damage.

Conclusion

Since the late 1980s many studies have been carried out on occult HBV. The detection of OBI in patients with chronic hepatitis in association or not with different risk factors such as HCV or alcohol abuse may identify individuals at higher risk of progression toward cirrhosis and possibly HCC. OBI detection may be recommended in patients undergoing chemotherapy and/or immunosuppressive treatments and most importantly blood and organ donors to undergo preventive treatment with antivirals. Unfortunately, until now, there is no standard method to detect OBI: the 'Statements from the Taormina expert meeting on occult hepatitis B virus infection' suggested to use the same oligonucleotide primers for detection of occult HBV DNA through 'nested' PCR amplification. The possible use of standardized tools for OBI detection is very interesting in terms of harmonization of all data to compare studies. Furthermore, it is clear in terms of OBI infection that searching anti-HBs/anti-HBc is not a discriminatory test. The development of molecular tests (HBV DNA) may be an important step towards a better understanding and detection of this type of infection.

References

[1] Glebe Dand Urban S, Viral and cellular determinants involved in hepadnaviral entry, *World J Gastroenterol*, 2007 Jan 7, 13(1), 22-38.

[2] Leistner CM, Gruen-Bernhard Sand Glebe D, Role of glycosaminoglycans for binding and infection of hepatitis B virus, *Cell Microbiol*, 2008 Jan, 10(1), 122-33.

[3] Kann M, Schmitz Aand Rabe B, Intracellular transport of hepatitis B virus, *World J Gastroenterol*, 2007 Jan 7, 13(1), 39-47.

[4] Hu Jand Lin L, RNA-protein interactions in hepadnavirus reverse transcription, *Front Biosci*, 2009, 14, 1606-18.

[5] Summers Jand Mason WS, Replication of the genome of a hepatitis B--like virus by reverse transcription of an RNA intermediate, *Cell*, 1982 Jun, 29(2), 403-15.

[6] Patient R, Hourioux Cand Roingeard P, Morphogenesis of hepatitis B virus and its subviral envelope particles, *Cell Microbiol*, 2009 Nov, 11(11), 1561-70.

[7] Glebe D, Recent advances in hepatitis B virus research: a German point of view, *World J Gastroenterol*, 2007 Jan 7, 13(1), 8-13.

[8] Hsieh YH, Su IJ, Wang HC, Chang WW, Lei HY, Lai MD, Chang WTand Huang W, Pre-S mutant surface antigens in chronic hepatitis B virus infection induce oxidative stress and DNA damage, *Carcinogenesis*, 2004 Oct, 25(10), 2023-32.

[9] Gunther S, Fischer L, Pult I, Sterneck Mand Will H, Naturally occurring variants of hepatitis B virus, *Adv Virus Res*, 1999, 52, 25-137.

[10] Fan YF, Lu CC, Chen WC, Yao WJ, Wang HC, Chang TT, Lei HY, Shiau ALand Su IJ, Prevalence and significance of hepatitis B virus (HBV) pre-S mutants in serum and

liver at different replicative stages of chronic HBV infection, *Hepatology*, 2001 Jan, 33(1), 277-86.

[11] Doria M, Klein N, Lucito Rand Schneider RJ, The hepatitis B virus HBx protein is a dual specificity cytoplasmic activator of Ras and nuclear activator of transcription factors, *EMBO J*, 1995 Oct 2, 14(19), 4747-57.

[12] Schek N, Bartenschlager R, Kuhn Cand Schaller H, Phosphorylation and rapid turnover of hepatitis B virus X-protein expressed in HepG2 cells from a recombinant vaccinia virus, *Oncogene*, 1991 Oct, 6(10), 1735-44.

[13] Sirma H, Weil R, Rosmorduc O, Urban S, Israel A, Kremsdorf Dand Brechot C, Cytosol is the prime compartment of hepatitis B virus X protein where it colocalizes with the proteasome, *Oncogene*, 1998 Apr 23, 16(16), 2051-63.

[14] Weil R, Sirma H, Giannini C, Kremsdorf D, Bessia C, Dargemont C, Brechot Cand Israel A, Direct association and nuclear import of the hepatitis B virus X protein with the NF-kappaB inhibitor IkappaBalpha, *Mol Cell Biol*, 1999 Sep, 19(9), 6345-54.

[15] Cha MY, Ryu DK, Jung HS, Chang HEand Ryu WS, Stimulation of hepatitis B virus genome replication by HBx is linked to both nuclear and cytoplasmic HBx expression, *J Gen Virol*, 2009 Apr, 90(Pt 4), 978-86.

[16] Henkler F, Hoare J, Waseem N, Goldin RD, McGarvey MJ, Koshy Rand King IA, Intracellular localization of the hepatitis B virus HBx protein, *J Gen Virol*, 2001 Apr, 82(Pt 4), 871-82.

[17] Arauz-Ruiz P, Norder H, Robertson BHand Magnius LO, Genotype H: a new Amerindian genotype of hepatitis B virus revealed in Central America, *J Gen Virol*, 2002 Aug, 83(Pt 8), 2059-73.

[18] Naumann H, Schaefer S, Yoshida CF, Gaspar AM, Repp Rand Gerlich WH, Identification of a new hepatitis B virus (HBV) genotype from Brazil that expresses HBV surface antigen subtype adw4, *J Gen Virol*, 1993 Aug, 74 (Pt 8), 1627-32.

[19] Norder H, Courouce AMand Magnius LO, Complete genomes, phylogenetic relatedness, and structural proteins of six strains of the hepatitis B virus, four of which represent two new genotypes, *Virology*, 1994 Feb, 198(2), 489-503.

[20] Okamoto H, Imai M, Tsuda F, Tanaka T, Miyakawa Yand Mayumi M, Point mutation in the S gene of hepatitis B virus for a d/y or w/r subtypic change in two blood donors carrying a surface antigen of compound subtype adyr or adwr, *J Virol*, 1987 Oct, 61(10), 3030-4.

[21] Stuyver L, De Gendt S, Van Geyt C, Zoulim F, Fried M, Schinazi RFand Rossau R, A new genotype of hepatitis B virus: complete genome and phylogenetic relatedness, *J Gen Virol*, 2000 Jan, 81(Pt 1), 67-74.

[22] Norder H, Courouce AM, Coursaget P, Echevarria JM, Lee SD, Mushahwar IK, Robertson BH, Locarnini Sand Magnius LO, Genetic diversity of hepatitis B virus strains derived worldwide: genotypes, subgenotypes, and HBsAg subtypes, *Intervirology*, 2004 Nov-Dec, 47(6), 289-309.

[23] Singh J, Dickens C, Pahal V, Kumar R, Chaudhary R, Kramvis Aand Kew MC, First report of genotype e of hepatitis B virus in an Indian population, *Intervirology*, 2009, 52(5), 235-8.

[24] Kumagai I, Abe K, Oikawa T, Sato A, Sato S, Endo R, Takikawa Y, Suzuki K, Masuda T, Sainokami S, Endo K, Takahashi Mand Okamoto H, A male patient with severe acute hepatitis who was domestically infected with a genotype H hepatitis B virus in Iwate, Japan, *J Gastroenterol*, 2007 Feb, 42(2), 168-75.
[25] Sanchez LV, Tanaka Y, Maldonado M, Mizokami Mand Panduro A, Difference of hepatitis B virus genotype distribution in two groups of mexican patients with different risk factors. High prevalence of genotype H and G, *Intervirology*, 2007, 50(1), 9-15.
[26] McMahon BJ, The influence of hepatitis B virus genotype and subgenotype on the natural history of chronic hepatitis B, *Hepatol Int*, 2009 Jun, 3(2), 334-42.
[27] Thakur V, Guptan RC, Kazim SN, Malhotra Vand Sarin SK, Profile, spectrum and significance of HBV genotypes in chronic liver disease patients in the Indian subcontinent, *J Gastroenterol Hepatol*, 2002 Feb, 17(2), 165-70.
[28] Kao JH, Hepatitis B virus genotypes and hepatocellular carcinoma in Taiwan, *Intervirology*, 2003, 46(6), 400-7.
[29] Kao JH, Chen PJ, Lai MYand Chen DS, Hepatitis B genotypes correlate with clinical outcomes in patients with chronic hepatitis B, *Gastroenterology*, 2000 Mar, 118(3), 554-9.
[30] Lee CM, Chen CH, Lu SN, Tung HD, Chou WJ, Wang JH, Chen TM, Hung CH, Huang CCand Chen WJ, Prevalence and clinical implications of hepatitis B virus genotypes in southern Taiwan, *Scand J Gastroenterol*, 2003 Jan, 38(1), 95-101.
[31] Tangkijvanich P, Mahachai V, Komolmit P, Fongsarun J, Theamboonlers Aand Poovorawan Y, Hepatitis B virus genotypes and hepatocellular carcinoma in Thailand, *World J Gastroenterol*, 2005 Apr 21, 11(15), 2238-43.
[32] Bonilla Guerrero Rand Roberts LR, The role of hepatitis B virus integrations in the pathogenesis of human hepatocellular carcinoma, *J Hepatol*, 2005 May, 42(5), 760-77.
[33] Minami M, Daimon Y, Mori K, Takashima H, Nakajima T, Itoh Yand Okanoue T, Hepatitis B virus-related insertional mutagenesis in chronic hepatitis B patients as an early drastic genetic change leading to hepatocarcinogenesis, *Oncogene*, 2005 Jun 23, 24(27), 4340-8.
[34] Murakami Y, Minami M, Daimon Yand Okanoue T, Hepatitis B virus DNA in liver, serum, and peripheral blood mononuclear cells after the clearance of serum hepatitis B virus surface antigen, *J Med Virol*, 2004 Feb, 72(2), 203-14.
[35] Ferber MJ, Montoya DP, Yu C, Aderca I, McGee A, Thorland EC, Nagorney DM, Gostout BS, Burgart LJ, Boix L, Bruix J, McMahon BJ, Cheung TH, Chung TK, Wong YF, Smith DIand Roberts LR, Integrations of the hepatitis B virus (HBV) and human papillomavirus (HPV) into the human telomerase reverse transcriptase (hTERT) gene in liver and cervical cancers, *Oncogene*, 2003 Jun 12, 22(24), 3813-20.
[36] Gozuacik D, Murakami Y, Saigo K, Chami M, Mugnier C, Lagorce D, Okanoue T, Urashima T, Brechot Cand Paterlini-Brechot P, Identification of human cancer-related genes by naturally occurring Hepatitis B Virus DNA tagging, *Oncogene*, 2001 Sep 27, 20(43), 6233-40.
[37] Horikawa Iand Barrett JC, cis-Activation of the human telomerase gene (hTERT) by the hepatitis B virus genome, *J Natl Cancer Inst*, 2001 Aug 1, 93(15), 1171-3.

[38] Paterlini-Brechot P, Saigo K, Murakami Y, Chami M, Gozuacik D, Mugnier C, Lagorce Dand Brechot C, Hepatitis B virus-related insertional mutagenesis occurs frequently in human liver cancers and recurrently targets human telomerase gene, *Oncogene*, 2003 Jun 19, 22(25), 3911-6.

[39] Liu XH, Lin J, Zhang SH, Zhang SM, Feitelson MA, Gao HJand Zhu MH, COOH-terminal deletion of HBx gene is a frequent event in HBV-associated hepatocellular carcinoma, *World J Gastroenterol*, 2008 Mar 7, 14(9), 1346-52.

[40] Slagle BL, Zhou YZand Butel JS, Hepatitis B virus integration event in human chromosome 17p near the p53 gene identifies the region of the chromosome commonly deleted in virus-positive hepatocellular carcinomas, *Cancer Res*, 1991 Jan 1, 51(1), 49-54.

[41] Zhou YZ, Slagle BL, Donehower LA, vanTuinen P, Ledbetter DHand Butel JS, Structural analysis of a hepatitis B virus genome integrated into chromosome 17p of a human hepatocellular carcinoma, *J Virol*, 1988 Nov, 62(11), 4224-31.

[42] Dejean A, Bougueleret L, Grzeschik KHand Tiollais P, Hepatitis B virus DNA integration in a sequence homologous to v-erb-A and steroid receptor genes in a hepatocellular carcinoma, *Nature*, 1986 Jul 3-9, 322(6074), 70-2.

[43] Wang J, Chenivesse X, Henglein Band Brechot C, Hepatitis B virus integration in a cyclin A gene in a hepatocellular carcinoma, *Nature*, 1990 Feb 8, 343(6258), 555-7.

[44] Wang J, Zindy F, Chenivesse X, Lamas E, Henglein Band Brechot C, Modification of cyclin A expression by hepatitis B virus DNA integration in a hepatocellular carcinoma, *Oncogene*, 1992 Aug, 7(8), 1653-6.

[45] Schluter V, Meyer M, Hofschneider PH, Koshy Rand Caselmann WH, Integrated hepatitis B virus X and 3' truncated preS/S sequences derived from human hepatomas encode functionally active transactivators, *Oncogene*, 1994 Nov, 9(11), 3335-44.

[46] Lupberger Jand Hildt E, Hepatitis B virus-induced oncogenesis, *World J Gastroenterol*, 2007 Jan 7, 13(1), 74-81.

[47] Hildt E, Munz B, Saher G, Reifenberg Kand Hofschneider PH, The PreS2 activator MHBs(t) of hepatitis B virus activates c-raf-1/Erk2 signaling in transgenic mice, *EMBO J*, 2002 Feb 15, 21(4), 525-35.

[48] Hildt E, Saher G, Bruss Vand Hofschneider PH, The hepatitis B virus large surface protein (LHBs) is a transcriptional activator, *Virology*, 1996 Nov 1, 225(1), 235-9.

[49] Chisari FV, Klopchin K, Moriyama T, Pasquinelli C, Dunsford HA, Sell S, Pinkert CA, Brinster RLand Palmiter RD, Molecular pathogenesis of hepatocellular carcinoma in hepatitis B virus transgenic mice, *Cell*, 1989 Dec 22, 59(6), 1145-56.

[50] Wang HC, Chang WT, Chang WW, Wu HC, Huang W, Lei HY, Lai MD, Fausto Nand Su IJ, Hepatitis B virus pre-S2 mutant upregulates cyclin A expression and induces nodular proliferation of hepatocytes, *Hepatology*, 2005 Apr, 41(4), 761-70.

[51] Balsano C, Avantaggiati ML, Natoli G, De Marzio E, Will H, Perricaudet Mand Levrero M, Full-length and truncated versions of the hepatitis B virus (HBV) X protein (pX) transactivate the cmyc protooncogene at the transcriptional level, *Biochem Biophys Res Commun*, 1991 May 15, 176(3), 985-92.

[52] Twu JS, Lai MY, Chen DSand Robinson WS, Activation of protooncogene c-jun by the X protein of hepatitis B virus, *Virology*, 1993 Jan, 192(1), 346-50.

[53] Avantaggiati ML, Natoli G, Balsano C, Chirillo P, Artini M, De Marzio E, Collepardo Dand Levrero M, The hepatitis B virus (HBV) pX transactivates the c-fos promoter through multiple cis-acting elements, *Oncogene*, 1993 Jun, 8(6), 1567-74.

[54] Diao J, Garces Rand Richardson CD, X protein of hepatitis B virus modulates cytokine and growth factor related signal transduction pathways during the course of viral infections and hepatocarcinogenesis, *Cytokine Growth Factor Rev*, 2001 Jun-Sep, 12(2-3), 189-205.

[55] Bouchard MJ, Wang Land Schneider RJ, Activation of focal adhesion kinase by hepatitis B virus HBx protein: multiple functions in viral replication, *J Virol*, 2006 May, 80(9), 4406-14.

[56] Martin-Lluesma S, Schaeffer C, Robert EI, van Breugel PC, Leupin O, Hantz Oand Strubin M, Hepatitis B virus X protein affects S phase progression leading to chromosome segregation defects by binding to damaged DNA binding protein 1, *Hepatology*, 2008 Nov, 48(5), 1467-76.

[57] Ma NF, Lau SH, Hu L, Xie D, Wu J, Yang J, Wang Y, Wu MC, Fung J, Bai X, Tzang CH, Fu L, Yang M, Su YAand Guan XY, COOH-terminal truncated HBV X protein plays key role in hepatocarcinogenesis, *Clin Cancer Res*, 2008 Aug 15, 14(16), 5061-8.

[58] Tu H, Bonura C, Giannini C, Mouly H, Soussan P, Kew M, Paterlini-Brechot P, Brechot Cand Kremsdorf D, Biological impact of natural COOH-terminal deletions of hepatitis B virus X protein in hepatocellular carcinoma tissues, *Cancer Res*, 2001 Nov 1, 61(21), 7803-10.

[59] Raimondo G, Allain JP, Brunetto MR, Buendia MA, Chen DS, Colombo M, Craxi A, Donato F, Ferrari C, Gaeta GB, Gerlich WH, Levrero M, Locarnini S, Michalak T, Mondelli MU, Pawlotsky JM, Pollicino T, Prati D, Puoti M, Samuel D, Shouval D, Smedile A, Squadrito G, Trepo C, Villa E, Will H, Zanetti ARand Zoulim F, Statements from the Taormina expert meeting on occult hepatitis B virus infection, *J Hepatol*, 2008 Oct, 49(4), 652-7.

[60] Torbenson Mand Thomas DL, Occult hepatitis B, *Lancet Infect Dis*, 2002 Aug, 2(8), 479-86.

[61] Raimondo G, Navarra G, Mondello S, Costantino L, Colloredo G, Cucinotta E, Di Vita G, Scisca C, Squadrito Gand Pollicino T, Occult hepatitis B virus in liver tissue of individuals without hepatic disease, *J Hepatol*, 2008 May, 48(5), 743-6.

[62] Song EY, Yun YM, Park MHand Seo DH, Prevalence of occult hepatitis B virus infection in a general adult population in Korea, *Intervirology*, 2009, 52(2), 57-62.

[63] Chemin I, Zoulim F, Merle P, Arkhis A, Chevallier M, Kay A, Cova L, Chevallier P, Mandrand Band Trepo C, High incidence of hepatitis B infections among chronic hepatitis cases of unknown aetiology, *J Hepatol*, 2001 Mar, 34(3), 447-54.

[64] Toyoda H, Hayashi K, Murakami Y, Honda T, Katano Y, Nakano I, Goto H, Kumada Tand Takamatsu J, Prevalence and clinical implications of occult hepatitis B viral infection in hemophilia patients in Japan, *J Med Virol*, 2004 Jun, 73(2), 195-9.

[65] Yeo W, Chan TC, Leung NW, Lam WY, Mo FK, Chu MT, Chan HL, Hui EP, Lei KI, Mok TSand Chan PK, Hepatitis B virus reactivation in lymphoma patients with prior

resolved hepatitis B undergoing anticancer therapy with or without rituximab, *J Clin Oncol*, 2009 Feb 1, 27(4), 605-11.

[66] Zoulim F, New insight on hepatitis B virus persistence from the study of intrahepatic viral cccDNA, *J Hepatol*, 2005 Mar, 42(3), 302-8.

[67] Raimondo G, Pollicino T, Cacciola Iand Squadrito G, Occult hepatitis B virus infection, *J Hepatol*, 2007 Jan, 46(1), 160-70.

[68] Pollicino T, Squadrito G, Cerenzia G, Cacciola I, Raffa G, Craxi A, Farinati F, Missale G, Smedile A, Tiribelli C, Villa Eand Raimondo G, Hepatitis B virus maintains its pro-oncogenic properties in the case of occult HBV infection, *Gastroenterology*, 2004 Jan, 126(1), 102-10.

[69] Pollicino T, Raffa G, Costantino L, Lisa A, Campello C, Squadrito G, Levrero Mand Raimondo G, Molecular and functional analysis of occult hepatitis B virus isolates from patients with hepatocellular carcinoma, *Hepatology*, 2007 Feb, 45(2), 277-85.

[70] Korba BE, Wells FV, Baldwin B, Cote PJ, Tennant BC, Popper Hand Gerin JL, Hepatocellular carcinoma in woodchuck hepatitis virus-infected woodchucks: presence of viral DNA in tumor tissue from chronic carriers and animals serologically recovered from acute infections, *Hepatology*, 1989 Mar, 9(3), 461-70.

[71] Ikeda K, Kobayashi M, Someya T, Saitoh S, Hosaka T, Akuta N, Suzuki F, Suzuki Y, Arase Yand Kumada H, Occult hepatitis B virus infection increases hepatocellular carcinogenesis by eight times in patients with non-B, non-C liver cirrhosis: a cohort study, *J Viral Hepat*, 2009 Jun, 16(6), 437-43.

[72] Potthoff A, Manns MPand Wedemeyer H, Treatment of HBV/HCV coinfection, *Expert Opin Pharmacother*, 2010 Apr, 11(6), 919-28.

[73] Schuttler CG, Fiedler N, Schmidt K, Repp R, Gerlich WHand Schaefer S, Suppression of hepatitis B virus enhancer 1 and 2 by hepatitis C virus core protein, *J Hepatol*, 2002 Dec, 37(6), 855-62.

[74] Shih CM, Lo SJ, Miyamura T, Chen SYand Lee YH, Suppression of hepatitis B virus expression and replication by hepatitis C virus core protein in HuH-7 cells, *J Virol*, 1993 Oct, 67(10), 5823-32.

[75] Pontisso P, Ruvoletto MG, Fattovich G, Chemello L, Gallorini A, Ruol Aand Alberti A, Clinical and virological profiles in patients with multiple hepatitis virus infections, *Gastroenterology*, 1993 Nov, 105(5), 1529-33.

[76] Bellecave P, Gouttenoire J, Gajer M, Brass V, Koutsoudakis G, Blum HE, Bartenschlager R, Nassal Mand Moradpour D, Hepatitis B and C virus coinfection: a novel model system reveals the absence of direct viral interference, *Hepatology*, 2009 Jul, 50(1), 46-55.

[77] Eyre NS, Phillips RJ, Bowden S, Yip E, Dewar B, Locarnini SAand Beard MR, Hepatitis B virus and hepatitis C virus interaction in Huh-7 cells, *J Hepatol*, 2009 Sep, 51(3), 446-57.

[78] Koike K, Yasuda K, Yotsuyanagi H, Moriya K, Hino K, Kurokawa Kand Iino S, Dominant replication of either virus in dual infection with hepatitis viruses B and C, *J Med Virol*, 1995 Feb, 45(2), 236-9.

[79] Cacciola I, Pollicino T, Squadrito G, Cerenzia G, Orlando MEand Raimondo G, Occult hepatitis B virus infection in patients with chronic hepatitis C liver disease, *N Engl J Med*, 1999 Jul 1, 341(1), 22-6.

[80] Koike K, Kobayashi M, Gondo M, Hayashi I, Osuga Tand Takada S, Hepatitis B virus DNA is frequently found in liver biopsy samples from hepatitis C virus-infected chronic hepatitis patients, *J Med Virol*, 1998 Apr, 54(4), 249-55.

[81] Matsuoka S, Nirei K, Tamura A, Nakamura H, Matsumura H, Oshiro S, Arakawa Y, Yamagami H, Tanaka Nand Moriyama M, Influence of occult hepatitis B virus coinfection on the incidence of fibrosis and hepatocellular carcinoma in chronic hepatitis C, *Intervirology*, 2008, 51(5), 352-61.

[82] Chemin Iand Trepo C, Clinical impact of occult HBV infections, *J Clin Virol*, 2005 Dec, 34 Suppl 1, S15-21.

[83] Alter MJ, Epidemiology of viral hepatitis and HIV co-infection, *J Hepatol*, 2006, 44(1 Suppl), S6-9.

[84] Sulkowski MS, Viral hepatitis and HIV coinfection, *J Hepatol*, 2008 Feb, 48(2), 353-67.

[85] Koblin BA, Taylor PE, Rubinstein Pand Stevens CE, Effect of duration of hepatitis B virus infection on the association between human immunodeficiency virus type-1 and hepatitis B viral replication, *Hepatology*, 1992 Apr, 15(4), 590-2.

[86] Bonacini M, Interaction between HIV and hepatitis B, *AIDS*, 1997 Nov 15, 11(14), 1789-90.

[87] Morsica G, Ancarani F, Bagaglio S, Maracci M, Cicconi P, Cozzi Lepri A, Antonucci G, Bruno R, Santantonio T, Tacconi L, Baldelli F, Piscopo R, Santoro D, Lazzarin Aand D'Arminio Monforte A, Occult hepatitis B virus infection in a cohort of HIV-positive patients: correlation with hepatitis C virus coinfection, virological and immunological features, *Infection*, 2009 Oct, 37(5), 445-9.

[88] Araujo NM, Branco-Vieira M, Silva AC, Pilotto JH, Grinsztejn B, de Almeida AJ, Trepo Cand Gomes SA, Occult hepatitis B virus infection in HIV-infected patients: Evaluation of biochemical, virological and molecular parameters, *Hepatol Res*, 2008 Dec, 38(12), 1194-203.

[89] Altfeld M, Rockstroh JK, Addo M, Kupfer B, Pult I, Will Hand Spengler U, Reactivation of hepatitis B in a long-term anti-HBs-positive patient with AIDS following lamivudine withdrawal, *J Hepatol*, 1998 Aug, 29(2), 306-9.

Section II. Promising New Biomarkers for Hepatocellular Carcinoma

In: Hepatocellular Carcionoma: A Global Challenge
Editor: Isabelle Chemin ISBN: 978-1-61470-644-1

Introduction to Section Two

H. E. Blum *
Department of Medicine II, University Hospital of Freiburg, Freiburg, Germany

Hepatocellular carcinoma (HCC) is one of the most common malignant tumors worldwide. The annual incidence ranges from <10 cases per 100,000 population in North America and Western Europe to 50-150 cases per 100,000 population in parts of Africa and Asia where HCC is responsible for a large proportion of cancer deaths. The major etiologies of HCC are well defined and include among others chronic viral hepatitis B, C and D, alcoholic, autoimmune and hereditary liver diseases, such as hemochromatosis, alpha-1-antitypsin deficiency and others. In addition, more recently identified risk factors for HCC development are non-alcoholic fatty liver disease (NAFLD) or non-alcoholic steatohepatitis (NASH) that are frequently associated with diabetes mellitus or other states of insulin resistance as well as obesity in men. These aspects are splendidly covered in first section on 'Epidemiology' of this book.

The second section addresses 'New Biomarkers' and focuses specifically in excellent, state-of-the-art contributions on the pathological aspects of HCCs, genetic and epigenetic aspects of the molecular pathogenesis of HCC development as well as the application of the 'omics' approach to the characterization of HCCs ('tumor profiling') aimed at predicting the natural course of the HCC, risk of metastasis or recurrence, as well as the response to therapy. More recently, the 'omics' analyses have been extended to the non-tumorous liver ('adjacent tumor profiling') aimed at predicting the risk of HCC development.

The molecular mechanisms of HCC development are not fully understood. As for most types of cancer, hepatocarcinogenesis is a multistep process involving different genetic and epigenetic alterations that ultimately lead to the malignant transformation of a hepatocyte. Malignant transformation of hepatocytes may occur regardless of the etiology through a pathway of increased liver cell turnover, induced by chronic liver injury and regeneration in a context of inflammation, immune response and oxidative DNA damage. This may result in genetic alterations, such as the activation of cellular oncogenes, the inactivation of tumor

* E-mail: hubert.blum@uniklinik-freiburg.de; Phone: 0049 761 2703404; Fax: 0049 761 2703610.

suppressor genes, possibly in cooperation with genomic instability, including DNA mismatch repair defects and impaired chromosomal segregation, overexpression of growth and angiogenic factors, and telomerase activation.

The molecular pathogenesis of HCCs is genetically very heterogeneous. Gene and gene expression profiles of HCCs increasingly allow to distinguish between dysplasia and neoplasia. In addition, transcriptome analyses of HCCs identified several genes that suggest a novel HCC classification with therapeutic implications. Microarray analyses of 6'000 genes in completely resected HCCs, for example, showed that 12 genes predict a high risk for an early intrahepatic recurrence. If validated by additional studies, it thus may become possible to preoperatively distinguish patients with a high risk of recurrence from those with a low risk of recurrence. Thus, the 'tumor profiling' may contribute to further optimize the therapeutic strategy for the individual patient.

Apart from clinical parameters and the gene or gene expression profiles of tumor-associated genes, such as glycipan-3 (GPC3), heat shock protein 70 (HSP70), survivin, LYVE1 and microRNA (miR) species in the tumor, there is increasing evidence that 'adjacent tumor profiling' may allow to predict the risk of HCC development and/ or HCC metastases.

In disease pathogenesis, incl. HCC development, miR species are increasingly attracting attention. The miR species are non-coding RNA molecules of 20-25 nucleotides length which suppress gene expression in the cell nucleus by complementary base-pairing with the 3'-non-translated region of mRNAs, thereby blocking translation. Based on this principle action, miR can function, among others, as tumor suppressor or oncogene. Analyses addressing the role of miR in HCC development revealed that females have a higher expression of miR-26a and miR-26b in the non-tumorous liver tissue adjacent to the HCC than males. Further, the expression of these miR species is lower in the HCC as compared to the adjacent non-tumorous liver and patients with a low miR expression in the HCC have a poorer prognosis but respond better to interferon treatment than patients with an high miR expression in the tumor. Other miR species have recently been identified that are involved in HCC development (miR221) HCC invasion and metastasis (miR-30d) as well as the prognosis of patients with this malignancy (miR-29).

The section on 'New Biomarkers' splendidly covers a broad spectrum of topics, ranging from the histopathology of HCC development to the molecular hepatocarcinogensis, incl. genetic and epigenetic events, signalling pathways and the contribution of miRNA. In addition, new technologies, such as gene or gene expression profiling, proteomic analyses and others are presented. These should allow to further elucidate the molecular events underlying the HCC development and to identify novel diagnostic markers as well as therapeutic and preventive targets.

In: Hepatocellular Carcionoma: A Global Challenge
Editor: Isabelle Chemin
ISBN: 978-1-61470-644-1

Chapter VI

Hepatocellular Carcinoma: Pathological Diagnosis

Valérie Paradis
Pathology Dpt Beaujon Hospital, Clichy, Paris, France

Introduction

HCC represents the first primary malignancy of the liver followed by cholangiocarcinoma. Its incidence is still increasing owe to the increased prevalence of the various risk factors of chronic liver diseases, mainly related to hepatitis infection with hepatitis C and B viruses, and more recently Fatty Liver Diseases which are mostly associated with metabolic syndrome [1]. Indeed, 60 to 90% of HCC occur in the setting of chronic liver diseases leading to cirrhosis. Still now, HCC carries a poor prognosis which is partly explained by its late diagnosis, the clinical context of the patient which may compromise potential therapeutic strategies, and also tumor itself which is prone to display angioinvasion.

HCC is a peculiar tumor for several aspects, especially for pathologists. It is admitted that HCC usually occurs after a mean delay of 10 years following the constitution of liver cirrhosis. This observation is highly consistent with the multistep process of liver cirrhosis that implies progressive malignant transformation of premalignant lesions. In addition, HCC may display various morphological patterns, beyond the usual classification based on growth pattern and tumor differentiation. At last, pathogenesis of HCC is complex, involving different molecular pathways that may reflect both underlying etiologies and biological behaviour. In addition, some molecular profiles of HCC have been recently associated with prognosis and the potential origin of the tumor. Thus, in the era of stem cells theory, HCC may have a specific place since it has been suggested that several forms of HCC may derive from hepatic stem cells proliferation.

Pathological Diagnosis

As already outlined, most of HCC are encountered in patients having chronic liver diseases and its development is considered as one of the main complications of cirrhosis, with an annual incidence of 3% [2]. In that setting, HCC arise through the malignant transformation of premalignant lesions, including dysplastic cirrhotic nodules.

Gross Macroscopy

Considerable diversity in the macroscopic appearances of HCC is observed. They could be single or multiple with a size ranging from less than 1 cm to over 30 cm. Usually on cirrhosis, size of HCC is smaller compared to those developed in non fibrotic liver, and HCC less than 2 cm are recognised as “early HCC” [3]. On cut sections, HCC typically form soft masses with an heterogeneous macroscopic appearance, polychrome with foci of hemorrhage or necrosis. Grossly, three main patterns are described [4]. The nodular (expanding) pattern, defined by multiple nodules with one dominant, frequently partly or totally limited by a fibrous capsule, throughout the cirrhotic tissue, is the most common observed. The infiltrative (massive) pattern is composed by a large poorly circumscribed single mass, usually encountered in a non-cirrhotic liver. The diffuse pattern represents a widespread infiltration by numerous small nodules that virtually replace the entire liver.

Histology

On histology, the main hallmark of HCC is its resemblance to the normal liver both in its plate-like growth and its cytology, which is usually observed at least in part of the tumor [5]. HCC may present varying degrees of hepatocellular differentiation, ranging from well to poorly-differentiated, that are based upon the architectural and cytologic features. Different histological patterns may be seen. The trabecular pattern of growth is defined by tumoral hepatocytes arranged in plates which vary in thickness from 2 to over 20 cells. They are separated by sinusoid vascular spaces lined by flat endothelial cells in which very few Kupffer cells may be observed. Compared to normal or adenomatous liver plates, the reticulin framework is commonly sparse or absent. The acinar or pseudoglandular pattern results either from gland-like dilatation of the canaliculi between tumor cells (lumens can contain bile) or central degeneration of trabeculae (lumen containing mainly fibrin). The compact or scirrhous pattern is composed of thick trabeculae that are compressed into a compact mass. The scirrhous HCC is a rare form characterized by a prominent and dense fibrous stroma [6].

Cytologically, tumoral hepatocytes may appear to be normal hepatocytes, with a polygonal shape displaying an eosinophilic granular cytoplasm, rounded nuclei and prominent nucleoli. The importance of cell pleomorphism varies according to the degree of differentiation. A clear cell variant of HCC is described. In that case, clear cells may contain fat or glycogen. Inside the tumor cell, globular hyaline bodies (weakly PAS positive) composed of α1-AT, albumin, fibrinogen and Mallory-Denk bodies may be observed, usually in well-differentiated HCC. Based on cytologic characterististics, several variants of HCC are described. In the scirrhous HCC, tumor cells are generally smaller in size, showing a granular eosinophilic cytoplasm, vesicular nuclei, and conspicuous nucleoli. [6] *Sarcomatoid HCC* is characterized by a sarcomatous-appearing component of spindle-shaped or giant tumor cells [7].

A large variety of immunophenotypical markers of HCC has been described. Some of them may help in the positive diagnosis of HCC, including Hep Par 1, albumin, fibrinogen and α1-AT. AFP, which is highly specific of HCC, lacks of sensitivity with only approximately 25% of HCC positive, usually weak and patchy. Noteworthy, in cases of poorly-differentiated tumors, such markers display insufficient performance. Therefore, additional markers, not specific for HCC, may be used, such as polyclonal CEA and CD10 which display a canalicular immunostaining. More recently, surrogate markers have been shown to be more relevant such as glypican-3, Glutamine synthetase and HSP70 [8-10]. Among them, GPC-3 seems to be the more performant with more than 80% of HCC immunopositive [8, 11]. Genomic studies provided molecular classifications of HCC based on gene expression [12, 13]. Such analysis allowed the identification of subgroups of patients according to etiological factors, stages of the disease, recurrence and survival [14-16]. Major classes of tumors emerging from these comprehensive analyses are also related to important carcinogenesis pathways such as activation of ß-catenin, AKT/mTOR, or inactivation of TP53 and RB1 [14, 17].

Grading and Histoprognostic Factors

Grading of HCC relies for many years on Edmondson & Steiner system which divided HCC into 4 grades from I to IV on the basis of histological differentiation [18]. Grade I is the best differentiated consisting of small tumor cells arranged in thin trabeculae. Cells in grade II are larger with abnormal nuclei and glandular structures may be present. In garade IV, tumor cells are much less differentiated with hyperchromatic nuclei and loss of trabecular pattern. In fact, most of HCC present as grade II or III. Compared to other carcinomas, there is a tendency to simplify the grading and use a 3-scale system including well-, moderately- and poorly-differentiated HCC.

Importantly, tumor grade appears as a weak independent predictor of the clinical course and conveys little prognostic information.The main prognostic factors of HCC are related to tumor stage (number and size of nodules, presence of vascular invasion, extrahepatic spread), liver function (defined by Child–Pugh's class, bilirubin, albumin, portal hypertension) and general health status. Among them, size is a major prognostic factor, with a very good prognosis for small or minute carcinomas Presence of vascular invasion and satellite nodules around the main tumor have also been recognized as predictors of recurrence and survival in several studies [19, 20].

Using microarray technology, recent studies have shown that a subset of adult HCC displays phenotypical traits of hepatoblasts. These tumors retent stem cells markers and express CK7 and CK19. Interestingly, worse survival was demonstrated for this subgroup [21] Although the significance of CK7 and CK19 expression in HCC is still unclear, this might represent a relevant prognostic factor although larger study with multidimensional analysis should be performed.

Preneoplastic Lesions

It is commonly accepted that in the context of cirrhosis, there is a stepwise progression from cirrhotic nodule to HCC. A unified nomenclature of such liver nodules has been recently reviewed [22]. According to such classification, one distinguished benign macroregenerative nodules that are histologically indistinguishable from the adjacent parenchymal cirrhotic nodules and dysplastic nodules (DN) further subdivided into low grade (LGDN) and high grade (HGDN), the latter being closer to HCC in the spectrum of hepatocarcinogenesis. The premalignant nature of DN is supported by different clues including the common association with HCC in cirrhotic livers, the presence of hepato-cellular cyto-architectural abnormalities and morphologic evidence of neoangiogenesis, the detection of both genetic and epigenetic changes close to overt HCC [23-26]. At the end of the spectrum, small HCC, defined as HCC with a maximum diameter of less than 2 cm, have been subdivided into 2 different entities: HCC of vaguely nodular type and HCC of distinctively nodular type) [22].

Specific Situations

Although the large majority of HCC arise in patients with advanced chronic liver diseases, HCC may be observed without advanced liver fibrosis or even in underlying normal liver.

HCC without Cirrhosis

HCC may occur early in the process of chronic liver diseases before the stage of cirrhosis. Although this situation may be observed whatever the etiological cause, it is especially encountered in the context of hepatitis B viral infection and metabolic syndrome [27-29]. Due to the increase prevalence of metabolic syndrome worldwide, HCC associated with metabolic syndrome will become a major concern. Occurrence of HCC in that setting is mainly related to development of metabolic fatty liver disorders, including steatosis and steato-hepatitis that may progress to fibrosis [30-32] Although, and as in other chronic liver diseases, the presence of cirrhosis may promote *per se* development of HCC in such patients, diabetes and obesity, as factors of metabolic syndrome, also appear to be independent risk factors in liver carcinogenesis [33, 34]. Interestingly, several studies reported significant number of cases of HCC in patients with non-advanced liver fibrosis [29, 35-37]. These data support the hypothesis that liver carcinogenesis related to metabolic syndrome may follow distinct molecular pathways of tumorigenesis, independently from the usual multistep process-fibrosis-cirrhosis-HCC at leat in some cases.

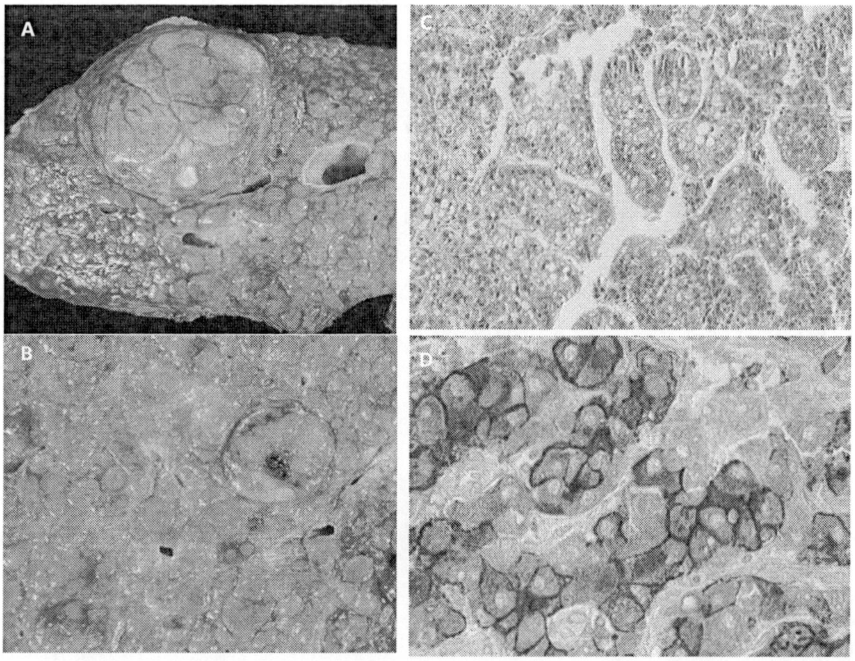

Figure 1. Hepatocellular carcinoma. A: Macroscopic view of a nodular HCC developed in a cirrhotic liver. B: Macroscopic view of an "early HCC" as a nodule of less than 2 cm in its largest size on a cirrhotic tissue. C: Histologically, HCC is made of large trabeculae of tumoral hepatocytes. D: Glypican staining of tumoral hepatocytes.

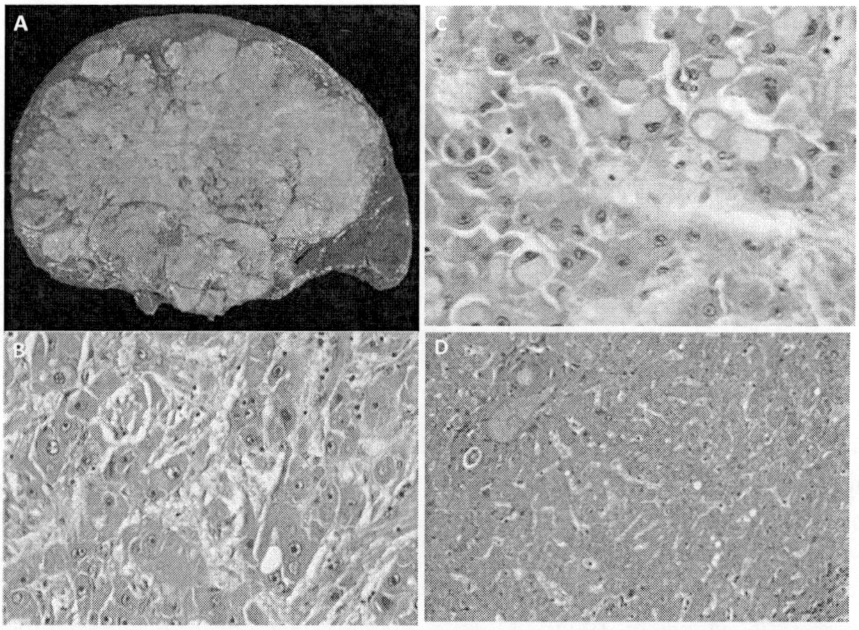

Figure 2. Fibrolamellar hepatocellular carcinoma. A: Macroscopic view showing a large well-limited tumor, polychrome with fibrous stroma. B: Histologically, tumoral cells are large, eosinophilic surrounded by hyaline fibrous bands. C: Presence of pale bodies inside the tumoral hepatocytes. D: Non tumoral liver displays a normal architecture without significant changes.

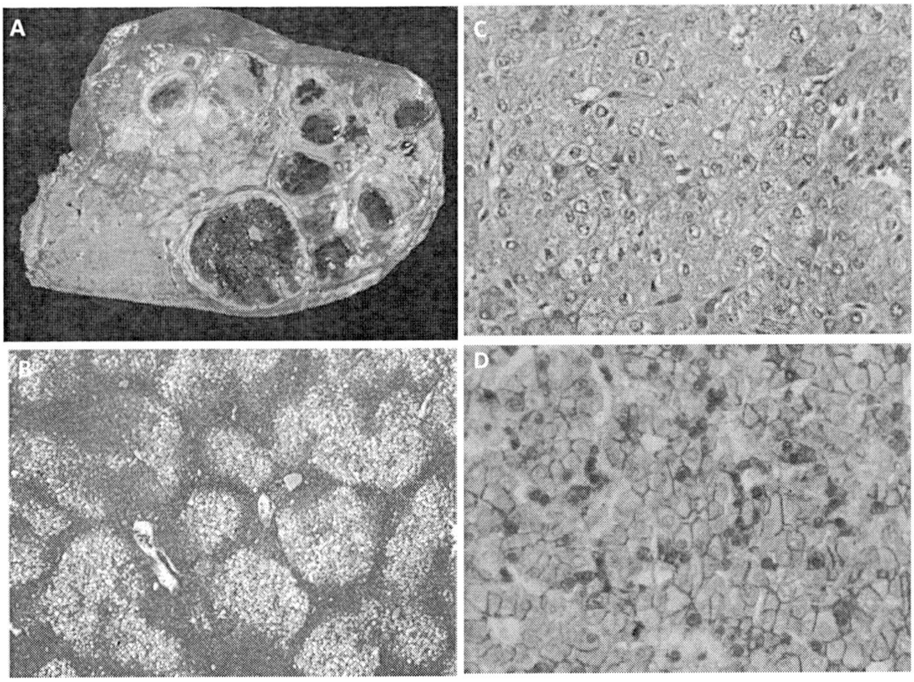

Figure 3. Hepatocellular carcinoma in metabolic syndrome. A/ Macroscopic view of a large heterogeneous hepatocellular tumor with hemorrhage. B: Adjacent non tumoral liver displays normal architecture with severe steatosis on trichtome staining. C: Inside the hepatocellular adenoma, presence foci of HCC proliferation of very-well differentiation grade. D: β-catenin staining shows a nuclear and cytoplasmic positivity suggestive of presence of β-catenin activation.

HCC on Normal Liver

Fibrolamellar Type of HCC

This entity, first described by Edmondson in 1980, is rare, accounting for < 1 % of all cases of primary liver cancer [38]. Such HCC is observed in young population without any association with chronic liver disease, or other known predisposing risk factors [39]. On gross examination, fibrolamellar HCC is firm, mostly well-defined single nodule ranging from 5 cm to over 20 cm. On cut section, prominent fibrous septa subdivide the mass and may connect with a central zone of scarring and calcifications may be observed. Histologically, the key-features include the presence of lamellar stromal bands surrounding nests of large polygonal eosinophilic tumor cells with proeminent nucleoli. Cytoplasmic inclusions of various types are common, including ground-glass pale bodies, eosinophilic cytoplasmic globules of variable PAS-positivity, and rarely, Mallory bodies. In contrast to most HCC, fibrolamellar HCC seems to express abundantly type 7 cytokeratin and, in some cells, biliary-type cytokeratin 19 [40]. Despite its large size at time of diagnosis, prognosis of fibrolamellar HCC is usually considered better than conventional HCC, especially due to the good shape clinical condition of the patient without chronic liver disease.

Malignant Transformation of Hepatocellular Adenomas

Hepatocellular adenomas (HCA) are rare benign neoplasms of the liver, mainly observed in young women, strongly associated with oral contraceptive use [41]. This tumor can also occur in men receiving anabolic steroids [42] or be associated with underlying metabolic diseases and metabolic syndrome [43, 44]. Malignant transformation into HCC is one of the most important complications of HCA, reported between 4 to 10% in the literature [44, 45, 46]. Several risk factors for malignant transformation are now recognized, including the gender (increased in male patients), the size (> 5 cm), and the subtype of HCA (especially those displaying β catenin activation) [44-47]. Malignancy commonly displays well differentiated HCC inside the HCA, with exceptional vascular invasion or satellite nodules [46].

Conclusion

Pathology of HCC is still evolving, mainly due to the significant advances in the molecular pathways of liver carcinogenesis and the relative changes in epidemiologic factors, with a noteworthy increase in metabolic syndrome. In that field, molecular pathology will play a key role for diagnostic and prognostic purposes.

References

[1] El-Serag HB. Epidemiology of hepatocellular carcinoma in USA. *Hepatol Res* 2007;37 Suppl 2:S88-94.

[2] Colombo M, de Franchis R, Del Ninno E, et al. Hepatocellular carcinoma in Italian patients with cirrhosis. *N Engl J Med.* 1991;325(1651452):675-680.

[3] Terminology of nodular hepatocellular lesions. International Working Party. *Hepatology.* Sep 1995;22(3):983-993.

[4] Okuda K, Peters RL, Simson IW. Gross anatomic features of hepatocellular carcinoma from three disparate geographic areas. Proposal of new classification. *Cancer.* 1984;54(6091861):2165-2173.

[5] Anthony PP. Primary carcinoma of the liver: a study of 282 cases in Ugandan Africans. *J Pathol.* 1973;110(4353217):37-48.

[6] Omata M, Peters RL, Tatter D. Sclerosing hepatic carcinoma: relationship to hypercalcemia. *Liver.* 1981;1(6294435):33-49.

[7] Kojiro M, Sugihara S, Kakizoe S, Nakashima O, Kiyomatsu K. Hepatocellular carcinoma with sarcomatous change: a special reference to the relationship with anticancer therapy. *Cancer Chemother Pharmacol.* 1989;23 Suppl(2466583):4-8.

[8] Wang XY et al. Glypican-3 expression in hepatocellular tumors: diagnostic value for preneoplastic lesions and hepatocellular carcinomas. *Human Pathol* 2006; 37:1435-1441.

[9] Shafizadeh N, et al. Utility and limitations of glypican-3 expression for the diagnosis of hepatocellular carcinoma at both ends of the differentiation spectrum. *Modern Pathol* 2008; 21:1011-1018.

[10] Di Tommaso L, et al. Diagnostic value of HSP70, Glypican 3 and Glutamine synthetase i hepatocellular nodules in cirrhosis. *Hepatology* 2007;45:725-737.

[11] Libbrecht L, et al. Glypican-3 expression distinguishes small hepatocellular carcinomas from cirrhosis, dysplastic nodules, and focal nodular hyperplasia-like nodules. *Am J Surg Pathol* 2006; 30:1405-1411.

[12] Villanueva A, Newell P, Chiang DY, Friedman SL, Llovet JM. Genomics and signaling pathways in hepatocellular carcinoma. *Semin Liver Dis* 2007;27:55-76.

[13] Chuma M, Sakamoto M, Yamazaki K, et al. Expression profiling in multistage hepatocarcinogenesis: identification of HSP70 as a molecular marker of early hepatocellular carcinoma. *Hepatology.* 2003;37(12500205):198-207.

[14] Villanueva A, Chiang DY, Newell P, et al. Pivotal role of mTOR signaling in hepatocellular carcinoma. *Gastroenterology.* 2008;135(18929564):1972-1983.

[15] Ladeiro Y, Couchy G, Balabaud C, et al. MicroRNA profiling in hepatocellular tumors is associated with clinical features and oncogene/tumor suppressor gene mutations. *Hepatology.* 2008;47(18433021):1955-1963.

[16] Boyault S, Rickman DS, de Reynies A, et al. Transcriptome classification of HCC is related to gene alterations and to new therapeutic targets. *Hepatology.* 2007;45(17187432):42-52.

[17] de La Coste A, Romagnolo B, Billuart P, et al. Somatic mutations of the beta-catenin gene are frequent in mouse and human hepatocellular carcinomas. *Proc Natl Acad Sci U S A.* 1998;95(9671767):8847-8851.

[18] Edmondson HA, Steiner PE. Primary carcinoma of the liver: a study of 100 cases among 48,900 necropsies. *Cancer* 1954;7:462-503.

[19] Nathan H, Schulick RD, Choti MA, Pawlik TM. Predictors of survival after resection of early hepatocellular carcinoma. *Ann Surg.* 2009;249(19387322):799-805.

[20] Pawlik TM, Delman KA, Vauthey JN, et al. Tumor size predicts vascular invasion and histologic grade: Implications for selection of surgical treatment for hepatocellular carcinoma. *Liver Transpl.* Sep 2005;11(9):1086-1092.

[21] Lee J-S, Chu I-S, Heo J, et al. Classification and prediction of survival in hepatocellular carcinoma by gene expression profiling. *Hepatology.* 2004;40 (15349906):667-676.

[22] Pathologic diagnosis of early hepatocellular carcinoma: a report of the international consensus group for hepatocellular neoplasia. *Hepatology.* Feb 2009;49(2):658-664.

[23] Theise ND, Schwartz M, Miller C, Thung SN. Macroregenerative nodules and hepatocellular carcinoma in forty-four sequential adult liver explants with cirrhosis. *Hepatology.* 1992;16(1328012):949-955.

[24] Ferrell L, Wright T, Lake J, Roberts J, Ascher N. Incidence and diagnostic features of macroregenerative nodules vs. small hepatocellular carcinoma in cirrhotic livers. *Hepatology.* 1992;16(1332923):1372-1381.

[25] Mion F, Grozel L, Boillot O, Paliard P, Berger F. Adult cirrhotic liver explants: precancerous lesions and undetected small hepatocellular carcinomas. *Gastroenterology.* Dec 1996;111(6):1587-1592.
[26] Takayama T, Makuuchi M, Hirohashi S, et al. Malignant transformation of adenomatous hyperplasia to hepatocellular carcinoma. *Lancet.* 1990;336(1978027): 1150-1153.
[27] Lam CM, Chan AO, Ho P, et al. Different presentation of hepatitis B-related hepatocellular carcinoma in a cohort of 1863 young and old patients - implications for screening. *Aliment Pharmacol Ther.* Apr 1 2004;19(7):771-777.
[28] Marrero JA, Fontana RJ, Su GL, Conjeevaram HS, Emick DM, Lok AS. NAFLD may be a common underlying liver disease in patients with hepatocellular carcinoma in the United States. *Hepatology.* Dec 2002;36(6):1349-1354.
[29] Paradis V, Zalinski S, Chelbi E, et al. Hepatocellular carcinomas in patients with metabolic syndrome often develop without significant liver fibrosis: a pathological analysis. *Hepatology.* Mar 2009;49(3):851-859.
[30] Angulo P. Non alcoloholic fatty liver diseases. *New Engl J Med* 2002;346:1221-1231.
[31] Adams LA, Lymp JF, Sauver JS, Sanderson SO, Lindor KD, Feldstein A, et al. The natural history of nonalcoholic fatty liver disease: a population-based cohort study. *Gastroenterology* 2005;129:113-121.
[32] Farrell GC, Larter CZ. Nonalcoholic fatty liver disease: from steatosis to cirrhosis. *Hepatology* 2006;43:S99-S112.
[33] El-Serag HB, Tran T, Everhart JE. Diabetes increases the risk of chronic liver disease and hepatocellular carcinoma. *Gastroenterology* 2004;126:460-468.
[34] Nair S, Mason A, Eason J, Loss G, Perillo RP. Is obesity an independent risk factor for hepatocellular carcinoma in cirrhosis ? *Hepatology* 2002;36:150-155.
[35] Cuadrado A, Orive A, García-Suárez C, Domínguez A, Fernández-Escalante JC, Crespo J. Pons-Romero F. Non-alcoholic steatohepatitis (Nash) and hepatocellular carcinoma. *Obesity Surgery* 2005; 15:442-446.
[36] Kawada N, Imanaka K, Kawaguchi T, Tamai C, Ishihara R, Matsunaga T, Gotoh K, Yamada T, Tomita Y. Hepatocellular carcinoma arising from non-cirrhotic nonalcoholic steatohepatitis. *J Gastroenterol* 2009; 44:1190-1194.
[37] Guzman G,Brunt,EM, Petrovic LM, Chejfec G, Layden TJ, Cotler SJ. Does nonalcoholic fatty liver disease predispose patients to hepatocellular carcinoma in the absence of cirrhosis? *Ach Pathol Lab Med* 2008; 132:1761-1766.
[38] Craig JR, Peters RL, Edmondson HA, Omata M. Fibrolamellar carcinoma of the liver: a tumor of adolescents and young adults with distinctive clinico-pathologic features. *Cancer.* 1980;46(6248194):372-379.
[39] El-Serag HB, Davila JA. Is fibrolamellar carcinoma different from hepatocellular carcinoma? A US population-based study. *Hepatology.* 2004;39(14999699):798-803.
[40] Van Eyken P, Sciot R, Brock P, Casteels-Van Daele M, Ramaekers FC, Desmet VJ. Abundant expression of cytokeratin 7 in fibrolamellar carcinoma of the liver. *Histopathology.* 1990;17(1699871):101-107.
[41] Rosenberg L. 1991. The risk of liver neoplasia in relation to combined oral contraceptive use.*Contraception*;43:643-52.

[42] Socas L, Zumbado M, Pérez-Luzardo O, et al. Hepatocellular adenomas associated with anabolic androgenic steroid abuse in bodybuilders: a report of two cases and a review of the literature. *Br J Sports Med* 2005;39:e27.

[43] Paradis V, Champault A, Ronot M, Deschamps L, Valla DC, Vidaud D, Vilgrain V, Belghiti J, Bedossa P. Telangiectatic adenomas: an entity associated with increased body mass index and inflammation. *Hepatology* 2007; 46:140-146.

[44] Dokmak S, Paradis V, Vilgrain V, Sauvanet A, Farges O, Valla D, Bedossa P, Belghiti J. A single-center surgical experience of 122 patients with single and multiple hepatocellular adenomas. *Gastroenterology* 2009; 137:1698-1705.

[45] Bioulac-Sage P, Laumonier H, Couchy G, Le Bail B, Sa Cunha A, Rullier A, Laurent C, Blanc JF, Cubel G, Trillaud H, Zucman-Rossi J, Balabaud C, Saric J. Hepatocellular adenoma management and phenotypic classification: the Bordeaux experience. *Hepatology*. 2009 Aug;50(2):481-9.

[46] Farges O, Ferreira N, Dokmak S, Belghiti J, Bedossa P, Paradis V. Changing trends in malignant transformation of hepatocellular adenoma. *Gut* 2011; 60:85-89.

[47] Deneve JL, Pawlik TM, Cunningham S, Clary B, Reddy S, Scoggins CR, Martin RCG, D'Angelica M et al. Liver Cell Adenoma: A Multicenter analysis of risk factors for rupture and malignancy. *Ann Surg Oncol* 2009 ; 16: 640-48.

In: Hepatocellular Carcionoma: A Global Challenge
Editor: Isabelle Chemin
ISBN: 978-1-61470-644-1

Chapter VII

Mutations of the Tumor Suppressor *TP53* as Hallmarks of Distinct Pathway of Progression towards Hepatocellular Carcinoma

Doriane Gouas*[1]*, Myriam Lereau*[1,2]*,
***Sandra Ortiz-Cuaran*[1] *and Pierre Hainaut*[1,*]**
[1]International Agency for Research on Cancer, Molecular Carcinogenesis Group, Lyon, France
[2]Université Lyon, Centre de Recherche en Lyon, France

Abstract

TP53 encodes a major tumor suppressor protein, which is mutated or otherwise inactivated in the majority of human cancers, including HepatoCellular Carcinoma (HCC). In HCC, the frequency and type of *TP53* mutation show striking geographic variations in relation with etiologic factors. In areas of high endemicity for Hepatitis B Virus (HBV) and of chronic exposure to Aflatoxin B_1 (AFB_1), a single mutation at codon 249 (*R249S*) occurs in at least half of HCC cases. In other etiological contexts (e.g. HCV, alcohol, iron overload, HBV without AFB_1 exposure), *TP53* mutation is less frequent (20-30%) and mutations are distributed throughout the central core domain of the p53 protein. This diversity in mutation patterns highlights the importance of p53 in managing the responses of hepatocytes to various forms of stress. In this chapter, we review recent evidence showing that p53 plays an important role as inducer of senescence of liver cells in response to DNA damage, oxidative stress or oncogene activation. We also discuss current data and hypotheses regarding how the HBx antigen may interfere or cooperate with wild-type and mutant p53 in hepatocarcinogenesis. Finally, we summarize the

* To whom correspondence should be addressed. Pierre Hainaut, e-mail: hainaut@iarc.fr; Telephone: +33 (0) 4.72.73.85.32.

evidence implicating the two members of the *TP53* family, *TP73* and *TP63*, in specific mechanisms of responses of hepatocytes to DNA damaging agents. Based on these considerations, we suggest a model of progression to liver cancer in which *TP53* mutation may represent either a primary or a secondary event, depending upon the etiological context.

Introduction

Mutations in the *TP53* tumor suppressor gene (located on Chromosome 17p13.1) are among the most common somatic alterations in human HepatoCellular Carcinomas (HCC). The p53 protein exerts multiple, coordinated activities in regulating cell cycle progression, cell survival, genome stability, cell metabolism and senescence in response to a wide variety of signals [1-5]. Long considered as a specific factor of response to DNA damage, p53 is now emerging as a critical factor in many physiological processes not directly linked to exposure to carcinogens. In particular, p53 is one of the factors that mediate cell senescence after telomere erosion and that also controls the maintenance of stem/progenitor cell status. These functions of p53 have long been underestimated because mice lacking *TP53* (p53-null mice) show overall normal development without major anomaly apart from increased risk of early cancer. More recently, however, it has become clear that p53-null mice display a number of subtle developmental, metabolic and ageing defects, underlying the role of p53 as a cross-road on several pathways essential for the regulation of cell fate [6].

One of the factors that may have obscured the role of p53 in mechanisms other than DNA damage is the fact that it belongs to a family that also contains two other genes, *TP73* and *TP63*, which retain the general transcription factor architecture of p53 but exert their main roles in stem cell regulation, epithelial or neuronal differentiation, and some very specific aspects of responses to stress [7]. These three distinct genes are found only in vertebrates. In invertebrates, only one "ancestor" gene is present, which resembles *TP63* more than *TP73* or *TP53*. Thus, the "*TP53* family" seems to have evolved by duplication of an ancestral gene to give rise to the two closely related forms *TP63* and *TP73*, followed by the emergence of a third form, *TP53*. The p53 protein may therefore be the product of a "retro-adaptative" mechanism in which the framework of an existing, old gene has been re-used in evolution to fulfill new functions associated with "vertebrate" status, namely, the regulation of stem cell pools and their protection against transformation and carcinogenesis.

Despite its frequent mutation in HCC, the involvement of p53 in liver carcinogenesis appears to be extremely dependent upon the etiological context. Notably, subjects who inherit a germline *TP53* mutation are not prone to HCC, suggesting that inactivation of p53 in itself is not sufficient for liver carcinogenesis. Mutations arise somatically and emerge as a genetic trait in clones of proliferative cells during the progression from chronic liver disease to cancer. Thus, p53 mutations might represent either a "founder event" (occurring very early in the carcinogenesis sequence and driving subsequent steps of cancer progression) or as a "secondary event", resulting from the selection pressures induced by the activation of several other oncogenic pathways. In this chapter, we discuss the diversity of *TP53* mutation patterns observed in human HCC in relation with different, viral and non-viral etiological risk factors.

Next, we summarize current knowledge on the roles of p53 in regulating cell proliferation, apoptosis and senescence in hepatocytes and we discuss how mutations in *TP53* may be informative as biomarkers in particular in the etiological context of joint exposure to chronic Hepatitis B Virus (HBV) infection and Aflatoxin B_1 (AFB_1). Finally, we show the structural and functional overlaps between p53, p63 and p73 and we discuss how the two latter proteins may exert specific functions, independently of p53. In conclusion, we propose a model of hepatocarcinogenesis in which mutation of *TP53* may arise in different pathways of progression to cancer.

Diversity of *TP53* Mutation Patterns in HCC

TP53 is the most commonly mutated tumor suppressor gene in human cancers with a mutational frequency of about 50% in most common cancers. More than 25,000 mutations are registered in the IARC *TP53* Mutation Database (http://www-p53.iarc.fr/), of which 80% are located in the DNA-binding domain, reflecting the selective effects of mutations that inactivate p53 by disrupting its capacity to bind DNA and transactivate multiple target genes. *TP53* is mutated in about 30% of liver cancers. However, this percentage highly depends on the etiology and the geographic region considered. In high incidence areas for HCC (mostly in tropical and sub-tropical areas), *TP53* is mutated in more than 50% of the cases. The mutation prevalence is somewhat lower in low incidence areas, although the full extent of the association between *TP53* mutations and diverse etiological conditions that prevail in most Western countries has not yet been described. Taking together all the mutations compiled in the IARC *TP53* database (which represents the data available in the current literature), the mutation pattern shows that more than 40% of mutations are G:C>T:A transversions (Figure 1A). Other mutation types such as A:T>G:C, A:T>T:A, G:C>A:T represent about 10% each, followed by deletions, G:C>A:T at CpG sites and G:C>C:G mutations (almost 7%). This general pattern is very different from the "average" pattern of *TP53* mutations in common cancers such as breast or colorectal cancer, in which G:C>A:T mutations at CpG sites are predominant. Interestingly, this type of mutation has been associated with inflammatory stress in many epithelial tumors. Their relative rarity in HCC, despite the important role of inflammation in hepatocarcinogenesis, is therefore a puzzle.

When broken down according to world regions and etiological risk factors, *TP53* mutation patterns show enormous disparities, unmatched in any other cancer type. In areas where HCC is extremely frequent due to high endemicity of HBV and to widespread exposure to AFB_1, mutations are almost exclusively G:C>T:A transversions located at the third base of codon 249 (AG<u>G</u> to AG<u>T</u>) and encoding serine instead of arginine (*R249S* mutations). These mutations represent 100% of the mutations identified to date in Western Africa and more than 60% in South-East Asia. The mechanism of formation and biological relevance of this *R249S* mutation will be discussed in the next part of this chapter. Assuming that the *R249S* mutation occurs in 50% of the patients in the joint HBV/AFB_1 exposure context, it may be estimated that this mutation arises in 3-400,000 new cases of liver cancer every year, making it one of the most, if not the most, single mutational event in the human population worldwide (Figure 1B). In contrast, in areas of the world where AFB_1 is not considered as a major risk factor for HCC, the *TP53* mutation pattern is much more heterogeneous, covering codons scattered throughout the coding sequence of the DNA-binding domain, with few specific hotspots. Most, if not all, of these mutations, have been experimentally shown to inactivate p53 transcriptional activity. However, the mechanisms of their formation are not precisely known.

p53 as Regulator of Hepatocyte Proliferation and Senescence

In most mature cell types, including hepatocytes, p53 levels are low and can be detected only with highly sensitive antibody-based techniques. This low expression is essentially due to the rapid turnover of the protein, which is constitutively expressed but does not accumulate because it is rapidly directed towards degradation by the proteasome. The protein does accumulate and exert its suppressor effects only after being stabilized by different types of exogenous or endogenous signals. Exogenous signals include a broad range of physical or chemical DNA damaging agents. Endogenous signals include hypoxia, oxidative stress, depletion of ribonucleotide pools and, significantly, excessive or untimely growth signals such as those generated by activated oncogenes (the latter defining "oncogenic stress"). In response to these stresses, p53 may mediate a wide range of cellular responses which depend upon the type of signals, its intensity, its consequence on cell physiological functions, as well as the status of the cell itself: the proliferative and differentiation status of the cell appear to be the most critical factor in determining how a given cell will respond to p53 activation.

p53 and Hepatocyte Differentiation

p53 on its own is not a central effector of hepatocyte differentiation. In p53-null mice, the liver develops normally and does not show major metabolic or physiological defects in adulthood. However, there is evidence that p53 may play a role as modulator, and possibly accelerator of hepatocyte differentiation in response to particular stress circumstances. Hepatocytes are the main cell type in the liver; along with biliary epithelial cells, they derive from the embryonic endoderm through a process involving the sequential expression of hepatocyte-specific markers, starting from mid-gestation. There is evidence that p53 may regulate the expression of several markers of hepatogenesis. A report on HepG2 cells (human HCC) and Hep1-6 cells (mouse hepatoma) revealed that p53 represses the transcription of the α-fetoprotein gene (*AFP*), an early hepatogenic differentiation marker [9]. On the other hand it has been reported that wild-type but not mutant p53 is able to repress the expression of the Hepatocyte Nuclear Factor 4 alpha (HNF4α), a transcription factor that binds to the promoter of nearly half of the genes involved in hepatocyte differentiation [10, 11]. Generally, $p21^{waf-1}$ is a target gene of p53, however in HepG2 cells, the effect of HNF4α appears to require $p21^{waf-1}$ in a p53-independent manner. This increase in $p21^{waf-1}$ may contribute to cell cycle arrest, thus allowing arrested cells to enter the hepatocyte differentiation program [12]. Although still fragmentary, these results suggest that activation of p53 in immature hepatocytes may contribute to enhance their differentiation, and that this effect may be hampered if cells harbor a mutant form of p53.

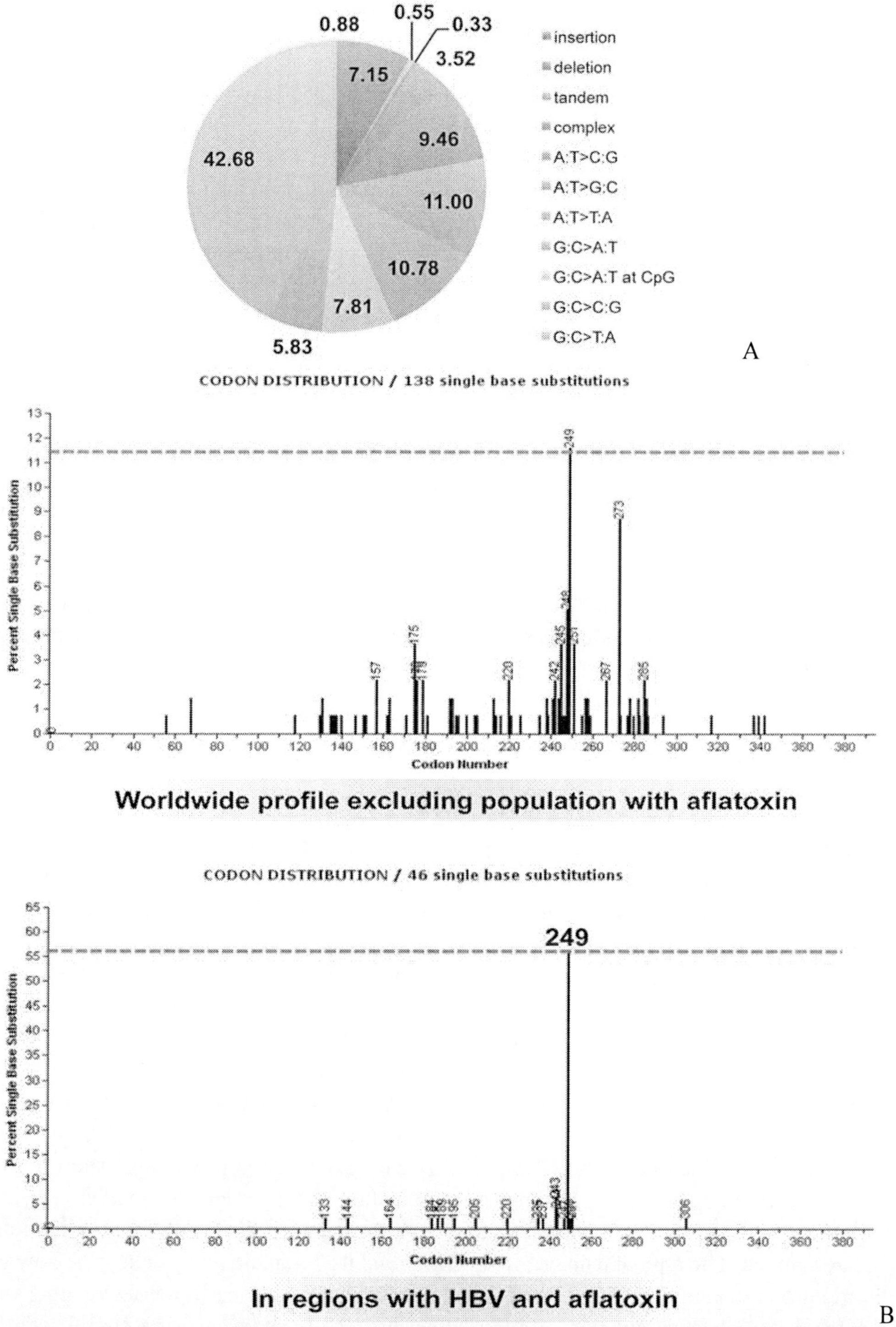

Figure 1. *TP53* mutation pattern in HCC. A: global mutation pattern in all cases of HCC listed in the IARC *TP53* database, irrespective of geographic origin and suspected etiology. B: Mutation distribution along the coding sequence in regions with HBV and AFB_1 (bottom) and in all other regions (excluding populations with high exposure to AFB_1; top). The high prevalence of *R249S* mutations is shown. Data from IARC *TP53* Mutation Database (http://www-p53.iarc.fr/, R14 version; [8]).

p53 and Response to DNA Damage

Under genotoxic stress, the tumor suppressor protein p53 plays a key role in genetic and genomic homeostasis through several mechanisms. The most extreme is induction of apoptosis in cells subjected to high levels of DNA damage. At lower levels of DNA damage, however, p53 operates as a facilitator of DNA repair. It has long been considered that induction of cell cycle arrest by p53 may represent a mechanism that allow cells additional time to repair their damaged DNA before resuming proliferation. This notion is certainly confirmed by observations in cultured, immortalized cells but it is not clear that it applies to primary, normal cells. Rather, in normal cells, p53-induced cell cycle arrest appears to be permanent, removing cells from the pool of cells capable of undergoing cell division. Nevertheless, p53 directly modulates the activity of several DNA repair systems [13]. Cells null for p53 show a decrease in nucleotide excision repair (NER) and base excision repair (BER) capacities. Among target genes activated by p53, several are directly involved in repair such as O^6MGMT, MSH2 and the gene encoding Ribonucleotide Reductase II. Moreover the C-terminus region of p53 binds directly to components of multi-molecular complexes of the DNA replication and repair machineries such as ERCC and RPA.

Reactive oxygen/nitrogen species are produced in large amounts during inflammatory stress. These species are detoxified by the cell redox machinery. However, their reactivity carries great risk of permanent damage to biomolecules including DNA. The p53 pathway is a key element of the cellular response towards such forms of stress [14]: DNA damage generated by $NO^{\bullet}$ leads to an accumulation of p53 and the induction of p53-dependent apoptosis; moreover, p53 has been shown to *trans*-repress *in vivo* the gene *NOS2* encoding the nitric oxide synthase 2 at the transcription level, thus decreasing the excessive production of $NO^{\bullet}$.

In hepatocytes, there is evidence that p53 is activated in response to a wide panel of genotoxic agents. This panel includes aromatic molecules forming bulky DNA adducts such as polycyclic aromatic hydrocarbons (PAH) and mycotoxins like aflatoxin B_1 (AFB_1). An AFB_1 dose-dependent accumulation of p53 phosphorylated on serine 15 has been observed *in vitro* at protein level after exposure to AFB_1, suggesting a specific accumulation in the presence of DNA damage [Lereau *et al.*, submitted]. As differentiated liver cells are extremely active in metabolizing these xenobiotics, they are one of the cell types that are the most exposed to their mutagenic effects. The same is true for co-factors that enhance the production of reactive oxygen species (ROS) such as metal ions, which specifically accumulate in liver cells. Iron overload is a well-known risk factor for HCC, as well as copper overload, which may lead to massive oxidative damage in the liver of subjects with Wilson disease, a rare syndrome leading to accumulation of copper ions in the liver [15].

Induction of p53 may be part of the protection mechanisms against these multiple forms of DNA damage. The type of damage, its intensity and its chronicity, may determine how p53 will orientate cell fate, selecting among a wide panel of suppressive responses ranging from DNA repair to enhanced apoptosis. In the latter case, the maintenance of a chronic state of stress activating p53 may play an important role in liver cell death that underlies chronic liver diseases such as cirrhosis. In mice fed with chronically damaging doses of ethanol, p53 deficiency abrogates liver cell death but predisposes to the early appearance of liver dysplasia [16].

p53 and Hepatocyte Senescence

Recent studies have underlined the role of p53 in the senescence of liver cancer cells. These findings (detailed below) indicate that p53 may be an important contender in the process of senescence of normal hepatocytes, a role that has not been formally demonstrated so far. Cell senescence is a process leading to permanent cell cycle and DNA replication arrest. Senescent cells display altered morphology and an altered pattern of gene expression. The final stage of this process is the resorption of senescent cells by the natural immune system. At the molecular level, senescence may result from several sets of signals such as telomere erosion, activated oncogenes, overproduction of ROS or persistent DNA damage. Two cyclin kinase inhibitors play central roles as effectors in senescence: $p16^{INK4a}$ and $p21^{Waf\text{-}1}$. Both lead to cell cycle arrest at the G1/S interface through control of the retinoblastoma protein (pRb) activation. After DNA damage, p53 activates $p21^{Waf\text{-}1}$, which will in turn prevents the release by pRb of transcription factors of the E2F family which are involved in the regulation of many effectors of S phase. In contrast to $p21^{waf\text{-}1}$, $p16^{INK4a}$ is not a direct transcriptional target of p53. This factor is however activated by multiple signals including in particular the TGF-ß pathway. Interestingly, the coding sequence of $p16^{INK4a}$ overlaps with the one of another gene, *ARF*, encoding the $p14^{arf}$ protein. The latter is a transcriptional target of E2F, and has several roles in DNA repair and cell cycle arrest. In particular, the $p14^{arf}$ protein binds Hdm2, the main regulator of p53 stability, thus tethering it into the nucleolus and preventing it to associate with p53. Therefore, $p14^{arf}$ provides a molecular link between excessive growth signaling (e.g. through activated oncogenes) and stabilization of p53. This stabilization and activation of p53 is, in turn a central mechanism in oncogene-induced senescence (for a recent review see [17]).

Using an elegant mouse model, Xue and collaborators have investigated the consequences of reactivating the p53 pathway in HCC. First, they have isolated liver progenitors from fetal cells and have engineered them to express a conditional interferent RNA (shRNA) targeting p53. The cells are re-implanted into the liver and the mice are allowed to grow until a time point when treatment with a drug activates the shRNA and leads to the down-regulation of p53 in these progenitors and their descents. In a matter of days, p53 abrogation results in the development of a characterized HCC, demonstrating the essential role of p53 in limiting the proliferative potential of liver progenitors. At this point, the drug can be removed, leading to the restoration of p53 status in HCC cells. As a consequence, the tumor mass shrinks into almost complete regression within 10-12 days. Using this protocol, they showed that even a brief reactivation (for 1 day) of endogenous p53 in p53-deficient tumors could produce complete tumor regression. The primary tumor suppressor response induced by p53 was not apoptosis, but cell senescence, as demonstrated by massive expression of senescence markers in HCC cells with re-activated p53 [18] (Figure 2). This study provides a convincing demonstration of both the role of p53 as a tumor suppressor in liver cells, and the primary implication of cell senescence as the suppressive response leading to p53-dependent regression of HCC. Whether this model accounts for the potential tumor suppressor role of p53 in human HCC should be taken with caution. Indeed, there are many molecular and pathological differences between rodent and human HCC, including in particular the absence of rodent equivalents to human HBV and HCV, and the fact that rodent *TP53* is rarely mutated in mouse or rat liver cancers.

It should be noted that p53 is not the only effector of cell senescence to be frequently targeted by molecular alterations in HCC cells. Although the *INK4a* gene, encoding p16, is rarely mutated in HCC, its epigenetic silencing by promoter methylation is observed in about 50% of HCC. This *de novo* methylation results in down-regulation of p16 protein expression. Overall, alterations in components of p53 and pRb pathways are commonly observed in HCC with different etiologies. Alterations of pRb pathway ($p16^{INK4a}$, $p15^{INK4b}$ or *RB1* genes), p53 pathway (*TP53* or *ARF* genes) and both pathways have been detected in 83%, 31% and 30% of HCC cases, respectively [19]. These observations are highly suggestive of the critical role of senescence-controlling pathways in hepatocarcinogenesis.

Inactivation of one or several effectors of cell senescence in liver cells may be of significance in promoting cancer in a context of chronic liver disease. In this context, chronic liver damage and cell death lead to compensatory liver cell regeneration by proliferation. Given the limited replication span of cells, determined by telomere erosion, cells that "switch off" senescence pathways would acquire a selective, proliferative advantage in such a context. Indeed, more than 80% of HCC display telomerase activity. However, cellular immortality is not sufficient for full malignancy [20]. Thus, senescence-related aberrations in HCC may confer a partial survival advantage.

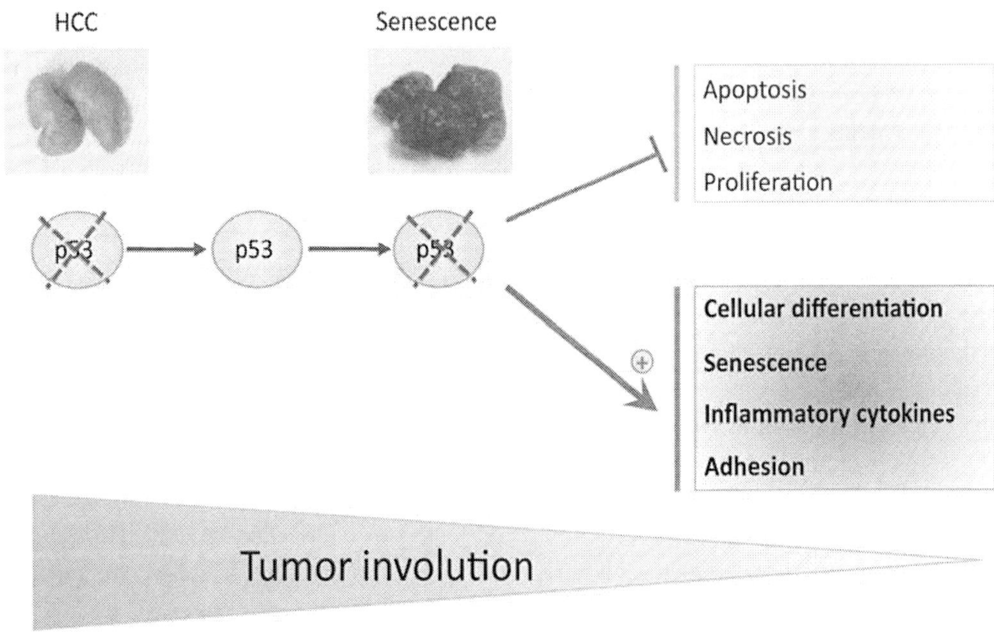

Figure 2: Irreversible effects of p53 reactivation in liver carcinomas. According to Xue *et al.* (2007) study, p53 can induce HCC involution through a process that, once activated, is irreversible. Surprisingly, the primary response to p53 reactivation was not apoptosis, nor necrosis. Instead, liver tumors showed a marked decrease in proliferation that was associated with signs of senescence (as shown by expression of ß-galactosidase throughout the tumor) [18].

Interactions between p53 and Hepatitis B Virus

Synergic Effects between Mutant p53 and Hepatitis B Virus

HBV chronic infection and exposure to AFB_1 are two known risk factors for HCC, which together, are responsible for about half of liver cancer worldwide. AFB_1 is a mycotoxin produced by *Aspergillus* species fungi, which contaminate food staples in hot and humid parts of the world such as Sub-Saharan Africa and South-East Asia. After ingestion of contaminated foodstuff, cytochromes P450 (CYP450) bio-activate AFB_1 in the liver into a highly reactive epoxide capable of forming adducts on the N7 position of Guanines. An inappropriate repair may lead to mutation formation. Studies in Sub-Saharan Africa and South-East Asia have extensively documented a hot spot mutation in *TP53* at the third base of the codon 249 (G to T transversion, *R249S*), which is characteristic of exposure to the mycotoxin. Whereas the etiological correlation between HBV endemicity, AFB_1 exposure and *R249S* mutation is well substantiated, the extent of their combined, synergistic action has been measured only in a small number of studies (Table 1).

Table 1. Relative risks for HCC after HBV infection and/or AFB_1 exposure

Country	HCC cases	Controls	Relative risk [95% CI]			Biomarkers of AFB_1 exposure	References
			HBV alone	AFB_1 alone	HBV + AFB_1		
China (Shangai)	22	140	4.8 [1.2-19.7]	1.9 [0.5-7.5]	60.1 [6.4-561.8]	Urinary AFB_1, metabolites and DNA adducts	[28]
	50	267	7.3 [2.2-24.4]	3.4 [1.1-10.0]	59.4 [15.6-212]		[27]
Taiwan	56	220	17.4 [3.7-81.9]	0.3 [0.0-3.6]	70.0 [11.8-415.4]	Albumin adducts in serum	[29]
			22.8 [3.6-143.4]	1.7 [0.3-10.8]	111.9 [13.8-905.0]	Urinary AFB_1 and metabolites	
	105	37	17.0 [2.8-103.9]	17.4 [3.4-90.3]	67.6 [12.2-373.2]	DNA adducts in liver	[26]
	230	1052	7.03 [4.45-11.09]	1.64 [0.89-3.03]	10.38 [5.73-18.82]	Albumin adducts in blood	[30]
			11.01 [5.79-20.92]	2.84 [1.44-5.57]	15.13 [7.83-29.25]	Urinary AFB_1 and metabolites	
The Gambia	186	348	10.0 [5.16-19.6]	13.2 [4.99-35.0]	399 [48.6-3270]	*R249S* in plasma	[24]

HBV infection was determined by HBsAg detection in serum.

The first experimental evidence for a synergy between AFB_1 and HBV in HCC development comes from transgenic mice studies in which the HBV surface protein was over-expressed [21]: animals fed with AFB_1-contaminated food developed more widespread and rapid hepatocyte dysplasia and HCC than non-exposed controls. A positive interaction in hepatocarcinogenesis between both HCC risk factors was also observed in woodchucks [22] and in Pekin ducks [23]. In human, epidemiological evidence for synergy have been obtained in studies performed in China, Taiwan and The Gambia [24-30]: the risk to develop HCC was found much higher in HBV chronic carriers exposed to AFB_1 than in HBV chronic carriers alone or individuals exposed to AFB_1 alone (Table 1). Overall, these studies show effects that are over-multiplicative, suggesting that each factor enhances the effect of the other.

From a DNA sequence viewpoint, there is now a good demonstration that metabolites of AFB_1 bind preferentially to guanines localized in the sequence AGGCC (the adducted guanine being underlined). This sequence context corresponds to codon 249 in *TP53* but not to any other codon where inactivating mutations might occur. This selectivity partially explains the uniqueness of the *TP53* mutation pattern in HCC occurring in a HBV/AFB_1 context. However, it does not explain the synergistic effects of the two factors. Several mechanisms have been proposed to explain this synergy [31-33]. First, it has been suggested that HBV chronic infection itself or HBV-induced chronic disease may sensitize hepatocytes to the mutagenic effects of AFB_1 by increasing AFB_1 metabolism and adduct formation. In HBV transgenic mice, induction of CYP450 was observed in association to the hepatic damage due to over-expression of HBsAg [34, 35]. In human cells, the necro-inflammatory chronic disease caused by persistent HBV infection may favor the formation of *R249S* through the production of oxygen/nitrogen species [36]. Second, HBV may favor the persistence of adducts on DNA and subsequent mutagenesis by altering DNA repair, in particular the NER pathway [37, 38]. Conversely, AFB_1 may modulate viral replication [39-41] and/or facilitate the integration of viral sequences into the host genome in particular at sites damaged by AFB_1 adducts or by oxidative DNA damage. The generation of AFB_1-induced mutations in HBV cccDNA is also a plausible hypothesis but has not been demonstrated so far. Finally, exposure to AFB_1 in infancy has been shown to induce growth retardation and immune deficiencies, which may enhance the acquisition of the chronic carrier status in children infected by HBV [42-45].

Interactions between Mutant p53 and Viral Antigens

Recently, another set of molecular information has shed a new light on the mechanisms underlying the synergistic effect discussed above. Indeed, even taking into account the preferential binding of AFB_1 adducts to codon 249 in *TP53*, it is difficult to explain why other mutations are so rare. The answer to this apparent paradox may lie in the capacity of p53, and in particular of the p.R249S mutant protein, to interact with HBx, a 17 KDa protein encoded by HBV. This protein has multiple and complex effects on signal transduction and proliferation in hepatocytes. First, it acts as an enhancer of transcription of many cellular genes. Second, it interacts with a range of cell proteins, including for example DDB1 (DNA-damage binding protein 1). Overall, there is evidence that HBx may exert oncogenic effects during HCC development, in particular after mutation and/or C-terminal truncation upon integration of HBV sequence in the host genome. On the other hand, wild-type HBx may also exert pro-apoptotic effects. In a symmetrical manner to this "double-faced" effect, the interactions of HBx with either wild-type or mutant p53 may have different impacts on the proliferation of hepatocytes and on HCC progression.

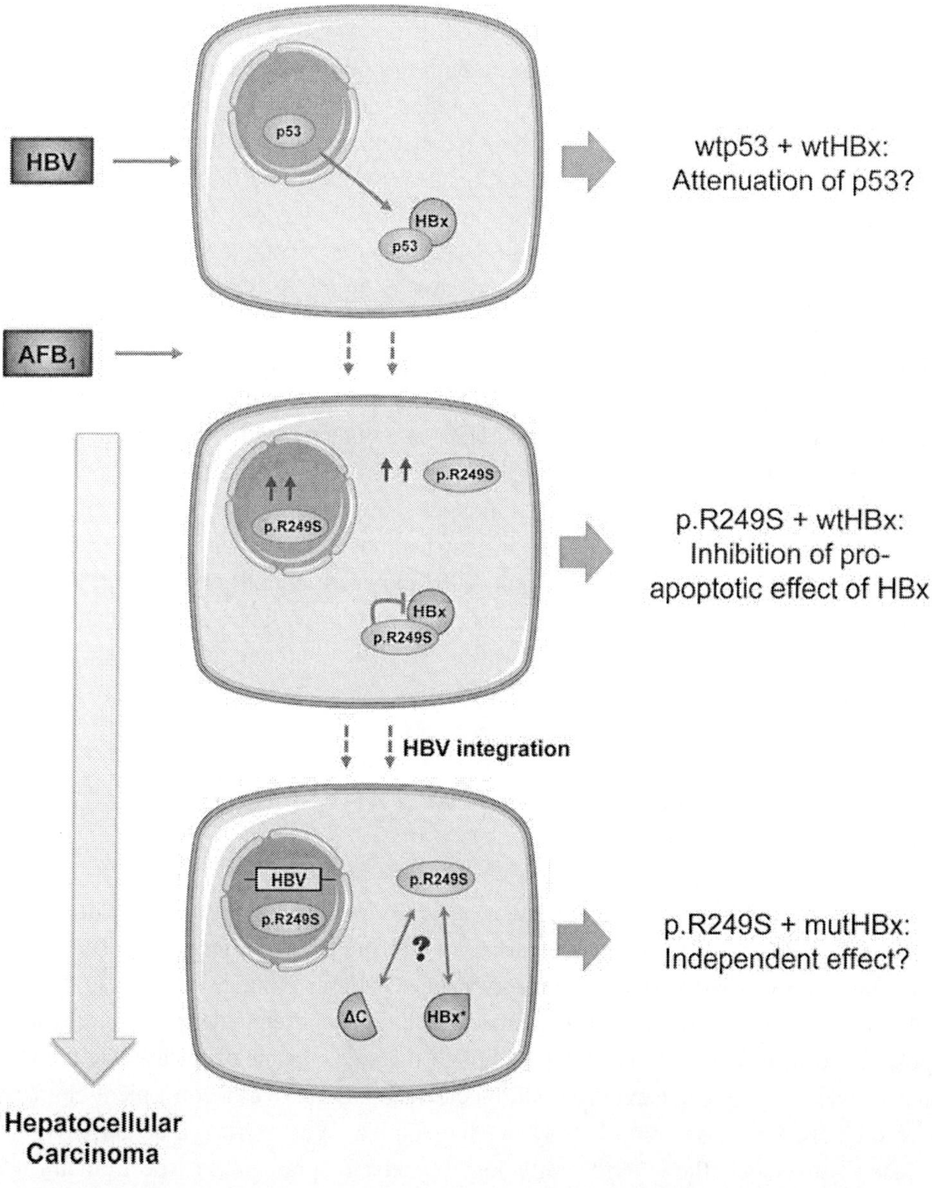

Figure 3. Model of cooperation between p53 and HBx in hepatocarcinogenesis. Three distinct situations are shown. Top: in hepatocytes infected by HBV, expression and binding of HBx may attenuate p53 suppressor effects, perhaps by maintaining it in the cytoplasm. Middle: in cells harbouring mutant p.R249S, the latter may bind to HBx and neutralize its pro-apoptotic effect. Bottom: in cells containing both p.R249S and mutant HBx (due to point mutations and/or 3'-truncation), the two proteins may act independently to promote oncogenesis [57, 58]. Model drawn thanks to Servier Medical Art (http://www.servier.fr/smart/ homesmart. asp).

In HBx transgenic mice, liver tumors were observed with a higher frequency compared to wild-type mice. It has been proposed that this effect may be due to the sequestration and the inactivation of wild-type p53 by excess HBx [46, 47]. *In vitro* studies have shown that HBx could induce the transformation of NIH3T3 fibroblasts in cooperation with oncogenes such as activated Ras and promote abnormal cell proliferation and abnormal mitosis [48-54]. Functional studies also revealed that HBx can bind directly to p53 and inhibit p53-mediated apoptosis [55].

Expression of HBx has been observed in both pre-malignant liver tissues and HCC [56]. Recently, several lines of evidence have provided support to a cooperation between the mutant p.R249S and HBx: (1) tumor-derived HBx mutants, but not their corresponding wild-type variants, could enhance cell proliferation and chromosome instability by cooperating with p.R249S in the hTERT-immortalized human hepatocyte cell line HHT4 [57]; (2) in HCC cells constitutively expressing p.R249S (PLC/PRF/5), a stable complex was identified between the mutant protein and HBx and this complex was shown to participate in maintaining a high proliferating rate [58].

Overall, these results support that HBx may provide a selective advantage for tumor progression in cooperation with p53. Two distinct situations may be identified. First, in chronically infected hepatocytes, wild-type HBx may interact with wild-type p53 and either attenuate or inhibit some of the suppressive effects of p53. This situation would however require that the two proteins are expressed in equivalent amounts and that HBx may sequester enough p53 to attenuate it, a phenomenon that has not been demonstrated in human cells. Second, after *TP53* mutation resulting from AFB_1 exposure the p.R249S mutant protein may bind to HBx and neutralize its pro-apoptotic capacities, providing a selective advantage for growth at least until mutation or 3'-truncation of HBx after integration turns HBx into a constitutively active oncogenic form (Figure 3).

Mutant p53 as Biomarker in HBV- and AFB_1-induced Hepatocarcinogenesis

The fact that AFB_1 induces a particular, specific mutation in *TP53* makes it possible to use that particular mutation as a biomarker of the mutagenic effect of AFB_1. Numerous studies have shown that plasma or serum of cancer patients contains significant amounts of circulating, cell-free DNA which often carries mutations and epigenetic alterations identical to those detected in tumor tissues [59]. Although the mechanisms of release and the stability of mutant DNA in the bloodstream are still unclear, it may serve as a convenient biomarker in cancer subjects. In a case-control study in The Gambia, West Africa, a quantitative method was used to detect the *R249S* mutation by electrospray mass spectrometry (Short Oligonucleotide Mass Analysis, SOMA): plasma concentrations of *R249S* were increased in HCC cases (median: 2,800 copies/mL, range 500-11,000) as compared to controls (median: 500 copies/mL, range 250-2,000). However, the detection of low levels of *R249S* (<500 copies/mL) in 46% of asymptomatic controls suggested that the mutation might also occur in the plasma as a marker of ongoing exposure to aflatoxin [60-62]. Indeed, in prospective studies in China, the *R249S* mutation was detected in the plasma of asymptomatic HBV carriers up to several years before HCC diagnosis [61, 63].

In The Gambia, chronic HBV carriage is endemic ranging from 11% to 16% in the adult population [64]. AFB_1 exposure is widespread and the incidence of HCC peaks at $80/10^5$ persons/year in 35-55 year-old males [65]. *R249S* is detectable in the plasma of 40% of HCC patients, with a concordance of 88% between plasma and tumor DNA [66]. *R249S* is also found in 15% of patients with liver cirrhosis and in 3% of control subjects with no detected liver disease [65]. These observations suggest that circulating *R249S* may be a biomarker of early liver disease, or alternatively, a biomarker of ongoing AFB_1 exposure.

The p53 Family: Roles of p63 and p73

Overlaps and Specificities among Members of the p53 Family

The discovery in the late nineties of two genes encoding proteins structurally related to p53 has led to re-examine many of the current knowledge on the functions of p53. Indeed, it was believed that a large deal of this knowledge was based on experimental studies in which p53 was overexpressed. Therefore, these high levels of p53 might have taken the roles normally assumed by the two homologs p63 and p73.

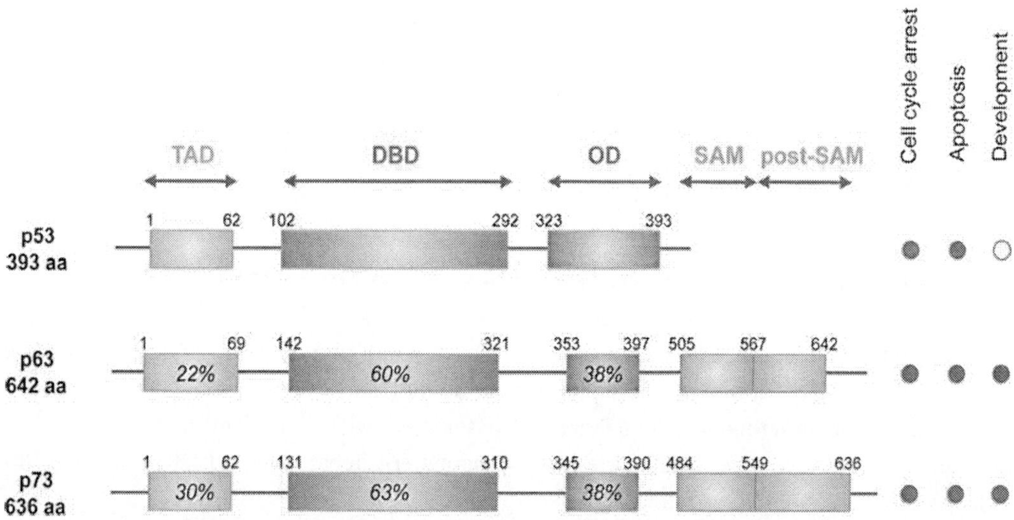

Figure 4. Schematic representation of protein structures of the p53 family members. The p53 family includes three genes that encode p53, p63 and p73 proteins. *TP53*, *TP63* and *TP73* are located on chromosomes 17, 3 and 1 and contain 11, 15 and 14 exons, respectively. The overall domain structure of p53, p63 and p73 is conserved and consists of an amino-terminal transactivation domain (TAD), a central DNA-binding domain (DBD) and a carboxy-terminal oligomerization domain (OD). In addition, p63 and p73 contain a carboxy-terminal sterile alpha motif (SAM) that corresponds to a putative protein-protein interaction domain, and a post-SAM domain. p63 and p73 play a role in cell cycle arrest and apoptosis as p53 and are both essential in development.

The p63 [67] and p73 [68, 69] proteins display a high degree of sequence and structural similarities with p53 (Figure 4). Their three major domains are highly conserved. The transactivation domains (TAD) of p63 and p73 are the least conserved with 22% and 30% of identity with p53, respectively. The DNA-binding domain (DBD) is the most conserved domain with 60% and 63% identity with p53 for p63 and p73, respectively, and therefore can bind the promoters of many p53-regulated genes. In addition, the residues of p53 that directly interact with DNA are identical in p63 and p73. Finally, the oligomerization domain (OD) is 38% identical with p63 and p73. Thus, p63 and p73 can form oligomers and can also interact with wild-type p53. Overall, the three proteins show considerable capacity to overlap in regulating cell cycle arrest, cellular senescence and apoptosis [67, 68, 70-72].

The main difference between p53 and its two cousins lies in its mechanisms of regulation. While p53 is highly stress-inducible and regulated at post-translational level, p63 and p73 are mainly regulated at transcriptional level and play important role in the regulation of differentiation and development. An important feature of p63 and p73 is that they are expressed as multiple isoforms, due to alternative splicing and/or distinct promoter usage. These alternatively spliced products retain the DNA-binding domain but show distinct N- and C-terminal regions [73-75]. In particular, the N-terminally truncated isoforms (termed DeltaNp63 or DeltaNp73) completely differ from p53 and their full-length counterpart in their capacity to transactivate target genes. Both DeltaNp63 and DeltaNp73 represent abundant forms of these proteins. Thus, p63 and p73 exhibit distinct and unique biological functions. p63 plays a major role in epithelium/mesenchyme interactions and in the development of squamous epithelia and their annexes, while p73 is indispensable for neuronal differentiation and the development of nervous and olfactory systems. Consistently, mice deficient for p63 present severe limb truncations and absence of skin, hair, teeth, mammary, lachrymal and salivary glands [76, 77], whereas p73-deficient mice show defects in neuronal development [78, 79].

p73, p63 and Responses of Hepatocytes to DNA Damage

To date, neither p63 nor p73 appear to play a vital role in liver organogenesis and differentiation. Mice deficient for either factor do not show major liver defects and, in human, germline mutations in *TP63* are not associated with liver malfunction. However, there is evidence that p73 plays a role in the response of hepatocytes to DNA-damage [80, 81].

The role of p73 in DNA damage is somehow parallel and complementary to the one of p53. The main difference between the two factors resides in their mechanism and timing of activation. In the case of p73, this mechanism involves both increased transcription of transactivation-competent isoforms and their activation through post-translational modifications. For example, it has been reported that p73 is phosphorylated during cisplatin-mediated apoptosis at Ser-47, Tyr-99 and Ser-289 by Chk1, c-Abl and PKCδ, respectively. Moreover, doxorubicin induces the acetylation of p73 at Lys-321, Lys-327 and Lys-331 by p300 [82]. The consequences of p73 activation include cell cycle arrest and apoptosis *via* both the extrinsic and the intrinsic signaling pathways [81]. p73 has been shown to be induced by a variety of chemotherapeutic agents in the liver cancer cell lines Hep3B (deficient for p53) and HepG2 (expressing wild-type p53). Treatment with bleomycin, doxorubicin and mitoxantrone resulted in p73 accumulation and in the induction of apoptosis in a dose and time-dependent manner. In addition, down-regulation of p53, p63 and p73 in these cells leads to chemoresistance [80].

The role of p63 in the response of liver cells to DNA damage is less clear. Levels of p63 expression are extremely low in hepatocytes and in HCC cell lines. However, the type of p63 isoform expressed is dependent on the p53 status in HCC cell lines. The DeltaNp63 isoform is detectable in Hep3B only (lacking p53). These results are in agreement with an inhibition of DeltaNp63 expression by p53. Overall, these results suggest that p63 may get involved in a kind of compensation mechanism, becoming expressed when p53 is absent or inactivated. However, the physiopathological relevance of these observations remains to be elucidated [74].

Conclusion

As in many human cancers, *TP53* appears to be an essential tumor suppressor in liver cells. However, in contrast to most tissues, p53 may be involved in hepatocarcinogenesis through very specific mechanisms. An important consideration is that the mature hepatocyte is a remarkable metabolic and detoxification machine. Its responses to stress are therefore different from those of many other cells and tissues which are not, by nature, equipped with such a high capacity to eliminate potentially damaging agents. In this particular physiological situation, p53 appears to be of central importance in the event of long-term, chronic injury. In the liver, chronic injury generally takes the form of combined exposure to hepatotropic viruses and to lifestyle or dietary toxic agents such as alcohol or AFB_1.

In this chapter, we have discussed how p53 may play a role in the suppression of hepatocyte growth, mainly through the induction of senescence. This suppression may represent an important molecular basis of chronic liver disease characterized by loss of liver cell function, such as liver cirrhosis. That loss of p53 (for example through mutation) may provide cells a selective survival advantage, resulting in their clonal expansion under detrimental conditions. In this context, hepatocytes would rapidly acquire additional genetic perturbations that would, in due course, result into their transformation.

In the case of HCC occurring in the etiological context of chronic HBV infection and AFB_1 exposure, it seems that these two factors have developed strong synergistic effects that accelerate and facilitate hepatocyte transformation, somehow bypassing the requirement for a protracted phase of pre-cancerous, chronic liver disease. This concept is illustrated in Figure 5. In other etiological contexts (e.g. chronic HCV infection, alcohol, iron overload), the occurrence of HCC is generally preceded by a long phase of chronic liver disease (e.g. liver cirrhosis, which is a precursor lesion in over 80% of HCC that develop in a context that does not involve AFB_1). The progression to cancer may primarily require the activation of a proliferative signaling pathway, such as the ß-catenin pathway. In turn, this oncogenic stress may activate the $p14^{arf}$/p53 connection and drive the cells into senescence, unless this connection is inactivated. This inactivation may occur through mutation of *TP53* (at multiple codons) or, in most instances, through inactivation of $p14^{arf}$ (mainly through promoter methylation). Having got rid of this suppressor mechanism, cells may rapidly progress towards malignancy. In contrast, in the case of widespread exposure to AFB_1, mutations in *TP53* may occur extremely early in life, and might be present in hepatocytes by the time they become chronically infected by HBV. In this context, the capacity of the p.R249S mutant to cooperate with HBx may have a dual effect: first, it may protect the hepatocytes from HBx-induced apoptotic effects. Second, it may induce a relaxation of the control exerted by wild-type p53 on genetic and genomic stability and thus enhance the probability of integration of HBV into the cell genome. These events would, together, launch cells on the path to cancer without going through a long, clinically symptomatic chronic liver disease. Indeed, in countries where HCC is mostly caused by HBV and AFB_1, liver cirrhosis is less frequently detected prior to HCC diagnosis than in countries where other etiologies predominate.

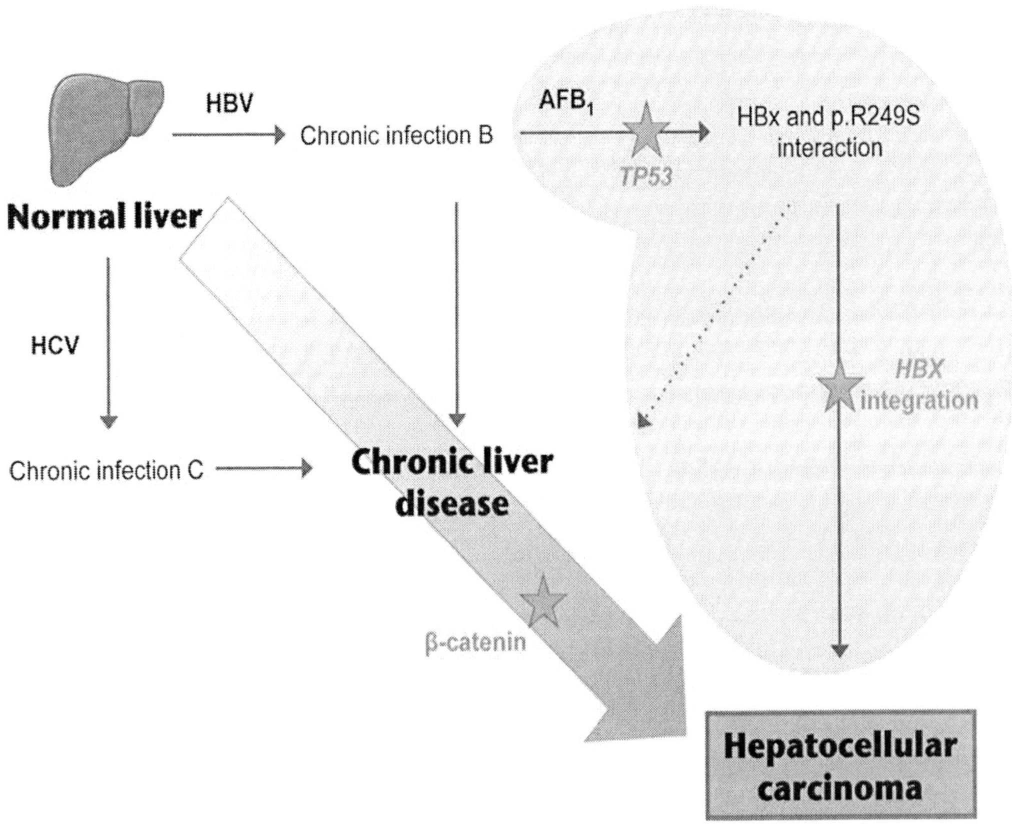

Figure 5. A model of hepatocarcinogenesis driven by different etiological contexts. The main route to HCC, represented by the large diagonal arrow, generally involves a long phase of precursor, chronic liver disease. Progression from chronic liver disease into HCC involves activation of oncogenic signals (e.g. ß-catenin) as primary mechanisms and inactivation of the suppressive response to oncogenic stress (e.g. inactivation of the $p53/p14^{arf}$ connection) as a secondary mechanism. In contrast, in the case of chronic exposure to AFB_1, the early formation of *R249S* mutations and the cooperation between HBx and the mutant p.R249S protein may enhance progression to HCC without the need for a protracted phase of chronic liver disease (pathway highlighted in green).

It is tempting to speculate that the particular synergistic mechanism between HBV and AFB_1 may have been selected through recent evolution as a mechanism that somehow protects subjects against the debilitating effects of chronic liver damage. By acquiring *R249S* mutations, chronically infected patients subjects may maintain liver functions despite chronic HBV infection, a situation that may have helped them to better survive in the extremely harsh environment that still prevails in many areas of HBV endemicity. Thus, early HCC might have represented the "price to pay" for this adaptation. Further studies are needed to better understand how this particular synergy has developed in many, but not all, areas of HBV endemicity.

References

[1] Vogelstein, B., Lane, D.& Levine, A. J. (2000). Surfing the p53 network. *Nature, 408*, 307-310.

[2] Levine, A. J., Feng, Z., Mak, T. W., You, H.& Jin, S. (2006). Coordination and communication between the p53 and IGF-1-AKT-TOR signal transduction pathways. *Genes Dev, 20*, 267-275.

[3] Levine, A. J.& Oren, M. (2009). The first 30 years of p53: growing ever more complex. *Nat Rev Cancer, 9*, 749-758.

[4] Vousden, K. H.& Prives, C. (2009). Blinded by the Light: The Growing Complexity of p53. *Cell, 137*, 413-431.

[5] Brown, C. J., Lain, S., Verma, C. S., Fersht, A. R.& Lane, D. P. (2009). Awakening guardian angels: drugging the p53 pathway. *Nat Rev Cancer, 9*, 862-873.

[6] Donehower, L. A. (2010). Using mice to examine p53 functions in cancer, aging, and longevity. In: A. J. Levine, & D. P. Lane (Eds.), *The p53 Family: A subject collection from Cold Spring Harbor Perspectives in Biology* (pp. 221-237). New York: Cold Spring Harbor Laboratory Press.

[7] Dötsch, V., Bernassola, F., Coutandin, D., Candi, E.& Melino, G. (2010). p63 and p73, the ancestors of p53. In: A. J. Levine, & D. P. Lane (Eds.), *The p53 Family: A subject collection from Cold Spring Harbor Perspectives in Biology* (pp. 49-62). New York: Cold Spring Harbor Laboratory Press.

[8] Petitjean, A., Mathe, E., Kato, S., Ishioka, C., Tavtigian, S. V., Hainaut, P.& Olivier, M. (2007). Impact of mutant p53 functional properties on TP53 mutation patterns and tumor phenotype: lessons from recent developments in the IARC TP53 database. *Hum Mutat, 28*, 622-629.

[9] Lee, K. C., Crowe, A. J.& Barton, M. C. (1999). p53-mediated repression of alpha-fetoprotein gene expression by specific DNA binding. *Mol Cell Biol, 19*, 1279-1288.

[10] Maeda, Y., Seidel, S. D., Wei, G., Liu, X.& Sladek, F. M. (2002). Repression of hepatocyte nuclear factor 4alpha tumor suppressor p53: involvement of the ligand-binding domain and histone deacetylase activity. *Mol Endocrinol, 16*, 402-410.

[11] Maeda, Y., Hwang-Verslues, W. W., Wei, G., Fukazawa, T., Durbin, M. L., Owen, L. B., Liu, X.& Sladek, F. M. (2006). Tumour suppressor p53 down-regulates the

expression of the human hepatocyte nuclear factor 4alpha (HNF4alpha) gene. *Biochem J, 400*, 303-313.

[12] Hwang-Verslues, W. W.& Sladek, F. M. (2008). Nuclear receptor hepatocyte nuclear factor 4alpha1 competes with oncoprotein c-Myc for control of the p21/WAF1 promoter. *Mol Endocrinol, 22*, 78-90.

[13] Liu, Y.& Kulesz-Martin, M. (2001). p53 protein at the hub of cellular DNA damage response pathways through sequence-specific and non-sequence-specific DNA binding. *Carcinogenesis, 22*, 851-860.

[14] Hussain, S. P., Schwank, J., Staib, F., Wang, X. W.& Harris, C. C. (2007). TP53 mutations and hepatocellular carcinoma: insights into the etiology and pathogenesis of liver cancer. *Oncogene, 26*, 2166-2176.

[15] Huster, D. (2010). Wilson disease. *Best Pract Res Clin Gastroenterol, 24*, 531-539.

[16] Pani, G., Fusco, S., Colavitti, R., Borrello, S., Maggiano, N., Cravero, A. A., Farre, S. M., Galeotti, T.& Koch, O. R. (2004). Abrogation of hepatocyte apoptosis and early appearance of liver dysplasia in ethanol-fed p53-deficient mice. *Biochem Biophys Res Commun, 325*, 97-100.

[17] Ozturk, M., Arslan-Ergul, A., Bagislar, S., Senturk, S.& Yuzugullu, H. (2009). Senescence and immortality in hepatocellular carcinoma. *Cancer Lett, 286*, 103-113.

[18] Xue, W., Zender, L., Miething, C., Dickins, R. A., Hernando, E., Krizhanovsky, V., Cordon-Cardo, C.& Lowe, S. W. (2007). Senescence and tumour clearance is triggered by p53 restoration in murine liver carcinomas. *Nature, 445*, 656-660.

[19] Edamoto, Y., Hara, A., Biernat, W., Terracciano, L., Cathomas, G., Riehle, H. M., Matsuda, M., Fujii, H., Scoazec, J. Y.& Ohgaki, H. (2003). Alterations of RB1, p53 and Wnt pathways in hepatocellular carcinomas associated with hepatitis C, hepatitis B and alcoholic liver cirrhosis. *Int J Cancer, 106*, 334-341.

[20] Hahn, W. C., Counter, C. M., Lundberg, A. S., Beijersbergen, R. L., Brooks, M. W.& Weinberg, R. A. (1999). Creation of human tumour cells with defined genetic elements. *Nature, 400*, 464-468.

[21] Sell, S., Hunt, J. M., Dunsford, H. A.& Chisari, F. V. (1991). Synergy between hepatitis B virus expression and chemical hepatocarcinogens in transgenic mice. *Cancer Res, 51*, 1278-1285.

[22] Bannasch, P., Khoshkhou, N. I., Hacker, H. J., Radaeva, S., Mrozek, M., Zillmann, U., Kopp-Schneider, A., Haberkorn, U., Elgas, M., Tolle, T.& et al. (1995). Synergistic hepatocarcinogenic effect of hepadnaviral infection and dietary aflatoxin B1 in woodchucks. *Cancer Res, 55*, 3318-3330.

[23] Cova, L., Wild, C. P., Mehrotra, R., Turusov, V., Shirai, T., Lambert, V., Jacquet, C., Tomatis, L., Trepo, C.& Montesano, R. (1990). Contribution of aflatoxin B1 and hepatitis B virus infection in the induction of liver tumors in ducks. *Cancer Res, 50*, 2156-2163.

[24] Kirk, G. D., Lesi, O. A., Mendy, M., Szymañska, K., Whittle, H., Goedert, J. J., Hainaut, P.& Montesano, R. (2005). 249(ser) TP53 mutation in plasma DNA, hepatitis B viral infection, and risk of hepatocellular carcinoma. *Oncogene, 24*, 5858-5867.

[25] Kirk, G. D., Lesi, O. A., Mendy, M., Szymanska, K., Whittle, H., Goedert, J. J., Hainaut, P.& Montesano, R. (2005). 249(ser) TP53 mutation in plasma DNA, hepatitis B viral infection, and risk of hepatocellular carcinoma. *Oncogene, 24*, 5858-5867.

[26] Lunn, R. M., Zhang, Y. J., Wang, L. Y., Chen, C. J., Lee, P. H., Lee, C. S., Tsai, W. Y.& Santella, R. M. (1997). p53 mutations, chronic hepatitis B virus infection, and aflatoxin exposure in hepatocellular carcinoma in Taiwan. *Cancer Res, 57*, 3471-3477.

[27] Qian, G. S., Ross, R. K., Yu, M. C., Yuan, J. M., Gao, Y. T., Henderson, B. E., Wogan, G. N.& Groopman, J. D. (1994). A follow-up study of urinary markers of aflatoxin exposure and liver cancer risk in Shanghai, People's Republic of China. *Cancer Epidemiol Biomarkers Prev, 3*, 3-10.

[28] Ross, R. K., Yuan, J. M., Yu, M. C., Wogan, G. N., Qian, G. S., Tu, J. T., Groopman, J. D., Gao, Y. T.& Henderson, B. E. (1992). Urinary aflatoxin biomarkers and risk of hepatocellular carcinoma. *Lancet, 339*, 943-946.

[29] Wang, L. Y., Hatch, M., Chen, C. J., Levin, B., You, S. L., Lu, S. N., Wu, M. H., Wu, W. P., Wang, L. W., Wang, Q., Huang, G. T., Yang, P. M., Lee, H. S.& Santella, R. M. (1996). Aflatoxin exposure and risk of hepatocellular carcinoma in Taiwan. *Int J Cancer, 67*, 620-625.

[30] Wu, H. C., Wang, Q., Yang, H. I., Ahsan, H., Tsai, W. Y., Wang, L. Y., Chen, S. Y., Chen, C. J.& Santella, R. M. (2009). Aflatoxin B1 exposure, hepatitis B virus infection, and hepatocellular carcinoma in Taiwan. *Cancer Epidemiol Biomarkers Prev, 18*, 846-853.

[31] Kew, M. C. (2003). Synergistic interaction between aflatoxin B1 and hepatitis B virus in hepatocarcinogenesis. *Liver Int, 23*, 405-409.

[32] Sylla, A., Diallo, M. S., Castegnaro, J.& Wild, C. P. (1999). Interactions between hepatitis B virus infection and exposure to aflatoxins in the development of hepatocellular carcinoma: a molecular epidemiological approach. *Mutat Res, 428*, 187-196.

[33] Wild, C. P.& Montesano, R. (2009). A model of interaction: aflatoxins and hepatitis viruses in liver cancer aetiology and prevention. *Cancer Lett, 286*, 22-28.

[34] Chemin, I., Takahashi, S., Belloc, C., Lang, M. A., Ando, K., Guidotti, L. G., Chisari, F. V.& Wild, C. P. (1996). Differential induction of carcinogen metabolizing enzymes in a transgenic mouse model of fulminant hepatitis. *Hepatology, 24*, 649-656.

[35] Kirby, G. M., Chemin, I., Montesano, R., Chisari, F. V., Lang, M. A.& Wild, C. P. (1994). Induction of specific cytochrome P450s involved in aflatoxin B1 metabolism in hepatitis B virus transgenic mice. *Mol Carcinog, 11*, 74-80.

[36] Hussain, S. P., Aguilar, F., Amstad, P.& Cerutti, P. (1994). Oxy-radical induced mutagenesis of hotspot codons 248 and 249 of the human p53 gene. *Oncogene, 9*, 2277-2281.

[37] Jia, L., Wang, X. W.& Harris, C. C. (1999). Hepatitis B virus X protein inhibits nucleotide excision repair. *Int J Cancer, 80*, 875-879.

[38] Madden, C. R., Finegold, M. J.& Slagle, B. L. (2002). Altered DNA mutation spectrum in aflatoxin b1-treated transgenic mice that express the hepatitis B virus x protein. *J Virol, 76*, 11770-11774.

[39] Banerjee, R., Caruccio, L., Zhang, Y. J., McKercher, S.& Santella, R. M. (2000). Effects of carcinogen-induced transcription factors on the activation of hepatitis B virus expression in human hepatoblastoma HepG2 cells and its implication on hepatocellular carcinomas. *Hepatology, 32*, 367-374.

[40] Barraud, L., Douki, T., Guerret, S., Chevallier, M., Jamard, C., Trepo, C., Wild, C. P., Cadet, J.& Cova, L. (2001). The role of duck hepatitis B virus and aflatoxin B1 in the induction of oxidative stress in the liver. *Cancer Detect Prev, 25*, 192-201.

[41] Barraud, L., Guerret, S., Chevallier, M., Borel, C., Jamard, C., Trepo, C., Wild, C. P.& Cova, L. (1999). Enhanced duck hepatitis B virus gene expression following aflatoxin B1 exposure. *Hepatology, 29*, 1317-1323.

[42] Bondy, G. S.& Pestka, J. J. (2000). Immunomodulation by fungal toxins. *J Toxicol Environ Health B Crit Rev, 3*, 109-143.

[43] Gong, Y., Hounsa, A., Egal, S., Turner, P. C., Sutcliffe, A. E., Hall, A. J., Cardwell, K.& Wild, C. P. (2004). Postweaning exposure to aflatoxin results in impaired child growth: a longitudinal study in Benin, West Africa. *Environ Health Perspect, 112*, 1334-1338.

[44] Gong, Y. Y., Cardwell, K., Hounsa, A., Egal, S., Turner, P. C., Hall, A. J.& Wild, C. P. (2002). Dietary aflatoxin exposure and impaired growth in young children from Benin and Togo: cross sectional study. *BMJ, 325*, 20-21.

[45] Turner, P. C., Moore, S. E., Hall, A. J., Prentice, A. M.& Wild, C. P. (2003). Modification of immune function through exposure to dietary aflatoxin in Gambian children. *Environ Health Perspect, 111*, 217-220.

[46] Kim, C. M., Koike, K., Saito, I., Miyamura, T.& Jay, G. (1991). HBx gene of hepatitis B virus induces liver cancer in transgenic mice. *Nature, 351*, 317-320.

[47] Yu, D. Y., Moon, H. B., Son, J. K., Jeong, S., Yu, S. L., Yoon, H., Han, Y. M., Lee, C. S., Park, J. S., Lee, C. H., Hyun, B. H., Murakami, S.& Lee, K. K. (1999). Incidence of hepatocellular carcinoma in transgenic mice expressing the hepatitis B virus X-protein. *J Hepatol, 31*, 123-132.

[48] Kim, Y. C., Song, K. S., Yoon, G., Nam, M. J.& Ryu, W. S. (2001). Activated ras oncogene collaborates with HBx gene of hepatitis B virus to transform cells by suppressing HBx-mediated apoptosis. *Oncogene, 20*, 16-23.

[49] Hodgson, A. J., Keasler, V. V.& Slagle, B. L. (2008). Premature cell cycle entry induced by hepatitis B virus regulatory HBx protein during compensatory liver regeneration. *Cancer Res, 68*, 10341-10348.

[50] Martin-Lluesma, S., Schaeffer, C., Robert, E. I., van Breugel, P. C., Leupin, O., Hantz, O.& Strubin, M. (2008). Hepatitis B virus X protein affects S phase progression leading to chromosome segregation defects by binding to damaged DNA binding protein 1. *Hepatology, 48*, 1467-1476.

[51] Kim, S., Park, S. Y., Yong, H., Famulski, J. K., Chae, S., Lee, J. H., Kang, C. M., Saya, H., Chan, G. K.& Cho, H. (2008). HBV X protein targets hBubR1, which induces dysregulation of the mitotic checkpoint. *Oncogene, 27*, 3457-3464.

[52] Wen, Y., Golubkov, V. S., Strongin, A. Y., Jiang, W.& Reed, J. C. (2008). Interaction of hepatitis B viral oncoprotein with cellular target HBXIP dysregulates centrosome dynamics and mitotic spindle formation. *J Biol Chem, 283*, 2793-2803.

[53] Forgues, M., Difilippantonio, M. J., Linke, S. P., Ried, T., Nagashima, K., Feden, J., Valerie, K., Fukasawa, K.& Wang, X. W. (2003). Involvement of Crm1 in hepatitis B virus X protein-induced aberrant centriole replication and abnormal mitotic spindles. *Mol Cell Biol, 23*, 5282-5292.

[54] Wang, W., Budhu, A., Forgues, M.& Wang, X. W. (2005). Temporal and spatial control of nucleophosmin by the Ran-Crm1 complex in centrosome duplication. *Nat Cell Biol, 7*, 823-830.

[55] Wang, X. W., Hussain, S. P., Huo, T. I., Wu, C. G., Forgues, M., Hofseth, L. J., Brechot, C.& Harris, C. C. (2002). Molecular pathogenesis of human hepatocellular carcinoma. *Toxicology, 181-182*, 43-47.

[56] Iavarone, M., Trabut, J. B., Delpuech, O., Carnot, F., Colombo, M., Kremsdorf, D., Brechot, C.& Thiers, V. (2003). Characterisation of hepatitis B virus X protein mutants in tumour and non-tumour liver cells using laser capture microdissection. *J Hepatol, 39*, 253-261.

[57] Jiang, W., Wang, X. W., Unger, T., Forgues, M., Kim, J. W., Hussain, S. P., Bowman, E., Spillare, E. A., Lipsky, M. M., Meck, J. M., Cavalli, L. R., Haddad, B. R.& Harris, C. C. (2010). Cooperation of tumor-derived HBx mutants and p53-249(ser) mutant in regulating cell proliferation, anchorage-independent growth and aneuploidy in a telomerase-immortalized normal human hepatocyte-derived cell line. *Int J Cancer, 127*, 1011-1020.

[58] Gouas, D. A., Shi, H., Hautefeuille, A. H., Ortiz-Cuaran, S. L., Legros, P. C., Szymanska, K. J., Galy, O., Egevad, L. A., Abedi-Ardekani, B., Wiman, K. G., Hantz, O., Caron de Fromentel, C., Chemin, I. A.& Hainaut, P. L. (2010). Effects of the TP53 p.R249S mutant on proliferation and clonogenic properties in human hepatocellular carcinoma cell lines: interaction with hepatitis B virus X protein. *Carcinogenesis, 31*, 1475-1482.

[59] Gormally, E., Caboux, E., Vineis, P.& Hainaut, P. (2007). Circulating free DNA in plasma or serum as biomarker of carcinogenesis: practical aspects and biological significance. *Mutat Res, 635*, 105-117.

[60] Lleonart, M. E., Kirk, G. D., Villar, S., Lesi, O. A., Dasgupta, A., Goedert, J. J., Mendy, M., Hollstein, M. C., Montesano, R., Groopman, J. D., Hainaut, P.& Friesen, M. D. (2005). Quantitative analysis of plasma TP53 249Ser-mutated DNA by electrospray ionization mass spectrometry. *Cancer Epidemiol Biomarkers Prev, 14*, 2956-2962.

[61] Jackson, P. E., Kuang, S. Y., Wang, J. B., Strickland, P. T., Munoz, A., Kensler, T. W., Qian, G. S.& Groopman, J. D. (2003). Prospective detection of codon 249 mutations in plasma of hepatocellular carcinoma patients. *Carcinogenesis, 24*, 1657-1663.

[62] Gormally, E., Vineis, P., Matullo, G., Veglia, F., Caboux, E., Le Roux, E., Peluso, M., Garte, S., Guarrera, S., Munnia, A., Airoldi, L., Autrup, H., Malaveille, C., Dunning, A., Overvad, K., Tjonneland, A., Lund, E., Clavel-Chapelon, F., Boeing, H., Trichopoulou, A., Palli, D., Krogh, V., Tumino, R., Panico, S., Bueno-de-Mesquita, H. B., Peeters, P. H., Pera, G., Martinez, C., Dorronsoro, M., Barricarte, A., Navarro, C., Quiros, J. R., Hallmans, G., Day, N. E., Key, T. J., Saracci, R., Kaaks, R., Riboli, E.&

Hainaut, P. (2006). TP53 and KRAS2 mutations in plasma DNA of healthy subjects and subsequent cancer occurrence: a prospective study. *Cancer Res, 66*, 6871-6876.

[63] Szymanska, K., Chen, J. G., Cui, Y., Gong, Y. Y., Turner, P. C., Villar, S., Wild, C. P., Parkin, D. M.& Hainaut, P. (2009). TP53 R249S mutations, exposure to aflatoxin, and occurrence of hepatocellular carcinoma in a cohort of chronic hepatitis B virus carriers from Qidong, China. *Cancer Epidemiol Biomarkers Prev, 18*, 1638-1643.

[64] Kirk, G. D., Bah, E.& Montesano, R. (2006). Molecular epidemiology of human liver cancer: insights into etiology, pathogenesis and prevention from The Gambia, West Africa. *Carcinogenesis, 27*, 2070-2082.

[65] Bah, E., Parkin, D. M., Hall, A. J., Jack, A. D.& Whittle, H. (2001). Cancer in the Gambia: 1988-97. *Br J Cancer, 84*, 1207-1214.

[66] Szymańska, K., Lesi, O. A., Kirk, G. D., Sam, O., Taniere, P., Scoazec, J. Y., Mendy, M., Friesen, M. D., Whittle, H., Montesano, R.& Hainaut, P. (2004). Ser-249TP53 mutation in tumour and plasma DNA of hepatocellular carcinoma patients from a high incidence area in the Gambia, West Africa. *Int J Cancer, 110*, 374-379.

[67] Yang, A., Kaghad, M., Wang, Y., Gillett, E., Fleming, M. D., Dotsch, V., Andrews, N. C., Caput, D.& McKeon, F. (1998). p63, a p53 homolog at 3q27-29, encodes multiple products with transactivating, death-inducing, and dominant-negative activities. *Mol Cell, 2*, 305-316.

[68] Jost, C. A., Marin, M. C.& Kaelin, W. G., Jr. (1997). p73 is a simian [correction of human] p53-related protein that can induce apoptosis. *Nature, 389*, 191-194.

[69] Kaghad, M., Bonnet, H., Yang, A., Creancier, L., Biscan, J. C., Valent, A., Minty, A., Chalon, P., Lelias, J. M., Dumont, X., Ferrara, P., McKeon, F.& Caput, D. (1997). Monoallelically expressed gene related to p53 at 1p36, a region frequently deleted in neuroblastoma and other human cancers. *Cell, 90*, 809-819.

[70] De Laurenzi, V., Costanzo, A., Barcaroli, D., Terrinoni, A., Falco, M., Annicchiarico-Petruzzelli, M., Levrero, M.& Melino, G. (1998). Two new p73 splice variants, gamma and delta, with different transcriptional activity. *J Exp Med, 188*, 1763-1768.

[71] Melino, G., Bernassola, F., Ranalli, M., Yee, K., Zong, W. X., Corazzari, M., Knight, R. A., Green, D. R., Thompson, C.& Vousden, K. H. (2004). p73 Induces apoptosis via PUMA transactivation and Bax mitochondrial translocation. *J Biol Chem, 279*, 8076-8083.

[72] Keyes, W. M., Wu, Y., Vogel, H., Guo, X., Lowe, S. W.& Mills, A. A. (2005). p63 deficiency activates a program of cellular senescence and leads to accelerated aging. *Genes Dev, 19*, 1986-1999.

[73] Machado-Silva, A., Perrier, S.& Bourdon, J. C. (2010). p53 family members in cancer diagnosis and treatment. *Semin Cancer Biol, 20*, 57-62.

[74] Petitjean, A., Cavard, C., Shi, H., Tribollet, V., Hainaut, P.& Caron de Fromentel, C. (2005). The expression of TA and DeltaNp63 are regulated by different mechanisms in liver cells. *Oncogene, 24*, 512-519.

[75] Murray-Zmijewski, F., Lane, D. P.& Bourdon, J. C. (2006). p53/p63/p73 isoforms: an orchestra of isoforms to harmonise cell differentiation and response to stress. *Cell Death Differ, 13*, 962-972.

[76] Mills, A. A., Zheng, B., Wang, X. J., Vogel, H., Roop, D. R.& Bradley, A. (1999). p63 is a p53 homologue required for limb and epidermal morphogenesis. *Nature, 398*, 708-713.

[77] Yang, A., Schweitzer, R., Sun, D., Kaghad, M., Walker, N., Bronson, R. T., Tabin, C., Sharpe, A., Caput, D., Crum, C.& McKeon, F. (1999). p63 is essential for regenerative proliferation in limb, craniofacial and epithelial development. *Nature, 398*, 714-718.

[78] Yang, A., Walker, N., Bronson, R., Kaghad, M., Oosterwegel, M., Bonnin, J., Vagner, C., Bonnet, H., Dikkes, P., Sharpe, A., McKeon, F.& Caput, D. (2000). p73-deficient mice have neurological, pheromonal and inflammatory defects but lack spontaneous tumours. *Nature, 404*, 99-103.

[79] Pozniak, C. D., Radinovic, S., Yang, A., McKeon, F., Kaplan, D. R.& Miller, F. D. (2000). An anti-apoptotic role for the p53 family member, p73, during developmental neuron death. *Science, 289*, 304-306.

[80] Seitz, S. J., Schleithoff, E. S., Koch, A., Schuster, A., Teufel, A., Staib, F., Stremmel, W., Melino, G., Krammer, P. H., Schilling, T.& Muller, M. (2010). Chemotherapy-induced apoptosis in hepatocellular carcinoma involves the p53 family and is mediated via the extrinsic and the intrinsic pathway. *Int J Cancer, 126*, 2049-2066.

[81] Irwin, M. S., Kondo, K., Marin, M. C., Cheng, L. S., Hahn, W. C.& Kaelin, W. G., Jr. (2003). Chemosensitivity linked to p73 function. *Cancer Cell, 3*, 403-410.

[82] Ozaki, T.& Nakagawara, A. (2005). p73, a sophisticated p53 family member in the cancer world. *Cancer Sci, 96*, 729-737.

In: Hepatocellular Carcionoma: A Global Challenge
Editor: Isabelle Chemin

ISBN: 978-1-61470-644-1

Chapter VIII

Hepatocellular Carcinoma: A Global Challenge. The Wnt Pathway

Anaïs Lopez[1] and Philippe Merle[1,2,*]
[1]Université Lyon 1, Inserm U1052, Centre de Recherche en Cancérologie de Lyon, Lyon, France
[2]Hospices Civils de Lyon, Service d'Hépatologie et de Gastroentérologie, Hôpital de la Croix-Rousse, Lyon, France

1. Introduction

Hepatocellular carcinoma (HCC) is a leading health problem worldwide. It is a poor prognosis tumor ranking third in terms of death by cancer [Parkin 2001]. This can be attributable to a common late diagnosis with advanced cancerous spread at presentation while patients have inoperable HCC. In this setting, therapies are mostly of modest benefit. Among systemic therapies, only sorafenib – i.e. the antiangiogenic and Ras-Raf-MAPK inhibitor - has been shown to significantly improve survival rates [Llovet 2008]. The growing incidence of HCC has generated intense research to understand its cellular and molecular mechanisms, with the hope of developing innovative therapies. Hepatocarcinogenesis is a complex process associating accumulation of genetic and epigenetic changes that occur during initiation, promotion and progression of the disease. Activation of oncogenes and the role of tumor suppressor genes have well been documented, and the signal transduction pathways implicated in HCC are being extensively studied [Hoshida 2008; Merle 2009]. Among these, evidence is accumulating that activation of the Wnt/Frizzled-mediated signaling could play a key role in HCC. The role of the Wnt pathway in liver biology has come to the forefront over the last several years. In the present paper, we'll aim at understanding the Wnt/Frizzled-mediated signaling and highlighting its deregulations encountered in hepatocarciniogenesis.

* Correspondence address to: Pr. Philippe Merle, M.D., Ph.D., INSERM U871, 151 Cours Albert Thomas, 69424 Lyon Cedex 03, France. Phone : 33 4 72 68 19 54; Fax: 33 4 72 68 19 71; E-mail: philippe.merle@inserm.fr.

Keywords: Hepatocellular carcinoma, Wnt, β-catenin, Jun-kinase, protein kinase C

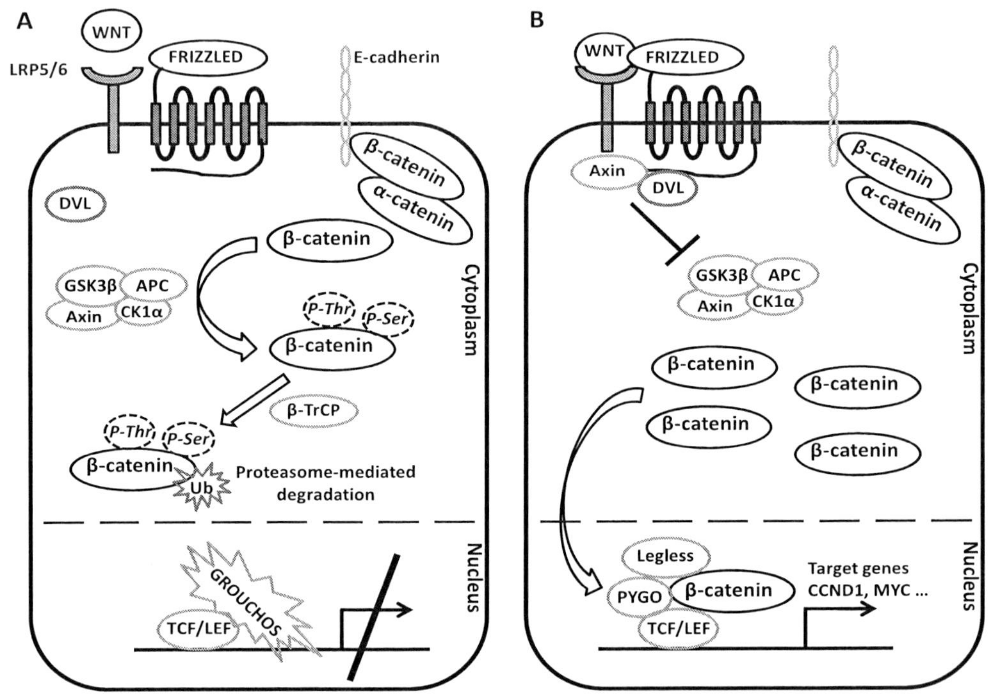

Figure 1. The canonical Wnt/β-catenin pathway. (A) In the absence of WNT ligand, soluble cytosolic β-catenin is phosphorylated on serin and threonin by a destruction complex comprising Axin1/2-APC-CK1α-GSK3β. CK1 phosphorylates β-catenin on Ser45. This event primes β-catenin for subsequent phosphorylation by GSK3β at Ser33, Ser37 and Thr41. These phosphorylations lead to its ubiquitination through β-TrCP and degradation by proteasome. (B) In context of active canonical signaling, Dishevelled (DVL) and axin are recruited to the membrane, that lead to avoid the formation of destruction complex. This results in accumulation of β-catenin into the cytoplasm and its translocation into the nucleus, and transactivation of β-catenin-targeted genes.

2. The Wnt Pathway

2.1. The Wnt/Frizzled-mediated Signaling

The human WNT gene family consists of 19 members, encoding extracellular soluble glycoproteins that interact with one over the ten known Frizzled family membrane receptors (FZD) in an auto-paracrine manner. Wnt signals are transduced through FZD to either the canonical in conjunction with LRP5/LRP6 co-receptors, or the noncanonical pathways thanks to ROR2 and RYK co-receptors (Figures 1 and 2). These pathways are able to control cell fate determination, survival, apoptosis, proliferation, differentiation, motility and tissue polarity. Wnt signals can transduce to one of both pathways, resulting from a complex network based on the cellular context, the expression profile pattern of WNT ligands, FZD receptors and co-receptors as well as extracellular secreted WNT inhibitors such as SFRP,

WIF and DKK [Oishi 2003; Lu 2004; Lu 2004 bis]. Classically but not being a rule since depending of many factors as mentioned above, WNT1/2/3/3a/8a/8b/10a/10b and FZD1/5/7/9 are regarded as the canonical complex receptor elements, whereas WNT4/5a/5b/6/7a/7b/11 and FZD2/3/4/6 appear as the non-canonicals, and WNT2b/9a/9b/16 and FZD8/10 remain undetermined [Huelsken 2001; Huelsken 2002]. SFRP family members and WIF are Wnt antagonists that inhibit WNT binding to FZD. DKK family members interact with LRP5/LRP6 co-receptors and trigger their endocytosis to prevent formation of the WNT-FZD-LRP5/LRP6 complex for the canonical Wnt signaling. Additionally, activity of intracellular Wnt signaling regulators can play a key role. APC, AXIN1, AXIN2, CKIα, GSK3β, NKD1, NKD2, ANKRD6, and NLK are negative regulators of the canonical Wnt pathway. APC, AXIN1, and AXIN2 are scaffold proteins of the β-catenin destruction complex, whereas CKIα and GSK3β are serine/threonine kinases that phosphorylate β-catenin to trigger its degradation by proteasome [Kawano 2003].

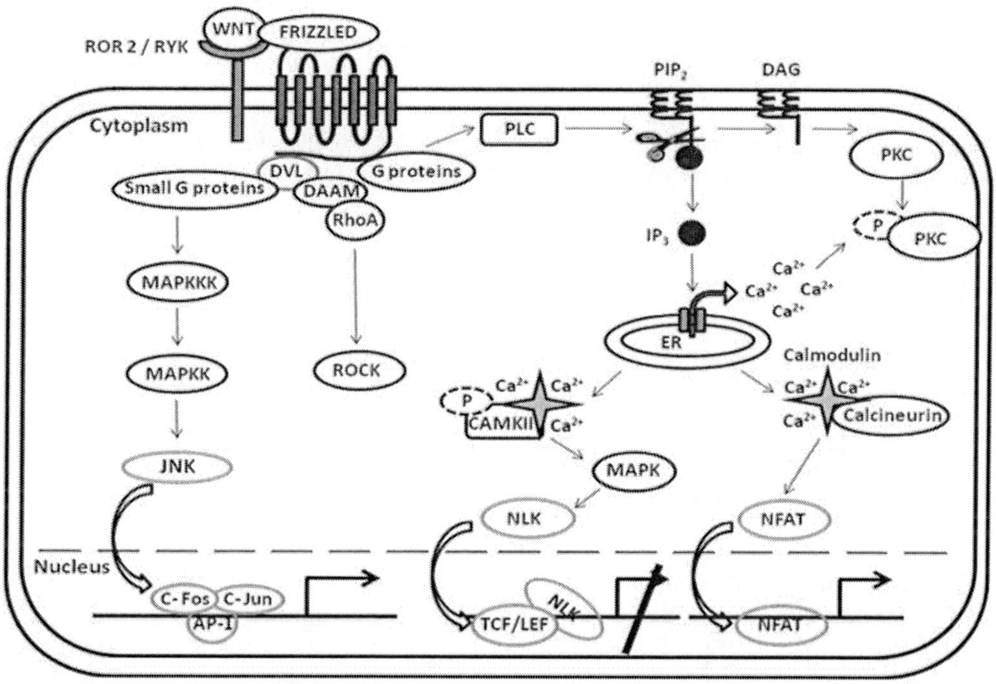

Figure 2. The non canonical Wnt pathways. *The WNT/Ca^{2+} pathway* (right panel): WNT/FRIZZLED interaction leads to activation of Phospholipase C (PLC) via G proteins, which cleave Phosphatidyl Inositol 4,5 bisphosphate (PIP2) into Diacylglycerol (DAG) and Inositol 1,4,5-trisphosphate (IP_3). DAG activates Protein Kinase C; while IP_3 increases the concentration of intracellular calcium from endoplasmic reticulum (ER) that can activate calmodulin. Activated calmodulin can either interact with calineurin to translocate the nuclear factor of activated T cells (NFAT) into the nucleus, or with calcium/calmodulin-dependent protein kinase II (CAMKII) to activate nemo-like kinase (NLK) which can repress canonical pathway by inhibiting TCF/LEF. *The WNT/Planar Cell Polarization (PCP) or WNT/JNK pathway* (left panel): WNT/FRIZZLED interaction leads to activation of Dishevelled protein (Dvl) which can either interact with small G proteins such as Rac to activate Jun-kinase (JNK) that lead to formation of transcription factor C-Jun/C-Fos on AP-1 promoter, or activate RhoA through Dishevelled-associated activator of morphogenesis (DAAM) that lead to ROCK signaling.

In the presence of canonical Wnt signal, Dishevelled (DVL) is phosphorylated by CKIα for high-affinity binding to FRAT. Because canonical Wnt signal induces the assembly of both FZD-DVL and LRP5/6-AXIN-FRAT complexes, β-catenin is released from phosphorylation by CKIα and GSK3β for stabilization, and thus is targeted towards nuclear translocation and accumulation [Wong 2003; Tolwinski 2003]. Small G proteins (RHOA, RHOU, RAC, and CDC42) and c-jun NH2-terminal kinase are the DVL-dependent effector molecules of the noncanonical pathway, whereas Nemo-like kinase (NLK) and nuclear factor of activated T cells (NFAT) are the Ca2+-dependent effector molecules. NLK phosphorylates TCF/LEF family transcription factors to inhibit the canonical Wnt signaling pathway [Ishitani 2003; Katoh 2005; Dejmek 2006].

Of evidence is that the Wnt-mediated signaling does not act alone in a given cell, but is involved in a complex network where it interplays with different pathways such as the *FGF-mediated signaling* through the phosphatidylinositol 3-kinase(PI3K)-AKT, Ca2+, and mitogen-activated protein kinase (MAPK) signaling cascades [Katoh 2006]. Although the mechanisms are not the same, FGF and canonical Wnt pathways inhibit GSK3β activity, and activate Ca2+ signaling. Cross-talk of FGF and Wnt pathways in tumors leads to more malignant phenotype through the potentiation of β-catenin, epithelial-mesenchymal transition (EMT), and NFAT signaling cascades. Regarding the *Notch signaling pathway*, it has been shown as synergizing with Wnt to inhibit terminal differentiation of epithelial cells partially through down-regulation of ATOH1/HATH1 βHLH transcription factor. Notch and Wnt signaling pathways keep the homeostasis of stem and progenitor (transit-amplifying) cells through the inhibition of terminal differentiation. The Wnt signaling also networks with *Eph*, *vascular endothelial growth factor (VEGF)*, *Hedgehog*, and *transforming growth factor β/bone morphogenetic protein (TGFβ/BMP)* pathways [Robbins 1992; Duncan 2005; Katoh 2006b].

2.2. The Canonical Wnt/β-catenin Pathway

The Wnt/β-catenin signaling pathway has a crucial role in the embryonic development of all animal species, in the regeneration of tissues in adult organisms and in numerous other processes controlling proliferation, survival, cell migration, differentiation, and patterning in the receiving cells and tissues. Deregulation of the canonical Wnt/β-catenin pathway can induce disease, most importantly cancer [Clevers 2006]. β-catenin is the central actor of the canonical Wnt/β-catenin pathway, being implicated in cell adhesion and Wnt signaling [White 1998]. Indeed, there is likely a crosstalk between β-catenin in two different compartments, the adhesion complex at the plasma membrane and a signaling complex in the nucleus. BCL9 proteins may act in the switch between cadherin-mediated cell adhesion and Wnt signaling [de la Roche 2008]. Unlike the multitude of cadherins and several tissue-specific α-catenin variants, a single β-catenin protein is present in vertebrates and insects. β-catenin is a 88 kDa protein encoded by the *CTNNB1* gene. Its primary structure comprises 781 amino acid consisting of an amino-terminal region of about 150 amino acids, a central ~520 residue domain composed of 12 armadillo (arm) repeats, and a carboxy-terminal 100 residue region [Hubert 1997; Graham 2000; Shapiro 2009]. As part of adherens junctions, the conserved cytoplasmic carboxyl terminus of the cell adhesion molecule E-cadherin binds three proteins: α-catenin, β-catenin, and plakoglobin (γ-catenin) [Ozawa 1989]. It joins classical cadherins to the actin cytoskeleton in cell adhesion, β-catenin binding to the cytoplasmic portion of cadherins by its arm domain, whereas α-catenin binds to residues 118-149, just before the start of the arm domain.

In the absence of canonical WNTs, cytoplasmic β-catenin is recruited into a destruction complex, in which it interacts with APC and the axins, and is amino-terminally phosphorylated by axin-bound CK1α and GSK3β. Following phosphorylation, β-catenin is targeted for proteasome-dependent degradation involving an interaction with β-TrCP (β-transducin repeat-containing protein), a component of the E3 ubiquitin ligase complex. Therefore, in the absence of canonical WNTs, cytoplasmic β-catenin levels remain low, and the transcription factors LEF1 and TCF interact with Grouchos in the nucleus to repress Wnt-specific target genes [Liu 2002]. In the presence of canonical WNTs, LRP5-LRP6 surface co-receptors are phosphorylated by CK1γ and GSK3β (and possibly further kinases), and DVL is recruited to the plasma membrane, where it interacts with FZD and polymerizes with other DVL molecules [Bilic 2007]. The inactivation of the destruction complex allows the cytoplasmic stabilization and translocation of β-catenin to the nucleus. Here, β-catenin forms a transcriptionally active complex with LEF1 and TCF transcription factors by displacing Grouchos and interacting with other coactivators [Klaus 2008].

β-catenin activity can be modulated by other signaling pathways. For instance, insulin-like growth factor II (IGF-II) leads to the internalization of E-cadherin/β-catenin and to E-cadherin degradation, leading to β-catenin activation [Morali 2001]. HGF/SF action on Met can result in β-catenin activation through tyrosine 142 phosphorylation of β-catenin [David 2008]. FGF and FGF receptor signaling also affects E-cadherin/β-catenin interaction and β-catenin/TCF signaling [Pai 2008]. EGF receptor signaling induces caveolin-mediated endocytosis of E-cadherin, resulting in β-catenin nuclear localization of β-catenin and therefore activation of the pathway [Lu 2003]. Recently, the tyrosine phosphatases PTPRK and PCP-2 have been shown to inhibit β-catenin signaling and increase E-cadherin-dependent adhesion [Novellino 2008]. The L1 adhesion system - i.e. transmembrane adhesion molecule with extracellular immunoglobulin-like domains and fibronectin type III repeats - has recently also been shown to affect cadherin-mediated cell adhesion and β-catenin signaling. L1 is up-regulated by Wnt/β-catenin signaling, it is expressed exclusively at the invasive front of colon cancer tissue, and its expression is correlated with tumor progression and metastasis [Gavert 2007]. It has now been shown that L1 disrupts the formation of adherent junctions by releasing E-cadherin, that it promotes epithelio-mesenchymal-like transition (EMT), and that it induces β-catenin cascade [Shtutman 2006].

The action of various serine/threonine and tyrosine kinases influences the function of β-catenin in adhesion and signaling [Daugherty 2007]. For instance, the carboxy-terminal phosphorylation of cadherins can strengthen or weaken interactions with β-catenin, depending on the sites of phosphorylation [Choi 2006]. β-catenin can be sequentially phosphorylated by different kinases, either promoting the degradation or the signaling activity of β-catenin. Phosphorylation at the amino terminus favors degradation, whereas phosphorylation in the armadillo domain changes the adhesiveness to cadherins and promotes nuclear localization [Roura 1999; Rhee 2007].

2.3. The Noncanonical Wnt/PKC Pathway

Non-canonical Wnt signaling does not operate through β-catenin. In some cases, it even inhibits nuclear β-catenin transactivity [Ishitani 2003]. Noncanonical Wnt signals can be classified by virtue of the several cascades they invoke, including Wnt/PCP (planar cell polarity), Wnt/JNK (c-Jun N-terminal kinase), Wnt/calcium and Wnt/Rho signalings [Liu 2008]. These pathways are initiated by the activation of FZD and co-receptors, such as ROR2 and RYK, and transduced through potentially diverse mechanisms which are either DVL-dependent or Ca2+-dependent. It has been suggested that the small GTPase RhoA and its effector ROK (Rho-associated kinase) are activated by DVL and function to regulate actin cytoskeleton in Wnt signaling [Winter 2001]. JNK is another downstream effector of DVL, and can be activated by RhoA to regulate PCP signaling during embryogenesis [Boutros 1998]. Noncanonical Wnt signals also operate through heterotrimeric G proteins which activate DVL and downstream calcium influx and/or PKC activity [Veeman 2003]. Nemo-like kinase (NLK) and the nuclear factor of activated T cells (NFAT) are the Ca2+-dependent effectors of the noncanonical pathway. NLK also phosphorylates TCF/LEF1 to inhibit the canonical Wnt signaling. Further insight into noncanonical Wnt signaling awaits the identification of the additional pathways and the mechanisms they invoke.

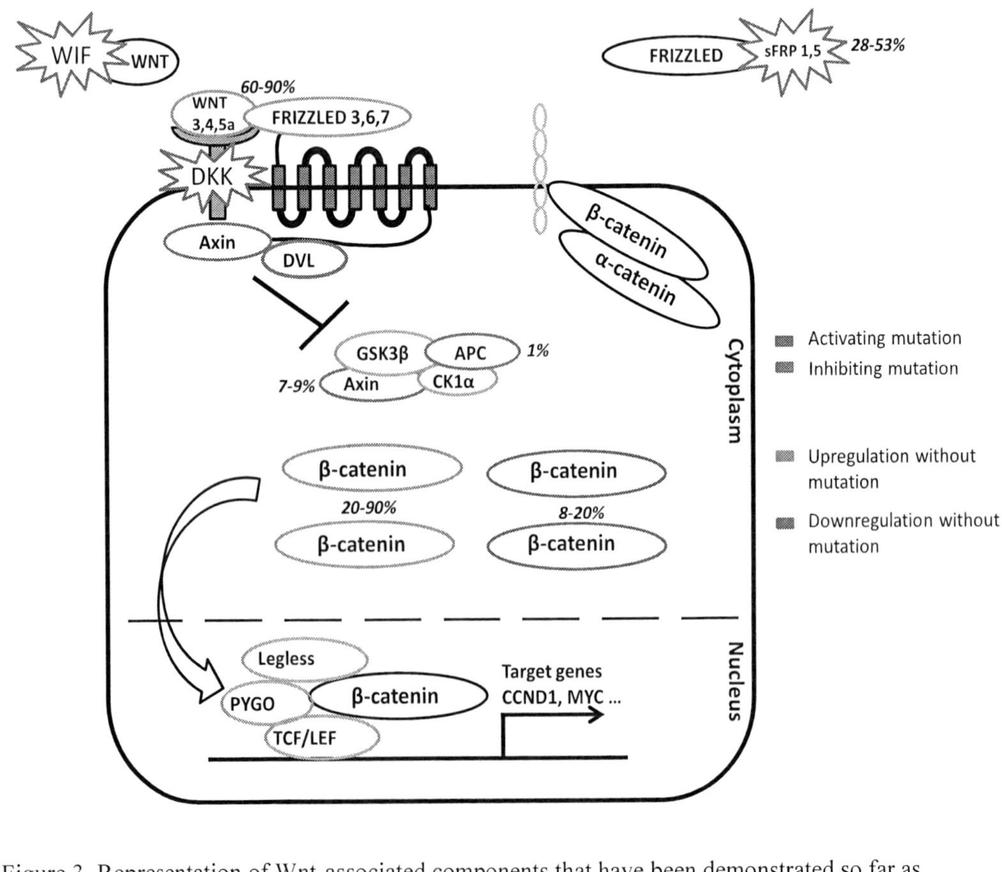

Figure 3. Representation of Wnt-associated components that have been demonstrated so far as deregulated in hepatocarcinogenesis.

3. Wnt Pathway and Hepatocarcinogenesis

The role of the canonical Wnt/β-catenin pathway has become identified as a key player in liver biology - i.e. in development, growth, regeneration, zonation, and metabolism. *Regarding the role of β-catenin in prenatal liver development*, liver derives from the foregut endoderm as a result of signaling from mesoderm in the form of FGF and BMP-4 which are both downstream targets of the Wnt pathway [Zaret 1998; Zaret 2000]. Active mesodermal WNT2b-mediated signaling has been identified at these stages in experimental models, and associated with β-catenin activation [Micsenyi 2004; Ober 2006]. Thus, β-catenin is likely playing an important role during early liver development in hepatocyte expansion *via* its transcriptional co-activator role. Interestingly, an overall decrease in total β-catenin levels occurs later on, when it begins localizing chiefly to the hepatocyte membrane. This membranous localization and functional complex with its partners E-cadherin and Met might be a hallmark of acquisition of hepatocytic maturation and polarity [Monga 2003]. *Regarding the role of β-catenin in normal liver growth*, β-catenin plays a pro-proliferative property in hepatocytes, especially evident in liver regeneration post-hepatectomy [Cadoret 2001; Tan 2006]. Additionally, HGF signaling is an important player in early liver regeneration, and an increase in levels of HGF and activation occurs early after partial hepatectomy, which may have consequences on the Met/β-catenin complex as well [Pediaditakis 2001]. *Finally, β-catenin acts on liver zonation and metabolism.* Indeed, interaction between β-catenin and APC may play a critical role in the zonation process in which APC is highly expressed in the periportal region, where β-catenin activation and signaling is quite low. In contrast, in the perivenous region, APC expression is absent and β-catenin activation is relatively high. Several genes involved in glutamine metabolism - i.e. encoding glutamine synthetase, ornithine aminotransferase, and the glutamate transporter GLT-1 - are targets of Wnt/β-catenin signaling [Cadoret 2002].

3.1. Canonical Wnt/β-catenin Pathway and Hepatocarcinogenesis

Assessing whether the β-catenin pathway is active or not, in a defined tissue or cell line, might be an issue. In tissues, β-catenin activation can be underlined by its nuclear and/or cytoplasmic accumulation as assessed by imunohistochemistry whereas a strict membrane accumulation would rather reflect a nonactive state. Others assimilate *CTNNB1* gene mutation, especially within its N-terminus portion, as witnessing activity of β-catenin although there is no strict correlation between *CTNNB1* gene mutation and β-catenin activity. Another way to ascertain β-catenin activity in a specific tissue is to show transactivation of β-catenin-target gene panels by transcriptomic analysis. In cell cultures, β-catenin transactivity can be more easily demonstrated by tranfection/transduction of reporter systems whose promoter is sensitive to the TCF/LEF/β-catenin complex. Nuclear and/or cytoplasmic accumulation of β-catenin is a frequent event in various human tumors including colorectal, lung, breast, cervix, skin, and liver [Candidus 1996; Rimm 1999; Johnsson 2000; Lin 2000; Chung 2000; Park 2001; Ueda 2001; Hommura 2002; Inagawa 2002]. During hepatocarcinogenesis, it has been reported that 8-20% of HCCs have β-catenin mutation(s), whereas 20% to 90% of HCCs display β-catenin activation [Hsu 2000; Devereux 2001; Wong 2001]. Among other candidate genes involved in stabilization of β-catenin, Axin-1 and Axin-2 were found mutated in a small fraction (7%-9%) of HCCs whereas APC mutations were found to be exceptionally rare [Huang 1999; Satoh 2000; Laurent-Puig 2001; Taniguchi 2002]. Thus, it is estimated that in 35%-80% of HCCs, the aberrant β-catenin cellular accumulation is not associated with a mutation affecting the β-catenin, Axin, or APC genes of the Wnt/β-catenin signal transduction cascade. Epigenetic deregulations of the pathway have been proposed. FZD7 receptor and/or its canonical activator - i.e. WNT3 - have been shown as overexpressed in 60%-90% of HCCs and 35%-60% of the surrounding peritumors. In addition, secreted Frizzled-receptors inhibitors sFRP have been found down-regulated in numerous HCCs [Merle 2004; Merle 2005; Kim 2008; Bengochea 2008; Takagi 2008]. Furthermore in human tissues, viral components may interfere with the Wnt/β-catenin pathway to activate β-catenin. In HBV-positive cases of HCC, hepatitis B virus encoded X antigen is associated with decreased expression of E-cadherin and activation of β-catenin, and upregulation of the hepatitis B virus encoded X antigen effector URG11 leads to increased activation of β-catenin [Lian 2006]. In HCV-related HCC, it's noteworthy that β-catenin gene mutation frequency is two-fold higher than in non-HCV-related HCCs [Huang 1999]. Although the mechanism of this predilection remains obscure, it has been shown that the HCV NS5A protein can stabilize β-catenin by direct binding and indirectly *via* activation of phosphoinositide-3 kinase (PI3K), Akt and GSK-3β [Milward 2010].

Evidence is accumulating to the fact that alterations of the Wnt/β-catenin pathway, due or unrelated to β-catenin gene mutation, is a common event in hepatocarcinogenesis and is associated with the clinical and pathological features of the disease [Hsu 2000; Devereux 2001; Wong 2001; Laurent-Puig 2001; Inagawa 2002]. However, β-catenin or APC gene mutation is a late event for malignant progression rather than an early genetic event involving the initiation of HCC development [Park 2005]. Although β-catenin activation is crucial for liver development and regeneration, it's not sufficient *per se* for hepatocarcinogenesis. Indeed, no study to date has shown spontaneous HCC in transgenic mice overexpressing wild-type or constitutively active mutated β-catenin [Cadoret 2001; Harada 2002; Tan 2005]. However, β-catenin overexpression/activation makes transgenic mice susceptible to H-Ras-related and chemical-induced HCCs, underlying the fact that β-catenin might rather play as a co-carcinogenic factor [Harada 2004; Nejak-Bowen 2010]. Interestingly, the animal model that succumbs to spontaneous HCC is the conditional APC deletion. However, APC deletions are not reported in HCC patients. By the way, APC has been shown to have direct DNA-binding functions through which it inhibits cell proliferation [Qian 2008]. Interestingly, β-catenin activation might be required for tumor initiation, but paradoxically its inactivation might accelerate tumor promotion. This was shown in a conditional β-catenin-deficient mouse model of chemically-induced HCC, in which chemicals could not promote HCC formation in β-catenin-deficient animals whereas the prevalence of tumors in β-catenin-deficient animals was much higher than in wild-type mice when the β-catenin gene was conditionnally invalidated after tumor initiation [Rignall 2010]. As β-catenin, Axin or APC gene mutations are a late event in hepatocarcinogenesis, it remains to be determined whether the Wnt/Frizzled-mediated signaling *per se*, in association or not with β-catenin activation, could play a prominent role in HCC initiation - i.e. in the very early steps of hepatocarcinogenesis.

3.2. Noncanonical Wnt/PKC and Wnt/JNK Pathways and Hepatocarcinogenesis

A very little is known about noncanonical Wnt pathways and HCC, and it remains questionable the accuracy of the role of these three FZD-potentially-dependent pathways in human hepatocarcinogenesis. As to the PKC and JNK pathways, their role and prevalence of activation remain poorly described in human hepatocarcinogenesis, although some studies have underlined their potentially oncogenic properties [Wu 2008; Delpuech 2002; Guo 2005]. It was reported that each of these pathways - i.e. PKC and JNK - can be found activated in a significant number of HCC tissues in conjunction with up-regulation of noncanonical WNT and FZD elements such as WNT4/5a and FZD3/6 [Bengochea 2008]. However, their specific role in HCC tumor phenotype remains obscure. Some have hypothesized that canonical and non canonical Wnt pathways might have complementary roles in HCC, where the canonical signaling contributes to tumor initiation, and non canonical to tumor progression. In HCC cell lines, *in vitro* studies showed that overexpression of the non canonical ligands WNT4/5a/5b/7b is specifically associated with poorly differentiated and aggressive phenotype [Yuzugullu 2009].

Regarding the role of JNK pathway, elevated JNK phosphorylation was found correlated with activation of AP-1 and HBV infection in human HCCs [Guo 2005]. JNK activity is involved *in vitro* for HCC cell line proliferation and *in vivo* for tumorigenesis of HCC cells xenografted in immunodeficient mice. In addition, JNK1$^{-/-}$ knock-out mice display decreased tumor cell proliferation in DEN-induced HCC [Hui 2008]. This pathway might even be involved in the very early steps of hepatocarcinogenesis since activation c-jun - i.e. a target of the JNK cascade - is a sufficient event to promote chemically induced HCC [Eferl 2003]. However, all these studies focusing on the pro-oncogenic power of JNK cascade did not assess its interplay with the noncanonical Wnt pathway and a lot of investigations remain to be done in this way.

Members of the protein kinase C (PKC) isoenzyme family plays a central role in the tumorigenesis of several tissues. However, little is known about the specific PKC specific isoforms expressed in human hepatocellular carcinomas, and there is a huge crosstalk between several pathways including the Wnt one, to activate PKC's. PKCβII and PKCθ were found down-regulated in human HCCs, correlating with the differentiation status [Lu 2010]. In contrast, it has been demonstrated that there was an up-regulation of PKCβ's in different metastatic HCC cells, and that both ERK and p38 MAPK are downstream signal molecules of PKCβ. Thus, it has been shown that inhibition of PKCβ activity, markedly reduced motility and invasion abilities of HCC cells [Guo 2008]. Another member of the PKC, the PKCα was found up-regulated at mRNA level in HCC specimens, and was significantly correlated with tumor size and high tumor grade [Wu 2007]. Recently, one correlation between PKCδ and WNT pathway has been demonstrated in HCC cell lines. It has been shown that inhibition of the Frizzled-7 mediating signaling, supposed to activate the canonical Wnt pathway, decreases cell viability and promotes apoptosis of HCC cells through β-catenin degradation and PKCδ activation [Beseme-Nambotin 2010]. These data support the idea of a very complex system, in which both canonical and noncanonical Wnt signals ascertain dual and opposite properties, depending on hepatocarcinogenesis step and in conjunction with other pathways.

Conclusion

Finally it is of evidence that Wnt signaling, key player in normal liver biology is also largely involved in hepatocarcinogenesis. It mainly acts on deregulated activation of the Wnt/β-catenin canonical pathway which mechanisms involve β-catenin or Axin gene mutation as well as up-regulation of specific WNT/FZD patterns. By contrast, little is known on the impact of the WNT/FZD-mediated PKC and JNK noncanonical cascades, and a lot of work remains to be done in the field. Regarding the role of Wnt signaling in very early steps of cancerous transformation and the specific subtype of liver cells that are permissive to its pro-oncogenic properties remains illusory, but in near future might help to set-up new biomarkers and define specific therapeutic targets.

References

Bengochea, A, de Souza, MM, Lefrancois, L, Le Roux, E, Galy, O, Chemin, I, Kim, M, Wands, JR, Trepo, C, Hainaut, P, Scoazec, JY, Vitvitski, L, Merle, P. Common dysregulation of Wnt/Frizzled receptor elements in human hepatocellular carcinoma. *Br J Cancer* 2008; 99: 143-50.

Beseme-Nambotin, S, Lefrancois, L, Sainsily, X, Berthillon, P, Kim, M, Wands, JR, Chevallier, M, Jalinot, P, Scoazec, JY, Trepo, C, Zoulim, F, Merle, P. Pharmacological inhibition of Frizzled-7 displays anti-tumor properties in hepatocellular carcinoma. *J Hepatol* 2011 (in press)

Bilic, J, Huang, YL, Davidson, G, Zimmermann, T, Cruciat, CM, Bienz M, Niehrs, C. Wnt induces LRP6 signalosomes and promotes dishevelled-dependent LRP6 phosphorylation. *Science* 2007; 316: 1619-22.

Boutros, M, Paricio, N, Strutt, DI, Mlodzik, M. Dishevelled activates JNK and discriminates between JNK pathways in planar polarity and wingless signaling. *Cell* 1998; 94: 109-18.

Cadoret, A, Ovejero, C, Saadi-Kheddouci, S, Souil, E, Fabre, M, Romagnolo, B, Kahn, A, Perret, C. Hepatomegaly in transgenic mice expressing an oncogenic form of β-catenin. *Cancer Res* 2001; 61: 3245-9.

Cadoret, A, Ovejero, C, Terris, B, Souil, E, Levy, L, Lamers, WH, Kitajewski, J, Kahn, A, Perret, C. New targets of β-catenin signaling in the liver are involved in the glutamine metabolism. *Oncogene* 2002; 21: 8293-301.

Candidus, S, Bischoff, P, Becker, KF, Hofler, H. No evidence for mutations in the α- and β-catenin genes in human gastric and breast carcinomas. *Cancer Res* 1996; 56: 49-52.

Choi, HJ, Huber, AH, Weis, WI. Thermodynamics of β-catenin-ligand interactions: the roles of the N- and C-terminal tails in modulating binding affinity. *J Biol Chem* 2006; 281: 1027-38.

Chung, DC. The genetic basis of colorectal cancer: insights into critical pathways of tumorigenesis. *Gastroenterology* 2000; 119: 854-65.

Clevers, H. Wnt/β-catenin signaling in development and disease. *Cell* 2006; 127: 469-80.

Daugherty, RL, Gottardi, CJ. Phospho-regulation of β-catenin adhesion and signaling functions. *Physiology* 2007; 22: 303-9.

David, MD, Yeramian, A, Dunach, M, Llovera, M, Canti, C, de Herreros, AG, Comella, JX, Herreros, J. Signaling by neurotrophins and hepatocyte growth factor regulates axon morphogenesis by differential β-catenin phosphorylation. *J Cell Sci* 2008; 121: 2718-30.

de la Roche, M, Worm, J, Bienz, M. The function of BCL9 in Wnt/β-catenin signaling and colorectal cancer cells. *BMC Cancer* 2008; 8: 199.

Dejmek, J, Safholm, A, Kamp-Nielsen, C, Andersson, T, Leandersson, K. Wnt-5a/Ca2+-induced NFAT activity is counteracted by Wnt-5a/Yes-Cdc42-casein kinase-Iα signaling in human mammary epithelial cells. *Mol Cell Biol* 2006; 26: 6024-36.

Delpuech, O, Trabut, JB, Carnot, F, Feuillard, J, Brechot, C, Kremsdorf, D. Identification, using cDNA macroarray analysis, of distinct gene expression profiles associated with pathological and virological features of hepatocellular carcinoma. *Oncogene* 2002; 21: 2926-37.

Devereux, TR, Stern, MC, Flake, GP, Yu, MC, Zhang, ZQ, London, SJ, Taylor, JA. *CTNNB1* mutations and β-catenin protein accumulation in human hepatocellular carcinomas associated with high exposure to aflatoxin B1. *Mol Carcinog* 2001; 31: 68-73.

Duncan, AW, Rattis, FM, DiMascio, LN, Congdon, KL, Pazianos, G, Zhao, C, Yoon, K, Cook, JM, Willert, K, Gaiano, N, Reya, T. Integration of Notch and Wnt signaling in hematopoietic stem cell maintenance. *Nat Immune* 2005; 6: 314-22.

Eferl, R, Ricci, R, Kenner, L, Zenz, R, David, JP, Rath, M, Wagner, EF. Liver tumor development. c-Jun antagonizes the proapoptotic activity of p53. *Cell* 2003; 112: 181-92.

Gavert, N, Sheffer, M, Raveh, S, Spaderna, S, Shtutman, M, Brabletz, T, Barany, F, Paty, P, Notterman, D, Domany, E, Ben-Ze'ev, A. Expression of L1-CAM and ADAM10 in human colon cancer cells induces metastasis. *Cancer Res* 2007; 67: 7703-12.

Graham, TA, Weaver, C, Mao, F, Kimelman, D, Xu, W. Crystal structure of a β-catenin/Tcf complex. *Cell* 2000; 103: 885-96.

Guo, L, Guo, Y, Xiao, S, Shi, X. Protein kinase p-JNK is correlated with the activation of AP-1 and its associated Jun family proteins in hepatocellular carcinoma. *Life Sci* 2005; 77: 1869-78.

Guo, K, Liu, Y, Zhou, H, Dai, Z, Zhang, J, Sun, R, Chen, J, Sun, Q, Lu, W, Kang, X, Chen, P. Involvement of protein kinase C β-extracellular signal-regulating kinase 1/2/p38 mitogen-activated protein kinase-heat shock protein 27 activation in hepatocellular carcinoma cell motility and invasion. *Cancer Sci* 2008: 99: 486-96.

Harada, N, Miyoshi, H, Murai, N, Oshima, H, Tamai, Y, Oshima, M, Taketo, MM. Lack of tumorigenesis in the mouse liver after adenovirus-mediated expression of a dominant stable mutant of β-catenin. *Cancer Res* 2002; 62: 1971-7.

Harada, N, Oshima, H, Katoh, M, Tamai, Y, Oshima, M, Taketo, MM. Hepatocarcinogenesis in mice with β-catenin and Ha-ras gene mutations. *Cancer Res* 2004; 64: 48-54.

Hommura, F, Furuuchi, K, Yamazaki, K, Ogura, S, Kinoshita, I, Shimizu, M, Moriuchi, T, Katoh, H, Nishimura, M, Dosaka-Akita, H. Increased expression of β-catenin predicts better prognosis in non-small cell lung carcinomas. *Cancer* 2002; 94: 752-8.

Hoshida, Y, Villanueva, A, Kobayashi, M, Peix, J, Chiang, DY, Camargo, A, Gupta, S, Moore, J, Wrobel, MJ, Lerner, J, Reich, M, Chan, JA, Glickman, JN, Ikeda, K, Hashimoto, M, Watanabe, G, Daidone, MG, Roayaie, S, Schwartz, M, Thung, S, Salvesen, HB, Gabriel, S, Mazzaferro, V, Bruix, J, Friedman, SL, Kumada, H, Llovet, JM, Golub, TR. Gene expression in fixed tissues and outcome in hepatocellular carcinoma. *N Engl J Med* 2008; 359: 1995-2004.

Hsu, HC, Jeng, YM, Mao, TL, Chu, JS, Lai, PL, Peng, SY. β-catenin mutations are associated with a subset of low-stage hepatocellular carcinoma negative for hepatitis B virus and with favorable prognosis. *Am J Pathol* 2000; 157: 763-70.

Huang, H, Fuji, H, Sankila, A, Mahler-Araujo, BM, Matsuda, M, Cathomas, G, Ohgaki, H. β-catenin mutations are frequent in human hepatocellular carcinomas associated with hepatitis C virus infection. *Am J Pathol* 1999; 155: 1795-801.

Huber, AH, Nelson, WJ, Weis, WI. Three-dimensional structure of the armadillo repeat region of β-catenin. *Cell* 1997; 90: 871-82.

Huelsken, J, Behrens, J. The Wnt signaling pathway. *J Cell Sci* 2002; 115, 3977-8.

Huelsken, J, Birchmeier, W. New aspects of Wnt signaling pathways in higher vertebrates. *Curr Opin Genet Dev* 2001; 11: 547-53.

Hui, L, Zatloukal, K, Scheuch, H, Stepniak, E, Wagner, EF. Proliferation of human HCC cells and chemically induced mouse liver cancers requires JNK1-dependent p21 downregulation. *J Clin Invest* 2008; 118: 3943-53.

Inagawa, S, Itabashi, M, Adachi, S, Kawamoto, T, Hori, M, Shimazaki, J, Yoshimi, F, Fukao, K. Expression and prognostic roles of β-catenin in hepatocellular carcinoma: correlation with tumor progression and postoperative survival. *Clin Cancer Res* 2002; 8: 450-6.

Ishitani, T, Kishida, S, Hyodo-Miura, J, Ueno, N, Yasuda, J, Waterman, M, Shibuya, H, Moon, RT, Ninomiya-Tsuji, J, Matsumoto, K. The TAK1-NLK mitogen-activated protein kinase cascade functions in the Wnt-5a/Ca2+ pathway to antagonize Wnt/β-catenin signaling. *Mol Cell Biol* 2003; 23: 131-9.

Johnsson, M, Borg, A, Nilbert, M, Andersson, T. Comments on involvement of adenomatous polyposis coli (APC) β-catenin signaling in human breast cancer. *Eur J Cancer* 2000; 36: 242-8.

Katoh, M. WNT/PCP signaling pathway and human cancer. *Oncol Rep* 2005; 14: 1583-8.

Katoh, M, Katoh, M. Cross-talk of Wnt and FGF signaling pathways at GSK3β to regulate β-catenin and Snail signaling cascades. *Cancer Biol Ther* 2006; 5: 1059-64.

Katoh, M, Katoh, M. Notch ligand, JAG1, is evolutionarily conserved target of canonical Wnt signaling pathway in progenitor cells. *Int J Mol Med* 2006b; 17: 681-5.

Kawano, Y, Kypta, R. Secreted antagonists of the Wnt signaling pathway. *J Cell Sci* 2003; 116: 2627-34.

Kim, M, Lee, HC, Tsedensodnom, O, Hartley, R, Lim, YS, Yu, E, Merle, P, Wands, JR. Functional interaction between Wnt3 and Frizzled-7 leads to activation of the Wnt/β-catenin signaling pathway in hepatocellular carcinoma cells. *J Hepatol* 2008; 48: 780-91.

Klaus, A, Birchmeier, W. Wnt signaling and its impact on development and cancer. *Nat Rev Cancer* 2008; 8: 387-98.

Laurent-Puig, P, Legoix, P, Bluteau, O, Belghiti, J, Franco, D, Binot, F, Mones, G, Thomas, G, Bioulac-Sage, P, Zucman-Rossi, J. Genetic alterations associated with hepatocellular carcinomas define distinct pathways of hepatocarcinogenesis. *Gastroenterology* 2001; 120: 1763-73.

Lian, Z, Liu, J, Li, L, Li, X, Clayton, M, Wu, MC, Wang, HY, Arbuthnot, P, Kew, M, Fan, D, Feitelson, MA. Enhanced cell survival of Hep3B cells by the hepatitis B x antigen effector, URG11, is associated with upregulation of β-catenin. *Hepatology* 2006; 43: 415-24.

Lin, SY, Xia, W, Wang, JC, Kwong, KY, Spohn, B, Wen, Y, Pestell, RG, Hung, MC. β-catenin, a novel prognostic marker for breast cancer: its roles in cyclin D1 expression and cancer progression. *Proc Natl Acad Sci USA* 2000; 7: 4262-6.

Liu, C, Li, Y, Semenov, M, Han, C, Baeg, GH, Tan, Y, Zhang, Z, Lin, X, He, X. Control of β-catenin phosphorylation/degradation by a dual-kinase mechanism. *Cell* 2002; 108: 837-47.

Liu, F, Kohlmeier, S, Wang, CY. Wnt signaling and skeletal development. *Cell Signal* 2008; 20: 999-1009.

Llovet, JM, Ricci, S, Mazzaferro, V, Hilgard, P, Gane, E, Blanc, JF, de Oliveira, AC, Santoro, A, Raoul, JL, Forner, A, Schwartz, M, Porta, C, Zeuzem, S, Bolondi, L, Greten, TF, Galle, PR, Seitz, JF, Borbath, I, Häussinger, D, Giannaris, T, Shan, M, Moscovici, M, Voliotis, D, Bruix, J; SHARP Investigators Study Group. Sorafenib in advanced hepatocellular carcinoma. *N Engl J Med* 2008; 359: 378-90.

Lu, Z, Ghosh, S, Wang, Z, Hunter, T. Downregulation of caveolin-1 function by EGF leads to the loss of E-cadherin, increased transcriptional activity of β-catenin, and enhanced tumor cell invasion. *Cancer cell* 2003; 4: 499-515.

Lu, X, Borchers, AG, Jolicoeur, C, et al. PTK7/CCK-4 is a novel regulator of planar cell polarity in vertebrates. *Nature* 2004b; 430: 93-8.

Lu, W, Yamamoto, V, Ortega, B, Baltimore, D. Mammalian Ryk is a Wnt co-receptor required for stimulation of neurite outgrowth. *Cell* 2004; 119: 97-108.

Lu, HC, Chou, FP, Yeh, KT, Chang, YS, Hsu, NC, Chang, JG. Expression of protein kinase C family in human hepatocellular carcinoma. *Pathol Oncol Res* 2010; 16: 385-91.

Merle, P, De la Monte, S, Kim, M, Herrmann, M, Tanaka, S, von dem Bussche, A, Kew, MC, Trepo, C, Wands, JR. Functional consequences of Frizzled-7 receptor overexpression in human hepatocellular carcinoma. *Gastroenterology* 2004; 127: 1110-22.

Merle, P, Kim, M, Herrmann, M, Gupte, A, Lefrançois, L, Califano, S, Trepo, C, Tanaka, S, Vitvitski, L, de la Monte, S, Wands, JR. Oncogenic role of the Frizzled-7/β-catenin pathway in hepatocellular carcinoma. *J Hepatol* 2005; 43: 854-62.

Merle, P, Trepo, C. Molecular mechanisms underlying hepatocellular carcinoma. *Viruses* 2009; 1: 852-72.

Micsenyi, A, Tan, X, Sneddon, T, Luo, JH, Michalopoulos, GK, Monga, SP. β-catenin is temporally regulated during normal liver development. *Gastroenterology* 2004; 126: 1134-46.

Milward, A, Mankouri, J, Harris, M. Hepatitis C virus NS5A protein interacts with β-catenin and stimulates its transcriptional activity in a phosphoinositide-3 kinase-dependent fashion. *J Gen Virol* 2010; 91: 373-81.

Monga, SP, Monga, HK, Tan, X, Mule, K, Pediaditakis, P, Michalopoulos, GK. β-catenin antisense studies in embryonic liver cultures: role in proliferation, apoptosis, and lineage specification. *Gastroenterology* 2003; 124: 202-16.

Morali, OG, Delmas, V, Moore, R, Jeanney, C, Thiery, JP, Larue, L. IGF-II induces rapid β-catenin relocation to the nucleus during epithelium to mesenchyme transition. *Oncogene* 2001; 20: 4942-50.

Nejak-Bowen, KN, Thompson, MD, Singh, S, Bowen, WC, Dar, MJ, Khillan, J, Dai, C, Monga, SPS. Accelerated liver regeneration and hepatocarcinogenesis in mice overexpressing serine-45 mutant β-catenin. *Hepatology* 2010; 51: 1603-13.

Novellino, L, De Filippo, A, Deho, P, Perrone, F, Pilotti, S, Parmiani, G, Castelli, C. PTPRK negatively regulates transcriptional activity of wild type and mutated oncogenic β-catenin and affects membrane distribution of b-catenin/E-cadherin complexes in cancer cells. *Cell Signal* 2008; 20: 872-83.

Ober, EA, Verkade, H, Field, HA, Stainier, DY. Mesodermal Wnt2b signaling positively regulates liver specification. *Nature* 2006; 442: 688-91.

Oishi, I, Suzuki, H, Onishi, N, Takada, R, Kani, S, Ohkawara, B, Koshida, I, Suzuki, K, Yamada, G, Schwabe, GC, Mundlos, S, Shibuya, H, Takada, S, Minami, Y. The receptor tyrosine kinase Ror2 is involved in non-canonical Wnt5a/JNK signaling pathway. *Genes Cells* 2003; 8: 645-54.

Ozawa, M, Baribault, H, Kemler, R. The cytoplasmic domain of the cell adhesion molecule uvomorulin associates with three independent proteins structurally related in different species. *EMBO J* 1989; 8: 1711-7.

Pai, R, Dunlap, D, Qing, J, Mohtashemi, I, Hotzel, K, French, DM. Inhibition of fibroblast growth factor 19 reduces tumor growth by modulating β-catenin signaling. *Cancer Res* 2008; 68: 5086-95.

Park, WS, Oh, RR, Park, JY, Kim, PJ, Shin, MS, Lee, JH, Kim, HS, Lee, SH, Kim, SY, Park, YG, An, WG, Kim, HS, Jang, JJ, Yoo, NJ, Lee, JY. Nuclear localization of β-catenin is an important prognostic factor in hepatoblastoma. *J Pathol* 2001; 193: 483-90.

Park, JY, Park, WS, Nam, SW, Kim, SY, Lee, SH, Yoo, NJ, Lee, JY, Park, CK. Mutations of β-catenin and Axin-I genes are a late event in human hepatocellular carcinogenesis. *Liver Int* 2005; 25: 70-6.

Parkin, DM, Bray, FI, Devesa, SS. Cancer burden in the year 2000. The global picture. *Eur J Cancer* 2001; 37 Suppl 8: S4-66.

Pediaditakis, P, Lopez-Talavera, JC, Petersen, B, Monga, SP, Michalopoulos, GK. The processing and utilization of hepatocyte growth factor/scatter factor following partial hepatectomy in the rat. *Hepatology* 2001; 34: 688-93.

Qian, J, Sarnaik, AA, Bonney, TM, Keirsey, J, Combs, KA, Steigerwald, K, Acharya, S, Behbehani, GK, Barton, MC, Lowy, AM, Groden, J. The APC tumor suppressor inhibits

DNA replication by directly binding to DNA via its carboxyl terminus. *Gastroenterology* 2008; 135: 152-62.

Rhee, J, Buchan, T, Zukerberg, L, Lilien, J, Balsamo, J. Cables links Robo-bound Abl kinase to N-cadherin bound β-catenin to mediate Slit-induced modulation of adhesion and transcription. *Nat Cell Biol* 2007; 9: 883-92.

Rignall, B, Braeuning, A, Buchmann, A, Schwarz, M. Tumor formation in liver of conditional β-catenin-deficient mice exposed to a diethylnitrosamine/phenobarbital tumor promotion regimen. *Carcinogenesis* 2010; 3.

Rimm, DL, Caca, K, Hu, G, Harrison, FB, Fearon, ER. Frequent nuclear/cytoplasmic localization of β-catenin without exon 3 mutations in malignant melanoma. *Am J Pathol* 1999; 154: 325-9.

Robbins, J, Blondel, BJ, Gallahan, D, Callahan, R. Mouse mammary tumor gene int-3: a member of the Notch gene family transforms mammary epithelial cells. *J Virol* 1992; 66: 2594-9.

Roura, S, Miravet, S, Piedra, J, Garcia de Herreros, A, Dunach, M. Regulation of E-cadherin/catenin association by tyrosine phosphorylation. *J Biol Chem* 1999; 274: 36734-40.

Satoh, S, Daigo, Y, Furukawa, Y, Kato, T, Miwa, N, Nishiwaki, T, Kawasoe, T, Ishiguro, H, Fujita, M, Tokino, T, Sasaki, Y, Imaoka, S, Murata, M, Shimano, T, Yamaoka, Y, Nakamura, Y. AXIN1 mutations in hepatocellular carcinomas, and growth suppression in cancer cells by virus-mediated transfer of AXIN1. *Nat Genet* 2000; 24: 245-50.

Shapiro, L, Weis, WI. Structure and biochemistry of cadherins and catenins. *Cold Spring Harb Perspect Biol* 2009; 1: 1-21.

Shtutman, M, Levina, E, Ohouo, P, Baig, M, Roninson, IB. Cell adhesion molecule L1 disrupts E-cadherin containing adherens junctions and increases scattering and motility of MCF7 breast carcinoma cells. *Cancer Res* 2006; 66: 11370-80.

Takagi, H, Sasaki, S, Suzuki, H, Toyota, M, Maruyama, R, Nojima, M, Yamamoto, H, Omata, M, Tokino, T, Imai, K, Shinomura, Y. Frequent epigenetic inactivation of SFRP genes in hepatocellular carcinoma. *J Gastroenterol* 2008; 43: 378-89.

Tan, X, Apte, U, Micsenyi, A, Kotsagrelos, E, Luo, JH, Ranganathan, S, Monga, DK, Bell, A, Michalopoulos, GK, Monga, SP. Epidermal growth factor receptor: a novel target of the Wnt/β-catenin pathway in liver. *Gastroenterology* 2005; 129: 285-302.

Tan, X, Behari, J, Cieply, B, Michalopoulos, GK, Monga, SP. Conditional deletion of β-catenin reveals its role in liver growth and regeneration. *Gastroenterology* 2006; 131: 1561-72.

Taniguchi, K, Roberts, LR, Aderca, IN, Dong, X, Qian, C, Murphy, LM, Nagorney, DM, Burgart, LJ, Roche, PC, Smith, DI, Ross, JA, Liu, W. Mutational spectrum of β-catenin, AXIN1, and AXIN2 in hepatocellular carcinomas and hepatoblastomas. *Oncogene* 2002; 21: 4863-71.

Tolwinski, NS, Wehrli, M, Rives, A, Erdeniz, N, DiNardo, S, Wieschaus, E. Wg/Wnt signal can be transmitted through arrow/LRP5, 6 and Axin independently of Zw3/Gsk3β activity. *Dev Cell* 2003; 4: 407-18.

Ueda, M, Gemmill, RM, Wset, J, Winn, R, Sugita, M, Tanaka, M, Ueki, M, Drabkin, HA. Mutations of the β- and γ-catenin genes are uncommon in human lung, breast, kidney, cervical and ovarian carcinomas. *Br J Cancer* 2001; 85: 64-8.

Veeman, MT, Axelrod, JD, Moon, RT. A second canon. Functions and mechanisms of β-catenin-independent Wnt signaling. *Dev Cell* 2003; 5: 367-77.

White, P, Aberle, H, Vincent, JP. Signaling and adhesion activities of mammalian β-catenin and plakoglobin in Drosophila. *J Cell Biol* 1998; 140: 183-95.

Winter, CG, Wang, B, Ballew, A, Royou, A, Karess, R, Axelrod, JD, Luo, L. Drosophila Rho-associated kinase (Drok) links Frizzled mediated planar cell polarity signaling to the actin cytoskeleton. *Cell* 2001; 105: 81-91.

Wong, CM, Fan, ST, Ng, IO. β-catenin mutation and overexpression in hepatocellular carcinoma: clinicopathologic and prognostic significance. *Cancer* 2001; 92: 136-45.

Wong, HC, Bourdelas, A, Krauss, A, Lee, HJ, Shao, Y, Wu, D, Mlodzik, M, Shi, DL, Zheng, J. Direct binding of the PDZ domain of Dishevelled to a conserved internal sequence in the C-terminal region of Frizzled. *Mol Cell* 2003; 12: 1251-60.

Wu, TT, Hsieh, YH, Wu, CC, Hsieh, YS, Huang, CY, Liu, JY. Overexpression of protein kinase C-α mRNA in human hepatocellular carcinoma: a potential marker of disease prognosis. *Clinica Chimica Acta* 2007; 382: 54-8.

Wu, TT, Hsieh, YH, Hsieh, YS, Liu, JY. Reduction of PKC-α decreases cell proliferation, migration, and invasion of human malignant hepatocellular carcinoma. *J Cell Biochem* 2008; 103: 9-20.

Yuzugullu, H, Benhaj, K, Ozturk, N, Senturk, S, Celik, E, Toylu, A, Tasdemir, N, Yilmaz, M, Erdal, E, Akcali, KC, Atabey, N, Ozturk, M. Canonical Wnt signaling is antagonized by noncanonical Wnt5a in hepatocellular carcinoma cells. *Molecular Cancer* 2009, 8: 1-20.

Zaret, K. Early liver differentiation: genetic potentiation and multi-level growth control. *Curr Opin Genet Dev* 1998; 8: 526-31.

Zaret, KS. Liver specification and early morphogenesis. *Mech Dev* 2000; 92: 83-8.

In: Hepatocellular Carcionoma: A Global Challenge
Editor: Isabelle Chemin
ISBN: 978-1-61470-644-1

Chapter IX

Toll Like Receptors and Hepatocellular Carcinoma

Claudia Zannetti and Uzma Hasan
Innate Immunity, Oncoviruses and Cancer,Faculte de Médecine,
Hopital Lyon Sud, Pierre Benite, France

Abstract

The innate immune response detects pathogen associated molecular patterns (PAMPs) via a panel of pattern recognition receptors (PRRs). Binding of PAMPs to PRRs expressed in a variety of cell types, initiates the innate inflammatory immune response. Hepatitis B virus (HBV) infection leads to chronicity in most cases in which inflammatory responses are some how deregulated.This chapter aims to summarize the different PRR currently identified and how HBV regulates their function post infection.

Innate Immune Receptors (CZ, UH)

The innate immune response is an evolutionally conserved mechanism whose role consists in sensing invading pathogenic microbes. Upon detection of the pathogen the innate system triggers an inflammatory response leading to the recruitment of phagocytes and to activation of dendritic cells (DC) which subsequently leads to the initiation of the adaptive immune response. Innate immune recognition is mediated by pattern recognition receptors (PRRs) which are germline encoded. PRRs have a broad specifity for conserved and invariant microbial motifs known as pathogen associated molecular patterns (PAMPs). These molecular motifs are shared by large groups of microbes, they are generally unique to microorganisms, allowing discrimination between self and non-self and they are essential components of the microbial metabolism, impairing the development of an evasion mechanism of the innate recognition system (Janeway, Jr., 1989).

Once pathogen molecules have been detected by PRRs e.g. in tissue-resident macrophages, an inflammatory response is elicited. Activation of PRRs leads to the production of several antimicrobial proteins, cytokines and chemokines such as type I Interferons (IFNs), tumor necrosis factor (TNF), IL-1, IL-6, IL-8. Type I IFNs (IFN-α and IFN-β) are mainly produced in response to a viral infection and trigger the expression of several proteins with antiviral activities. TNF and IL-1β trigger vasodilatation of the local endothelium, an increase of the permeability of the blood vessels and activation of the endothelial cells to express adhesion molecules allowing the adherence of circulating leucocytes. IL-8 acts as chemotactic factor to recruit neutrophils to the site of infection. TNF triggers immature DCs to mature into fully active antigen presenting cells (APC), to express on the cell surface the co-stimulatory molecules (CD80, CD86) and to migrate to lymph nodes where they can activate naive CD4 T cells to start the adaptive immune response. TNF and IL-1β exert effects also at the systemic level by acting as pyrogens by inducing fever. Moreover TNF-α, IL-1β and IL-6 act within hours on the liver and trigger the hepatocytes to produce acute phase proteins, including the C-reactive proteins and the mannose binding lectin (MBL). These proteins mimic the action of antibodies but have broad specificity for PAMPs since they are able to opsonize the bacteria through the recognition of conserved molecular motifs on the bacterial cell walls, such as phosphocolins and mannose residues respectively. These proteins also induce the activation of the complement cascade, a system of plasma proteins which are able to bind to pathogens and trigger their elimination. Among the acute phase response protein there are the pulmonary surfactant proteins SP-A and SP-D which are found in the alveolar fluid of the lung and which promote the phagocytosis of respiratory pathogens through opsonization. Overall PRRs play a crucial role in the response against pathogens by rapidly eliciting an inflammatory response which is then very important for the activation of the adaptive one.

Over the past fifteen years a vast number of studies led to a more complete characterization of the innate immune receptors. In this part of the chapter we will look more closely at the main characteristics of each receptor class and at the proinflammatory signalling pathways elicited in response to microbial infections.

Toll-like Receptors

Toll-like receptors (TLRs) are the best characterized family of PRRs. They are type I transmembrane glycoproteins, with an ectodomain at the N-terminal that contains several leucine reach repeat (LRR) domains and a cytoplasmic domain with a Toll/IL-1 receptor (TIR) domain. Christallography studies revealed that the LRR region has a horse-shoe shape and that this region is responsible for binding the ligand (Choe et al., 2005; Jin et al., 2007). TLRs are expressed mostly on tissues with a role in immune surveillance (spleen) and on the interfaces between the host and the external environments (mucosal epithelia and skin). TLR have been detected in various immune cells, including macrophages, monocytes, DC, neutrophils, T cells and B cells and also in nonimmune cells including fibroblasts and epithelial cells (Akira et al., 2006). In humans 10 TLRs have been characterized, TLR1 to TLR10. TLR1, 2, 4, 5, and 6 are expressed on the cell surface and recognize mainly constituents of the bacterial cell wall (Akira et al., 2006). TLR2 can form homodimers or heterodimers with TLR1 or TLR6 and plays a major role in recognizing Gram-positive bacteria through the detection of lipoproteins, lipomannans and lipoteichoic acids. TLR4 is classically activated by LPS from Gram-negative bacteria. However a large number of studies demonstrated the role of TLR2 and TLR4 in the detection of PAMPs derived from the cell walls of mycobacteria, fungi and from the capsids of viral origins (Thoma-Uszynski et al., 2001; Netea et al., 2004; Compton et al., 2003). TLR5 detects the bacterial flagellin. TLR3, 7, 8 and 9 are localized intracellularly in the endosomes and they play a crucial role in detecting viral infections through the recognition of nucleic acids. TLR3 is activated by dsRNA, TLR7 and 8 by ssRNA and TLR9 by unmethylated dsDNA (Kawai and Akira, 2006). Upon ligand binding TIR domains undergo conformational change and recruit a set of adaptor molecules including MyD88, TIRAP, TRIF and TRAM. MyD88, essential to all TLRs but TLR3 for signalling transduction, triggers the activation of NF-κB and ATF2-cjun transcription factors and the subsequent expression of inflammatory genes including IL-6, IL-12p40, TNF-α, IL-8. These cytokines are produced in large quantity in response to a bacterial infection. However in the case of viral infection protective responses rely principally on the production of type I IFNs. In pDC, a restricted subset of DCs specialized in secreting high doses of type I IFN, TLR7 and 9 elicit IFN-α production through the activation of IRF7 in a MyD88 dependent pathway (Colonna et al., 2004). Activation of TLR3 through dsRNA involves activation of NF-κB and IRF3 transcription factors via the adaptor molecule TRIF and elicit IFN-β secretion (Alexopoulou et al., 2001).

RLH

RIG-like Helicase receptors, (RLHs) constitute a family of cytoplasmic sensors for viral RNA released in the cytosol of infected cells. TLR3, 7 and 8 expression is largely restricted to immune cells such as DCs that detect infection through the endocytosis of apoptotic bodies of infected cells. Despite them, RLH are found ubiquitously expressed in all cell types and play a crucial role in the direct detection of actively replicating viruses. The best characterized members of this family are RIG-I and MDA-5 (Yoneyama et al., 2008). They share at the N-terminal two caspase recruitment domains (CARD) which are important for signal transduction, a RNA helicase domain with ATPase activity and a zinc binding domain at the C-terminal which is essential for ligand binding. RIG-I recognizes 5' triphosphate ssRNA and short dsRNA while MDA-5 binds to longer dsRNA. These ligands present features that are absent from the host cellular RNA allowing the activation of the antiviral response only in the case of infection. Once activated RIG-I and MDA-5 are recruited to the mitochondria outer membrane and bind to the adaptor protein IPS-1 which triggers the production of IFN-β and the setting of the antiviral response through the activation of the NF-κB and IRF3 pathways. LGP2 is the third member of the RLH family. This receptor lacks the CARD domain and it was shown to act as the negative regulator of RIG-I and MDA-5 signaling. However its role remains controversial, since a positive role against encephalomyocarditis virus (EMCV) infection has been demonstrated (Venkataraman et al., 2007).

A physiological importance of the RLH has been documented by a large court of studies: both RIG-I and MDA-5 are reported to play a protective role against the Newcastle disease virus, Sendai virus, ECMV, Vesicular Stomatitis Virus (VSV) (Yoneyama et al., 2004; Yoneyama et al., 2005).

On the other hand viruses have developed different strategy to counteract the IFN response triggered by RLHs. NS3-4A protease of hepatitis C virus (HCV) cleaves IPS-1 blocking signal transduction (Meylan et al., 2005). V protein from Paramyxovirus associates with MDA-5 and inhibits the downstream signal (Andrejeva et al., 2004).

Nod-like Receptors and the Inflammasome

NOD-like receptors (NLRs) constitute a family of intracellular PRRs of more than 20 members in mammals. Although the ligands and the functions for several of these receptors remain unknown, they have been shown overall to elicit a proinflammatory response upon detection of PAMPs and host danger signals also known as danger associated molecular patterns (DAMPs).

NLR genes consists of three domains with 1) a C-terminal LRR domain for microbial sensing; 2) a nucleotide binding oligomerization domain (NOD); 3) a N-terminal effector region containing a protein-protein interaction domain such as CARD, PYRIN or BIR. NLRs have been classified into three subfamilies according to the effector region composition: the NOD subfamily containing CARD domains, the NALP family with the PYRIN domain and the NAIP family comprising the BIR domain (Fritz et al., 2006; Inohara et al., 2005). NOD1 and NOD2 are the first NLR members reported to respond to cytoplasmic PAMPs by sensing specific elements of the peptidoglycan (PGN) of bacterial cell walls such as iE-DAP and MDP respectively. Upon ligand binding NOD1 and 2 promote NF-κB- and MAPK-dependent gene expression, the production of cytokines and chemokines, the recruitment of neutrophils and the secretion of anti-microbial peptides such as defensins (Inohara et al., 2005). In addition the NOD response has been involved in the onset of the adaptive immune response (Fritz et al., 2006). The response triggered by the NOD proteins appears to be physiologically important since several mutations in their genes have been linked to inflammatory diseases, such as the Crohn's disease (Eckmann et al., 2005).

Recently some members of the NALP subfamily have been reported to sense pathogens and to induce the activation of caspase-1 through the assembly of a multiprotein complex known as inflammasome (Martinon et al., 2002). Caspase-1 activity is responsible for the maturation of IL-1β and IL-18. These cytokines once secreted bind to their receptors and trigger NF-κB and MAPK pathways leading to the activation of several effector pathways. Their activity has been associated to inflammation, induction of immune response and autoimmune diseases. IL-1β effects comprise the induction of fever, the activation of lymphocytes, the recruitment of leukocytes to the site of infection and production of other inflammatory cytokines. IL-18 activates lymphocytes and NK cell and induces IFN-γ which triggers the expression of interferon stimulated genes (ISG) with antiviral functions (Martinon and Tschopp, 2004). *In vitro* studies showed that the production of mature IL-1*β* and IL-18 through the inflammasome requires a multi step mechanism: 1) the transcription of pro-IL-1β and pro-IL-18 triggered by TLR signalling through NF-κB pathway activation; 2) the formation of the inflammasome platform. There are several types of inflammasome, classified according to the NLR family member involved in its composition. The NALP3 inflammasome is the best characterized and comprises NALP3, the adaptor ASC, the protein CARDINAL and the caspase-1. The production of IL-1β and IL-18 cytokines is achieved in vitro supplying macrophages with PAMPs and ATP, which triggers the formation of inflammasome by eliciting the opening of a transmembrane pore and a rapid K^+ efflux from the cytosol. The same effect is triggered with bacterial toxins such as nigericin and maitotoxin, capable of forming holes in the cellular membrane (Mariathasan et al., 2006). Bacterial RNA has been also individuated as a NALP3 inflammasome inducer (Kanneganti et al., 2006).

In addition recent studies showed that NALP3 inflammasome can be triggered in response to molecules produced by the host itself in stress conditions, known as DAMPS. Accumulation of monosodium urate (MSU) and calcium phosphate diydrate (CPPD) christals causes auto-inflammatory diseases known as gout and pseudogout respectively (Martinon et al., 2006). It has been proposed that the inflammasome pathway is involved in the aetiology of these diseases: NALP3 activation is due to phagocytosis of christals which leads eventually to lysosomal rupture and to the consequent presence in the cytosol of lysosomal protease cathepsin B, the molecule sensed by NALP3. Other molecules such as silica and asbestos christals have been shown to activate NALP3 inflammasome with a similar mechanism (Hornung et al., 2008).

Other stimuli such as MDP and the anthrax toxin have been involved in the NALP1 inflammasome activation (Boyden and Dietrich, 2006). Two other NLR family members, IPAF and NAIP5 have been shown to induce inflammasome activation in response to cytosolic flagellin (Franchi et al., 2006; Ren et al., 2006).

The inflammasome activation has been described in a first moment in response to bacterial infections. However several studies showed later the NALP3-dependent IL-1β secretion in response to adenovirus and influenza virus (Muruve et al., 2008; Thomas et al., 2009).

Recently a new PRR has been identified, Absent in Melanoma 2 (AIM2) which detects cytoplasmic dsDNA. Once activated it triggers the formation of an inflammasome with ASC and caspase-1. The AIM-2 inflammasome responds to vaccinia virus infection and triggers the production of IL-1β and a new form of cellular death known as pyroptosis (Hornung et al., 2009; Fernandes-Alnemri et al., 2009).

Overall is becoming clear that inflammasome activity is of central role in innate immunity by mounting an important inflammatory response upon bacterial and viral infections and danger signals. The physiological importance of the inflammasomes is highlighted in *in vivo* studies which show the protective role of the inflammasome response against bacterial and viral injuries (Fernandes-Alnemri et al., 2010; Allen et al., 2009). On the other hand it's becoming evident the link between the inflammasome response and the autoinflammatory diseases (Petrilli and Martinon, 2007). Therefore further investigations are needed to provide new elements on the mechanisms of host defense and the pathogenesis of autoimmunodiseases.

CLRs

C-type lectin receptors (CLRs) constitute a large family of PRRs with an important antifungal function. These proteins are characterized by conserved carbohydrate-recognition domains (CRD) which are important for the recognition of pathogens and the immunoreceptor tyrosin-based activation-like (ITAM-like) domain which is important for signal transduction. CLR are expressed in a large variety of cells including macrophages and DCs.

Dectin-1 is the primary transmembrane receptor on macrophages which mediates phagocytosis of fungi upon detection of β-glucan, an important component of fungal cell walls (Brown et al., 2003). Following Dectin-1 activation phagocytosis is elicited and the ITAM-like domain engages syk kinase. The activity of syk triggers the activation of the NF-κB pathway, the secretion of inflammatory cytokines and the production of reactive O species (ROS) which cause pathogen destruction. It has been reported that dectin-1 and TLR2 work synergistically since they both recognize fungal PAMPs (Gantner et al., 2003). This cooperation is important for an optimal activation of the innate immunity response and the clearance of the infection.

Another member of the CLRs family is the DC-specific intercellular adhesion molecule grabbing nonintegrin (DC-SIGN). This transmembrane receptor not only plays a role in the recognition and phagocytosis of fungal pathogens but is also capable of recognizing viral species including HIV and Ebola virus (den et al., 2009).

The mannose binding lectin (MBL) belongs to the CLR family but despite the members described above is a soluble receptor produced by the liver in the acute phase response. MBL plays a major role in innate immunity against yeast. Its main role consists in the opsonization of pathogens through the binding of repetitive mannose residues on the microbial cell wall leading to opsonization of the pathogen, activation of the complement system and induction of phagocytosis by polymorphonuclear cells (van Asbeck et al., 2008).

HBV and Immune Deregulation (UH)

HBV is a DNA virus characterized by a small genome size and unique replication via reverse transcription. The circular genome has been well exploited, thus limiting genome variation, and leaves no possibility for genes in addition to those essentially needed during the viral live cycle. Hepatitis B viruses are prototype non-cytopathic viruses causing persistent infection. Because infection usually persists for many years, if not lifelong, hepatitis B viruses need efficient mechanisms to hide from the immune response of the host. To escape the immune response, they exploit different strategies in relation to infection of the host cell, hepatocytes. Firstly, they use their structural and non-structural proteins in conjunction to alter the immune response. Secondly, HBV replicates by establishing a pool of stable extrachromosomal transcription templates, which allow the virus to react sensitively to changes in its microenvironment by up- or downregulating gene expression. Thirdly, hepatitis B viruses replicate in the liver which is an immunopriviledged site. These three elements already set the basis for successful immune evasion, yet the host attacks HBV infection by mounting innate and adaptive immune responses. In most cases the viral infection is cleared by the immune response but in certain cases HBV induces cellular transformation of the host cell as well as immune deregulation to persist and promote cancer. The focus in this section is to update our understanding in terms of how can HBV deregulate the first line of immune defence termed the innate immune response. As described previously, innate immune responses consist principally of complement activation, inflammation and anti-viral production of IFN.

The current view is that HBV is a stealth virus, which does not induce innate immunity neither during the acute or chronic phase. This concept was largely established following experiments performed in chimpanzees (Wieland et al., 2004), but also after observations made in human experiencing an acute HBV infection (Stacey et al., 2009; Dunn et al., 2009). In the latter studies, authors monitored the production of cytokine/chemokines in blood (systemic and not intra liver production) and the activation/inhibition of NK and T cell functions. They found that HBV, in contrast to HIV (and HCV to a lesser extent) does not seem to elicit in the majority of patients a strong production of type-I/III IFN, TNF-α, IL-15, IL-6, IL-1β within 10 days after initiation of viral expansion (i.e. increase of DNA level in serum). However the production of IL-10, an NK inhibitory cytokine, was documented in one of the two studies. It was proposed that, in addition to failing to induce some immune mechanisms, HBV could use an immunosuppressive strategy to actively inhibit immune functions (Dunn et al., 2009).

The weak induction of an innate immune response by HBV may be due to poor sensing by the host or potent inhibition by the viral escape strategies. There is increasing evidence which suggests that HBV can inhibit innate responses in chronic hepatitis B (CHB) patients in particular by deregulating TLRs or TLR signalling. A reduction of TLR9 levels (mRNA) which correlated to impaired IFN-α production by pDCs, was observed in CHB patients (Xie et al., 2009). Remarkably, TLR9 but not TLR7 ability to induce secrection of IFN-α in a dose dependent manner was affected. Recently Xu et al., showed that treatment of pDCs with 25 μg of HBsAg led to the secretion of less IFN-α than control cells stimulated with the TLR9 ligand CpG 2216 (Xu et al., 2009). Furthermore, suppression was specific for TLR9, with no effects upon TLR7-mediated IFN-α secretion. Similarly, HIV gp120 and HCV virions have also been shown to suppress TLR9-mediated IFN-α induction without any effect on TLR7 signaling, suggesting that both TLR pathways might differ at yet unidentified levels (Martinelli et al., 2007; Shiina and Rehermann, 2008). Therefore, additional studies are required to clarify the mechanisms involved in HBV specific disruption of TLR9- but not TLR7-mediated activation of pDCs. While several non-viral negative regulators of TLR-mediated immune responses have been identified, only Epstein-Barr and Kaposi's sarcoma viruses were shown to down regulate IFN-α response in pDCs by blocking IRF7 (Cao and Liu, 2007; Liew et al., 2005). Recently shown is the ability of HBsAg to inhibit TLR9 -mediated IRF-7 expression and nuclear translocation which are important for induction of IFN-α gene expression (Xu et al., 2009). Work in our lab has shown that suppression occurred early after CpG stimulation and was associated with a decrease in TLR9 transcription. Furthermore neutralising CpG motifs were found to suppress TLR9 immune activation (Vincent et al submitted). Indeed, HBV has been shown to interfere with the IFN-α signaling pathway in HBV-expressing hepatocytes (Christen et al., 2007), and a recent study by Wang et al showed that HBV polymerase has the ability to down-regulate the transcription of the IFN-β gene by inhibiting the interaction between IKKε and DDX3 DEAD box known to enhance IFN-β production (Wang and Ryu, 2010). HBV has been also shown to suppress poly(deoxyadenylate-thymidylate)-activated IFN-β production in hepatocytes. Specifically, hepatitis B virus X (HBX) interacted with MAVS and promoted the degradation of MAVS through Lys^{136} ubiquitin in MAVS protein, thus preventing the induction of IFN-β (Wei et al., 2010). Thus distinct mechanisms may be involved in hepatocytes and pDCs, which, respectively, do not express TLR9 and are not permissive to HBV infection (Untergasser et al., 2006).

Due to the abundance of Kupffer cells (i.e. liver-specific macrophages; KC), natural killer (NK) cells, and natural killer T (NKT), the liver is considered as an organ with innate immune features and is therefore thought to play an active role in the first line host defense against pathogens. In addition parenchymal (i.e. hepatocytes) and non-parenchymal cell types (e.g. LSEC) can also have immuno-regulatory functions, by secreting cytokines in response to infection. Infected cells can detect the presence of viral components or PAMPs (pathogen associated molecular patterns) via cellular sensors or PRRs. Engagement of those innate immune receptors can lead to production of antiviral type-I (and typeIII) IFNs, as well as other pro-inflammatory cytokines (e.g. IL-1β, IL-6…). Down regulation of TLR2 in PBMCs as well as kupffer cells and hepatocytes were observed in HBeAg positive patients (Visvanathan et al., 2007). This may suggest an immunomoduloatory role for this secreted viral protein. Observed in a murine model the only TLR ligand that did induce an anti-HBV effect was a TLR2 ligand (Isogawa et al., 2005), suggesting suppression of TLR2 expression. These hypothesis were corroborated in PBMCs from CHB patients whom expressed lower levels of TLR1, 2 4 and 6 mRNA Vs healthy donors. In addition the cytokine levels produced when TLR2 or 4 ligands were added dropped in CHB patients (Chen et al., 2008). Finally, using the HBV transgenic mouse model, it was also demonstrated that HBV (either purified virions, HBeAg or HBsAg) suppresses the innate response elicited by TLR3 and TLR4 stimulation of hepatocytes and non parenchymal liver cells (Wu et al., 2009). This correlated with the suppression of IFN-β production and subsequent decrease in the activation of interferon-stimulated genes (*e.g.*, MxA, IP-10, NFκB, or pERK) (Wu et al., 2009).

References

Akira,S., Uematsu,S., and Takeuchi,O. (2006). Pathogen recognition and innate immunity. *Cell 124*, 783-801.

Alexopoulou,L., Holt,A.C., Medzhitov,R., and Flavell,R.A. (2001). Recognition of double-stranded RNA and activation of NF-kappaB by Toll-like receptor 3. *Nature 413*, 732-738.

Allen,I.C., Scull,M.A., Moore,C.B., Holl,E.K., Elvania-TeKippe,E., Taxman,D.J., Guthrie,E.H., Pickles,R.J., and Ting,J.P. (2009). The NLRP3 inflammasome mediates in vivo innate immunity to influenza A virus through recognition of viral RNA. *Immunity. 30*, 556-565.

Andrejeva,J., Childs,K.S., Young,D.F., Carlos,T.S., Stock,N., Goodbourn,S., and Randall,R.E. (2004). The V proteins of paramyxoviruses bind the IFN-inducible RNA helicase, mda-5, and inhibit its activation of the IFN-beta promoter. *Proc. Natl. Acad. Sci. U. S. A 101*, 17264-17269.

Boyden,E.D. and Dietrich,W.F. (2006). Nalp1b controls mouse macrophage susceptibility to anthrax lethal toxin. *Nat. Genet. 38*, 240-244.

Brown,G.D., Herre,J., Williams,D.L., Willment,J.A., Marshall,A.S., and Gordon,S. (2003). Dectin-1 mediates the biological effects of beta-glucans. *J. Exp. Med. 197*, 1119-1124.

Cao,W. and Liu,Y.J. (2007). Innate immune functions of plasmacytoid dendritic cells. *Curr. Opin. Immunol. 19*, 24-30.

Chen,Z., Cheng,Y., Xu,Y., Liao,J., Zhang,X., Hu,Y., Zhang,Q., Wang,J., Zhang,Z., Shen,F., and Yuan,Z. (2008). Expression profiles and function of Toll-like receptors 2 and 4 in peripheral blood mononuclear cells of chronic hepatitis B patients. *Clin. Immunol. 128*, 400-408.

Choe,J., Kelker,M.S., and Wilson,I.A. (2005). Crystal structure of human toll-like receptor 3 (TLR3) ectodomain. *Science 309*, 581-585.

Christen,V., Duong,F., Bernsmeier,C., Sun,D., Nassal,M., and Heim,M.H. (2007). Inhibition of alpha interferon signaling by hepatitis B virus. *J. Virol. 81*, 159-165.

Colonna,M., Trinchieri,G., and Liu,Y.J. (2004). Plasmacytoid dendritic cells in immunity. *Nat. Immunol. 5*, 1219-1226.

Compton,T., Kurt-Jones,E.A., Boehme,K.W., Belko,J., Latz,E., Golenbock,D.T., and Finberg,R.W. (2003). Human cytomegalovirus activates inflammatory cytokine responses via CD14 and Toll-like receptor 2. *J. Virol. 77*, 4588-4596.

den,D.J., Gringhuis,S.I., and Geijtenbeek,T.B. (2009). Innate signaling by the C-type lectin DC-SIGN dictates immune responses. *Cancer Immunol. Immunother. 58*, 1149-1157.

Dunn,C., Peppa,D., Khanna,P., Nebbia,G., Jones,M., Brendish,N., Lascar,R.M., Brown,D., Gilson,R.J., Tedder,R.J., Dusheiko,G.M., Jacobs,M., Klenerman,P., and Maini,M.K. (2009). Temporal analysis of early immune responses in patients with acute hepatitis B virus infection. *Gastroenterology 137*, 1289-1300.

Eckmann,L., Karin,M., Fritz,J.H., Le,B.L., Sellge,G., Magalhaes,J.G., Fsihi,H., Kufer,T.A., Collins,C., Viala,J., Ferrero,R.L., Girardin,S.E., and Philpott,D.J. (2005). NOD2 and Crohn's disease: loss or gain of function? Nod1-mediated innate immune recognition of peptidoglycan contributes to the onset of adaptive immunity. *Immunity. 22*, 661-667.

Fernandes-Alnemri,T., Yu,J.W., Datta,P., Wu,J., and Alnemri,E.S. (2009). AIM2 activates the inflammasome and cell death in response to cytoplasmic DNA. *Nature 458*, 509-513.

Fernandes-Alnemri,T., Yu,J.W., Juliana,C., Solorzano,L., Kang,S., Wu,J., Datta,P., McCormick,M., Huang,L., McDermott,E., Eisenlohr,L., Landel,C.P., and Alnemri,E.S. (2010). The AIM2 inflammasome is critical for innate immunity to Francisella tularensis. *Nat. Immunol. 11*, 385-393.

Franchi,L., Amer,A., Body-Malapel,M., Kanneganti,T.D., Ozoren,N., Jagirdar,R., Inohara,N., Vandenabeele,P., Bertin,J., Coyle,A., Grant,E.P., and Nunez,G. (2006). Cytosolic flagellin requires Ipaf for activation of caspase-1 and interleukin 1beta in salmonella-infected macrophages. *Nat. Immunol. 7*, 576-582.

Fritz,J.H., Ferrero,R.L., Philpott,D.J., and Girardin,S.E. (2006). Nod-like proteins in immunity, inflammation and disease. *Nat. Immunol. 7*, 1250-1257.

Gantner,B.N., Simmons,R.M., Canavera,S.J., Akira,S., and Underhill,D.M. (2003). Collaborative induction of inflammatory responses by dectin-1 and Toll-like receptor 2. *J. Exp. Med. 197*, 1107-1117.

Hornung,V., Ablasser,A., Charrel-Dennis,M., Bauernfeind,F., Horvath,G., Caffrey,D.R., Latz,E., and Fitzgerald,K.A. (2009). AIM2 recognizes cytosolic dsDNA and forms a caspase-1-activating inflammasome with ASC. *Nature 458*, 514-518.

Hornung,V., Bauernfeind,F., Halle,A., Samstad,E.O., Kono,H., Rock,K.L., Fitzgerald,K.A., and Latz,E. (2008). Silica crystals and aluminum salts activate the NALP3 inflammasome through phagosomal destabilization. *Nat. Immunol. 9*, 847-856.

Inohara, Chamaillard, McDonald,C., and Nunez,G. (2005). NOD-LRR proteins: role in host-microbial interactions and inflammatory disease. *Annu. Rev. Biochem. 74*, 355-383.

Isogawa,M., Robek,M.D., Furuichi,Y., and Chisari,F.V. (2005). Toll-like receptor signaling inhibits hepatitis B virus replication in vivo. *J. Virol. 79*, 7269-7272.

Janeway,C.A., Jr. (1989). Approaching the asymptote? Evolution and revolution in immunology. *Cold Spring Harb. Symp. Quant. Biol. 54 Pt 1*, 1-13.

Jin,M.S., Kim,S.E., Heo,J.Y., Lee,M.E., Kim,H.M., Paik,S.G., Lee,H., and Lee,J.O. (2007). Crystal structure of the TLR1-TLR2 heterodimer induced by binding of a tri-acylated lipopeptide. *Cell 130*, 1071-1082.

Kanneganti,T.D., Ozoren,N., Body-Malapel,M., Amer,A., Park,J.H., Franchi,L., Whitfield,J., Barchet,W., Colonna,M., Vandenabeele,P., Bertin,J., Coyle,A., Grant,E.P., Akira,S., and Nunez,G. (2006). Bacterial RNA and small antiviral compounds activate caspase-1 through cryopyrin/Nalp3. *Nature 440*, 233-236.

Kawai,T. and Akira,S. (2006). Innate immune recognition of viral infection. *Nat. Immunol. 7*, 131-137.

Liew,F.Y., Xu,D., Brint,E.K., and O'Neill,L.A. (2005). Negative regulation of toll-like receptor-mediated immune responses. *Nat. Rev. Immunol. 5*, 446-458.

Mariathasan,S., Weiss,D.S., Newton,K., McBride,J., O'Rourke,K., Roose-Girma,M., Lee,W.P., Weinrauch,Y., Monack,D.M., and Dixit,V.M. (2006). Cryopyrin activates the inflammasome in response to toxins and ATP. *Nature 440*, 228-232.

Martinelli,E., Cicala,C., Van,R.D., Goode,D.J., Macleod,K., Arthos,J., and Fauci,A.S. (2007). HIV-1 gp120 inhibits TLR9-mediated activation and IFN-{alpha} secretion in plasmacytoid dendritic cells. *Proc. Natl. Acad. Sci. U. S. A 104*, 3396-3401.

Martinon,F., Burns,K., and Tschopp,J. (2002). The inflammasome: a molecular platform triggering activation of inflammatory caspases and processing of proIL-beta. *Mol. Cell 10*, 417-426.

Martinon,F., Petrilli,V., Mayor,A., Tardivel,A., and Tschopp,J. (2006). Gout-associated uric acid crystals activate the NALP3 inflammasome. *Nature 440*, 237-241.

Martinon,F. and Tschopp,J. (2004). Inflammatory caspases: linking an intracellular innate immune system to autoinflammatory diseases. *Cell 117*, 561-574.

Meylan,E., Curran,J., Hofmann,K., Moradpour,D., Binder,M., Bartenschlager,R., and Tschopp,J. (2005). Cardif is an adaptor protein in the RIG-I antiviral pathway and is targeted by hepatitis C virus. *Nature 437*, 1167-1172.

Muruve,D.A., Petrilli,V., Zaiss,A.K., White,L.R., Clark,S.A., Ross,P.J., Parks,R.J., and Tschopp,J. (2008). The inflammasome recognizes cytosolic microbial and host DNA and triggers an innate immune response. *Nature 452*, 103-107.

Netea,M.G., Van der,G.C., Van der Meer,J.W., and Kullberg,B.J. (2004). Recognition of fungal pathogens by Toll-like receptors. *Eur. J. Clin. Microbiol. Infect. Dis. 23*, 672-676.

Petrilli,V. and Martinon,F. (2007). The inflammasome, autoinflammatory diseases, and gout. *Joint Bone Spine 74*, 571-576.

Ren,T., Zamboni,D.S., Roy,C.R., Dietrich,W.F., and Vance,R.E. (2006). Flagellin-deficient Legionella mutants evade caspase-1- and Naip5-mediated macrophage immunity. *PLoS. Pathog. 2*, e18.

Shiina,M. and Rehermann,B. (2008). Cell culture-produced hepatitis C virus impairs plasmacytoid dendritic cell function. *Hepatology 47*, 385-395.

Stacey,A.R., Norris,P.J., Qin,L., Haygreen,E.A., Taylor,E., Heitman,J., Lebedeva,M., DeCamp,A., Li,D., Grove,D., Self,S.G., and Borrow,P. (2009). Induction of a striking systemic cytokine cascade prior to peak viremia in acute human immunodeficiency virus type 1 infection, in contrast to more modest and delayed responses in acute hepatitis B and C virus infections. *J. Virol. 83*, 3719-3733.

Thoma-Uszynski,S., Stenger,S., Takeuchi,O., Ochoa,M.T., Engele,M., Sieling,P.A., Barnes,P.F., Rollinghoff,M., Bolcskei,P.L., Wagner,M., Akira,S., Norgard,M.V., Belisle,J.T., Godowski,P.J., Bloom,B.R., and Modlin,R.L. (2001). Induction of direct antimicrobial activity through mammalian toll-like receptors. *Science 291*, 1544-1547.

Thomas,P.G., Dash,P., Aldridge,J.R., Jr., Ellebedy,A.H., Reynolds,C., Funk,A.J., Martin,W.J., Lamkanfi,M., Webby,R.J., Boyd,K.L., Doherty,P.C., and Kanneganti,T.D. (2009). The intracellular sensor NLRP3 mediates key innate and healing responses to influenza A virus via the regulation of caspase-1. *Immunity. 30*, 566-575.

Untergasser,A., Zedler,U., Langenkamp,A., Hosel,M., Quasdorff,M., Esser,K., Dienes,H.P., Tappertzhofen,B., Kolanus,W., and Protzer,U. (2006). Dendritic cells take up viral antigens but do not support the early steps of hepatitis B virus infection. *Hepatology 43*, 539-547.

van Asbeck,E.C., Hoepelman,A.I., Scharringa,J., Herpers,B.L., and Verhoef,J. (2008). Mannose binding lectin plays a crucial role in innate immunity against yeast by enhanced complement activation and enhanced uptake of polymorphonuclear cells. *BMC. Microbiol. 8*, 229.

Venkataraman,T., Valdes,M., Elsby,R., Kakuta,S., Caceres,G., Saijo,S., Iwakura,Y., and Barber,G.N. (2007). Loss of DExD/H box RNA helicase LGP2 manifests disparate antiviral responses. *J. Immunol. 178*, 6444-6455.

Visvanathan,K., Skinner,N.A., Thompson,A.J., Riordan,S.M., Sozzi,V., Edwards,R., Rodgers,S., Kurtovic,J., Chang,J., Lewin,S., Desmond,P., and Locarnini,S. (2007). Regulation of Toll-like receptor-2 expression in chronic hepatitis B by the precore protein. *Hepatology 45*, 102-110.

Wang,H. and Ryu,W.S. (2010). Hepatitis B virus polymerase blocks pattern recognition receptor signaling via interaction with DDX3: implications for immune evasion. *PLoS. Pathog. 6*, e1000986.

Wei,C., Ni,C., Song,T., Liu,Y., Yang,X., Zheng,Z., Jia,Y., Yuan,Y., Guan,K., Xu,Y., Cheng,X., Zhang,Y., Yang,X., Wang,Y., Wen,C., Wu,Q., Shi,W., and Zhong,H. (2010). The hepatitis B virus X protein disrupts innate immunity by downregulating mitochondrial antiviral signaling protein. *J. Immunol. 185*, 1158-1168.

Wieland,S., Thimme,R., Purcell,R.H., and Chisari,F.V. (2004). Genomic analysis of the host response to hepatitis B virus infection. *Proc. Natl. Acad. Sci. U. S. A 101*, 6669-6674.

Wu,J., Meng,Z., Jiang,M., Pei,R., Trippler,M., Broering,R., Bucchi,A., Sowa,J.P., Dittmer,U., Yang,D., Roggendorf,M., Gerken,G., Lu,M., and Schlaak,J.F. (2009). Hepatitis B virus suppresses toll-like receptor-mediated innate immune responses in murine parenchymal and nonparenchymal liver cells. *Hepatology 49*, 1132-1140.

Xie,Q., Shen,H.C., Jia,N.N., Wang,H., Lin,L.Y., An,B.Y., Gui,H.L., Guo,S.M., Cai,W., Yu,H., Guo,Q., and Bao,S. (2009). Patients with chronic hepatitis B infection display deficiency of plasmacytoid dendritic cells with reduced expression of TLR9. *Microbes. Infect. 11*, 515-523.

Xu,Y., Hu,Y., Shi,B., Zhang,X., Wang,J., Zhang,Z., Shen,F., Zhang,Q., Sun,S., and Yuan,Z. (2009). HBsAg inhibits TLR9-mediated activation and IFN-alpha production in plasmacytoid dendritic cells. *Mol. Immunol. 46*, 2640-2646.

Yoneyama,M., Kikuchi,M., Matsumoto,K., Imaizumi,T., Miyagishi,M., Taira,K., Foy,E., Loo,Y.M., Gale,M., Jr., Akira,S., Yonehara,S., Kato,A., and Fujita,T. (2005). Shared and unique functions of the DExD/H-box helicases RIG-I, MDA5, and LGP2 in antiviral innate immunity. *J. Immunol. 175*, 2851-2858.

Yoneyama,M., Kikuchi,M., Natsukawa,T., Shinobu,N., Imaizumi,T., Miyagishi,M., Taira,K., Akira,S., and Fujita,T. (2004). The RNA helicase RIG-I has an essential function in double-stranded RNA-induced innate antiviral responses. *Nat. Immunol. 5*, 730-737.

Yoneyama,M., Onomoto,K., and Fujita,T. (2008). Cytoplasmic recognition of RNA. Adv. *Drug Deliv. Rev. 60*, 841-846.

In: Hepatocellular Carcionoma: A Global Challenge
Editor: Isabelle Chemin
ISBN: 978-1-61470-644-1

Chapter X

Epigenetic Changes in Hepatocellular Carcinoma

Anupam Paliwal[1,2] ***and Zdenko Herceg***[1,*]
[1]Epigenetics Group, International Agency for Research on Cancer (IARC), Lyon, France
[2]Institute for Cancer Genetics, Columbia University Medical Center, New York, NY, US

Abstract

Epigenetic mechanisms can be viewed as an interface between the genome and environmental influences. Aberrant epigenetic events associated with viral infection and various environmental factors are likely to play an important role in the onset and progression of different human cancers, including hepatocellular carcinoma (HCC). At the cellular level, aberrant epigenetic events may deregulate critical cellular events, such as gene expression, DNA damage response and DNA repair, cell cycle checkpoints, and carcinogen detoxification, all of which may contribute to the initiation and progression of liver cancer. In this review, we summarize recent progress in our understanding of epigenetic mechanisms by which viral agents and environmental factors may promote hepatocarcinogenesis. Although we focus on epigenetic changes and risk factors involved in liver cancer, similar mechanisms may operate in the development of other cancer types.

Hepatocellular Carcinoma

Hepatocellular carcinoma (HCC) accounts for 85–90% of all primary liver cancers and is the third most common cause of cancer-related death worldwide. Annually, more than

* Correspondence: Dr Zdenko Herceg, PhD. Epigenetics Group, International Agency for Research on Cancer (IARC), 150 cours Albert Thomas, 69372 Lyon cedex 08, France. Phone: +33 4 72 73 83 98 ; Fax: +33 4 72 73 83 29 ; Email: herceg@iarc.fr.

620,000 new patients are diagnosed with HCC, and approximately the same number, 600,000, die because of the disease. The general prognosis is poor with overall survival rates of 3–5% [1,2,3]. The development and progression of HCC is typical of a multistage process. The transformation begins in the liver tissue undergoing chronic hepatitis or cirrhosis caused by risk factor(s) (hepatitis B virus (HBV) or hepatitis C virus HCV infection, intake of aflatoxin B1 or alcohol abuse), progresses through a series of hyperplastic and dysplastic stages, and ultimately acquires the malignant phenotype [1,2,3,4,5]. The incidence and progression of HCC involve the deregulation of critical cellular genes by both genetic and epigenetic mechanisms (Figure 1). Moreover, from recent reports it is becoming increasingly evident that aberrant epigenetic states may predispose genetic changes and the disrupted genetic architecture may further initiate the series of aberrant epigenetic events.

Epigenetic Modifications

The field of epigenetics has been receiving remarkable attention over recent years, owing to the awareness that epigenetic mechanisms are essential for normal development and maintenance of tissue-specific gene expression patterns in mammals. Disruption of epigenetic processes can lead to altered gene function and malignant cellular transformation. The term "epigenetics" defines studies of heritable changes in gene expression and chromatin organization that are not encoded in the genomic DNA itself. This heritability of gene expression patterns is mediated by epigenetic modifications, which include methylation of cytosine bases in DNA, posttranslational modifications of histone proteins, RNA-interference as well as the positioning of nucleosomes along the DNA. The complement of these modifications, collectively referred to as the epigenome, provides a mechanism for cellular diversity by regulating what genetic information can be accessed by cellular machinery [3,4,6,7,8].

DNA Methylation in HCC

Aberrant DNA methylation is an epigenetic mechanism of gene silencing in a wide range of human cancers, including liver cancer. This epigenetic silencing, either alone or in combination with genetic changes, may lead to the inactivation of tumor suppressor genes and other cancer-associated genes promoting hepatocarcinogenesis. Several recent studies have identified aberrant CpG methylation of many genes in HCC. Abnormal DNA methylation for RASSF1A, p16, SYK, CRABP1, GSTP1, SFRP1, GAAD45a and p15 tumor suppressor genes, is associated with HCC, while those at the *CHFR (checkpoint with forkhead associated and ring finger)* and *SKY (spleen tyrosine kinase)*, are detected specifically in advanced stages of HCC [4,9,10]. Moreover, HCC tumors exhibit specific DNA methylation signatures associated with major risk factors and tumor progression stage, indicating potential clinical applications of these epigenetic changes in diagnosis and prognosis of HCC [9,11].

In addition to altering promoter specific methylation patterns, HCC onset and progression induces genomic instability, activation of oncogenes or transposons and promotes tumorigenesis by altering methylation states of repetitive sequences. Cancer cell genomes undergo global hypomethylation, with malignant cells having 20–60% less genomic 5-methylcytosine than their normal counterparts. This loss is accomplished mainly by hypomethylation of the repetitive DNA sequences, which account for 20–30% of the human genome. The methylation level of LINE1 repetitive element and satellite 2 (SAT2) in pericentromeric satellite regions reportedly decreases along with the progression of chronic hepatitis and HCC [9,12,13].

DNA methylation is also used as a common cellular defense mechanism to silence invading foreign DNA and viral genomes. Investigations show that the HBV genome is hypermethylated in both premalignant (cirrhosis) and malignant (HCC) tissues, compared to nontumor liver tissues, suggesting that hypermethylation of the viral genome must also be strongly associated with the malignant process. However, the exact biological significance of the observed methylation in the HBV genome and its role in HCC remain unclear [14,15].

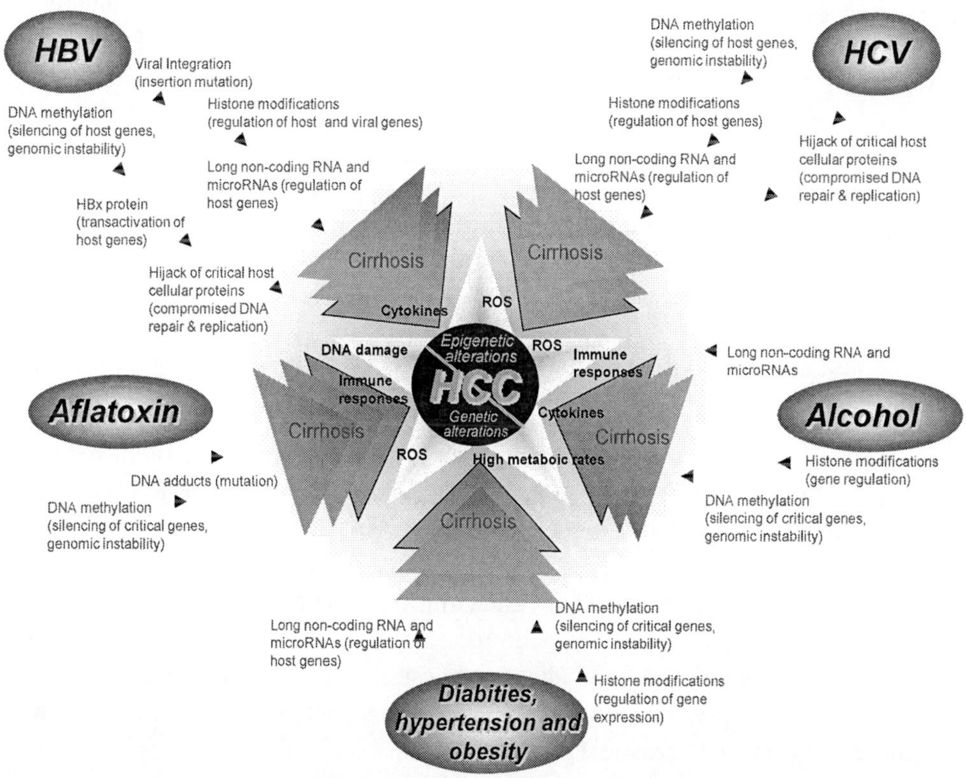

Figure 1. Genetic and epigenetic events associated with the main risk factors in the onset of hepatocellularcarcinoma.

Histone Modification in HCC

Histone (chromatin) modifications define covalent posttranslational modifications of histone proteins. The fundamental unit of chromatin is the nucleosome, which consists of 146 base pairs of genomic DNA wrapped around an octamer of 4 core histones. The N-terminal tails of nucleosomal histones are subject to different modifications including acetylation, methylation, phosphorylation and ubiquitination [8]. HCC's have been reported to display altered histone modification machinery and as a result an altered cellular epigenetic state. Patt1 (a GNAT family acetyltransferase) is highly expressed in a normal healthy liver and is downregulated in hepatocellular carcinoma. Similarly, a histone-modification, dimethylation of histone H3 at lysine 4 (H3K4diMe) remains almost undetectable in HCC [4,16]. Certain histone code alterations exhibit risk-factor specificity, e.g., HCV infection induces methylation of histone H4 on arginine 3 and plays an important role in DNA repair by dephosphorylating the damage-induced phosphorylation of H2AX (γ-H2AX). In fact alteration of these important histone marks is considered to be a very critical early event in hepatocarcinogenesis, in the context of chronic viral hepatitis [4,8,17]. Similarly, HBV encoded protein X (HBx), has been reported to directly interact with CBP/P300 complex possessing histone acetyltransferase activity, resulting in an acetylated (active) histone state of the target cellular genes [3,15,18,19]. HBx has also been reported to result in repressive marks via its interaction with a histone deacetylase (HDAC) [20]. However, it remains possible that different risk-factor exposures and life-style or environmental cues may affect different histone modifications, which may ultimately modulate the HCC initiation and progression.

Noncoding RNA in HCC

Another mechanism of epigenetic inheritance involved in HCC is micro and long noncoding RNA mediated RNA interference. Micro or long noncoding RNA can interfere with transcription or translation of target gene mRNA via RNA interference, altering the gene expression states [4,6,7]. In HCC several miRNAs are deregulated. Some function as oncogenes (miR-221), promote cell invasion (miR-9), inhibit migration and proliferation (miR23b) or act as tumor suppressors (miR-101, 195, 122, 338). miR-122, in HCC, regulates the metastatic properties. These findings suggest that RNA interference, mediated via different RNA could play important roles in HCC and thus may serve as potential novel molecular targets for HCC treatment [4,6,21].

Conclusion

Being specific to different risk-factor exposures epigenetic events (DNA methylation, histone modifications and RNA interference) form a signature (epigenetic signature), which holds the potential to serve as an important biomarker for early detection and prevention of

HCC [4,7,9]. Moreover, unlike genetic changes, epigenetic changes are reversible and hence many efforts and resources have been mobilized in the development of different therapeutic approaches that are known as "epigenetic therapies" [3]. However, it needs to be emphasized that although different epigenetic events have been described/studied separately, to better understand them, all epigenetic events are interdependent and they collectively define the epigenetic state of an individual cell in a given tissue for each individual. Examples of the crosstalk between different epigenetic modifications and their roles in the regulation of cellular processes and tumorigenesis are becoming more evident and remain important towards understanding and developing better epigenetics based theraputic regimes.

References

[1] K. Schutte, J. Bornschein, P. Malfertheiner, Hepatocellular carcinoma--epidemiological trends and risk factors, *Dig Dis* 27 (2009) 80-92.

[2] H.B. El-Serag, K.L. Rudolph, Hepatocellular carcinoma: epidemiology and molecular carcinogenesis, *Gastroenterology* 132 (2007) 2557-2576.

[3] N.I. Herath, B.A. Leggett, G.A. MacDonald, Review of genetic and epigenetic alterations in hepatocarcinogenesis, *J Gastroenterol Hepatol* 21 (2006) 15-21.

[4] J. Huang, Current progress in epigenetic research for hepatocarcinomagenesis, *Sci China C Life Sci* 52 (2009) 31-42.

[5] H. Nordenstedt, D.L. White, H.B. El-Serag, The changing pattern of epidemiology in hepatocellular carcinoma, *Dig Liver Dis 42 Suppl* 3 S206-214.

[6] Z. Herceg, Epigenetics and cancer: towards an evaluation of the impact of environmental and dietary factors, *Mutagenesis* 22 (2007) 91-103.

[7] P.A. Jones, S.B. Baylin, The epigenomics of cancer, *Cell* 128 (2007) 683-692.

[8] C. Sawan, T. Vaissiere, R. Murr, Z. Herceg, Epigenetic drivers and genetic passengers on the road to cancer, *Mutat Res* 642 (2008) 1-13.

[9] I. Tischoff, A. Tannapfe, DNA methylation in hepatocellular carcinoma, *World J Gastroenterol* 14 (2008) 1741-1748.

[10] N. Nishida, T. Nagasaka, T. Nishimura, I. Ikai, C.R. Boland, A. Goel, Aberrant methylation of multiple tumor suppressor genes in aging liver, chronic hepatitis, and hepatocellular carcinoma, *Hepatology* 47 (2008) 908-918.

[11] H. Hernandez-Vargas, M.P. Lambert, F. Le Calvez-Kelm, G. Gouysse, S. McKay-Chopin, S.V. Tavtigian, J.Y. Scoazec, Z. Herceg, Hepatocellular carcinoma displays distinct DNA methylation signatures with potential as clinical predictors, *PLoS One* 5 e9749.

[12] D.F. Calvisi, S. Ladu, A. Gorden, M. Farina, J.S. Lee, E.A. Conner, I. Schroeder, V.M. Factor, S.S. Thorgeirsson, Mechanistic and prognostic significance of aberrant methylation in the molecular pathogenesis of human hepatocellular carcinoma, *J Clin Invest* 117 (2007) 2713-2722.

[13] S.B. Baylin, DNA methylation and gene silencing in cancer, *Nat Clin Pract Oncol* 2 Suppl 1 (2005) S4-11.

[14] P. Kaur, A. Paliwal, D. Durantel, P. Hainaut, J.Y. Scoazec, F. Zoulim, I. Chemin, Z. Herceg, DNA methylation of hepatitis B virus (HBV) genome associated with the development of hepatocellular carcinoma and occult HBV infection, *J Infect Dis* 202 700-704.

[15] A.F. Fernandez, M. Esteller, Viral epigenomes in human tumorigenesis, *Oncogene* 29 1405-1420.

[16] C. Magerl, J. Ellinger, T. Braunschweig, E. Kremmer, L.K. Koch, T. Holler, R. Buttner, B. Luscher, I. Gutgemann, H3K4 dimethylation in hepatocellular carcinoma is rare compared with other hepatobiliary and gastrointestinal carcinomas and correlates with expression of the methylase Ash2 and the demethylase LSD1, *Hum Pathol* 41 181-189.

[17] F.H. Duong, V. Christen, S. Lin, M.H. Heim, Hepatitis C virus-induced up-regulation of protein phosphatase 2A inhibits histone modification and DNA damage repair, *Hepatology* 51 741-751.

[18] J. Lupberger, E. Hildt, Hepatitis B virus-induced oncogenesis, *World J Gastroenterol* 13 (2007) 74-81.

[19] Z. Herceg, A. Paliwal, HBV protein as a double-barrel shot-gun targets epigenetic landscape in liver cancer, *J Hepatol* 50 (2009) 252-255.

[20] D.L. Zheng, L. Zhang, N. Cheng, X. Xu, Q. Deng, X.M. Teng, K.S. Wang, X. Zhang, J. Huang, Z.G. Han, Epigenetic modification induced by hepatitis B virus X protein via interaction with de novo DNA methyltransferase DNMT3A, *J Hepato*l 50 (2009) 377-387.

[21] L. Gramantieri, F. Fornari, E. Callegari, S. Sabbioni, G. Lanza, C.M. Croce, L. Bolondi, M. Negrini, MicroRNA involvement in hepatocellular carcinoma, *J Cell Mol Med* 12 (2008) 2189-2204.

In: Hepatocellular Carcionoma: A Global Challenge
Editor: Isabelle Chemin
ISBN: 978-1-61470-644-1

Chapter XI

MicroRNAs in Liver Cancer

Pascal Pineau*
Unité d'Organisation Nucléaire et Oncogenèse, INSERM U993, Institut Pasteur, Paris, France

Introduction

Hepatocellular carcinoma (HCC) is a highly malignant tumor that invariably kills patients not eligible for surgical procedures [1]. This appalling situation is primarily due to the late detection of patients with a locally advanced tumor. Furthermore, hepatocytes, the transformed cells that form the tumor, are specialized in detoxification, an originally beneficial function that makes them almost naturally resistant to anticancer chemotherapy [2]. Since decades, HCC incidence is steadily increasing worldwide and the tumor represents now a serious concern for public health [3].

The recent progress of genomics and genetics stimulate an intense research aiming at the identification of suitable therapeutic targets in HCC. However, contrasting with the situation prevailing in other major human cancers, the proportion of HCC devoid of any mutations targeting oncogenes or oncosuppressors remains high. In European patients, for example, p53 and beta-catenin mutations barely affect, in any populations, half of the samples analyzed, leaving investigators without any clues about the molecular alterations present in a large proportion of tumor specimens [4]. Gene expression profiling appeared once as useful tool to proceed beyond the shortcomings of genomic DNA analysis as HCC transcriptome is usually characterized by aberrant expressions of thousands of genes [5]. For a small subset of affected genes, de novo DNA methylation represents an important mechanism underlying a decrease of gene expression. However, the molecular bases driving most changes are still poorly understood [6].

* Pascal Pineau, pascal.pineau@pasteur.fr, tel : 33 1 45 68 88 24, fax : 33 1 45 68 89 43.

These disappointing observations provide a rationale for the rush toward microRNAs, a new and potentially « drugable » class of major players in liver tumorigenesis. MicroRNAs, are a highly conserved class of non coding RNA present in all metazoans, endowed of the capacity to destabilize messenger RNAs (mRNA) through Watson-Crick interaction with the 3' untranslated region of messengers [7]. In the liver cells, microRNAs may find potential targets among some major but paucimutated or never mutated tumor suppressor genes endowed with long 3' untranslated regions (e.g. PTEN, RB1, APC, SMAD4). On the opposite, protooncogenes almost never mutated in liver cells, as RAS-RAF or MYC genes may be preserved by the downregulation of their primary foes belonging to the lethal-7 family of microRNAs. The aim of the present chapter is to summarize our current knowledge about microRNAs in HCC.

The Cell: A World of Small Non Coding RNAs

Mammalian cells are roamed by different families of endogenous small non coding RNAs (ncRNAs). Most of them are housekeeping RNAs such as rRNA, tRNA, snRNA (among them snoRNA), and SRP RNA [8].

Ribosomal RNAs (rRNAs) represent the RNA component of ribosomes and tRNA or Transfer RNA are the 74-95 nucleotides RNA molecules that transfer amino acid during translation. SRP RNA is the RNA component of the Signal recognition ribonucleoprotein complex that directs the traffic of proteins within cells. Small nuclear RNA (snRNAs) are involved in RNA splicing, regulation of certain transcription factors and RNA polymerase II or maintenance of the telomeres. They are included in ribonucleoproteic complexes. The most important class of snRNA are the Small Nucleolar RNAs (SnoRNAs) a class of RNA molecules that catalyzes the maturation (methylation, pseudoridylation) of ribosomal RNAs.

Centromeric heterochromatin is composed of highly repetitive DNA (satellite) that produce small non-coding RNA molecules required for maintaining the heterochromatin state and centromeric stability. Abnormal epigenetic marks and subsequent alterations of protein recruitment in these regions are suspected to represent major causes of chromosomal instability and aneuploidy in tumors. However, experimental data about this class of nc RNAs, of potential major importance in liver cancer, is scarce [9]. Furthermore, a large fraction of genomic ultraconserved regions encode a particular set of ncRNAs whose expression is altered in human cancers. Genome-wide profiling revealed that UCRs have distinct signatures in human leukemias and carcinomas. It has been shown that the inhibition of a selected UCR expression induces apoptosis in colon cancer cells [10].

The last category of ncRNA is composed of two subsets of small regulatory RNAs found in mammalian cells. The largest class is the Piwi-interacting RNA or piRNA a group of 26-31 nucleotides RNAs without sequence conservation involved in the transcriptional silencing of retrotransposons in germline cells [11, 12].

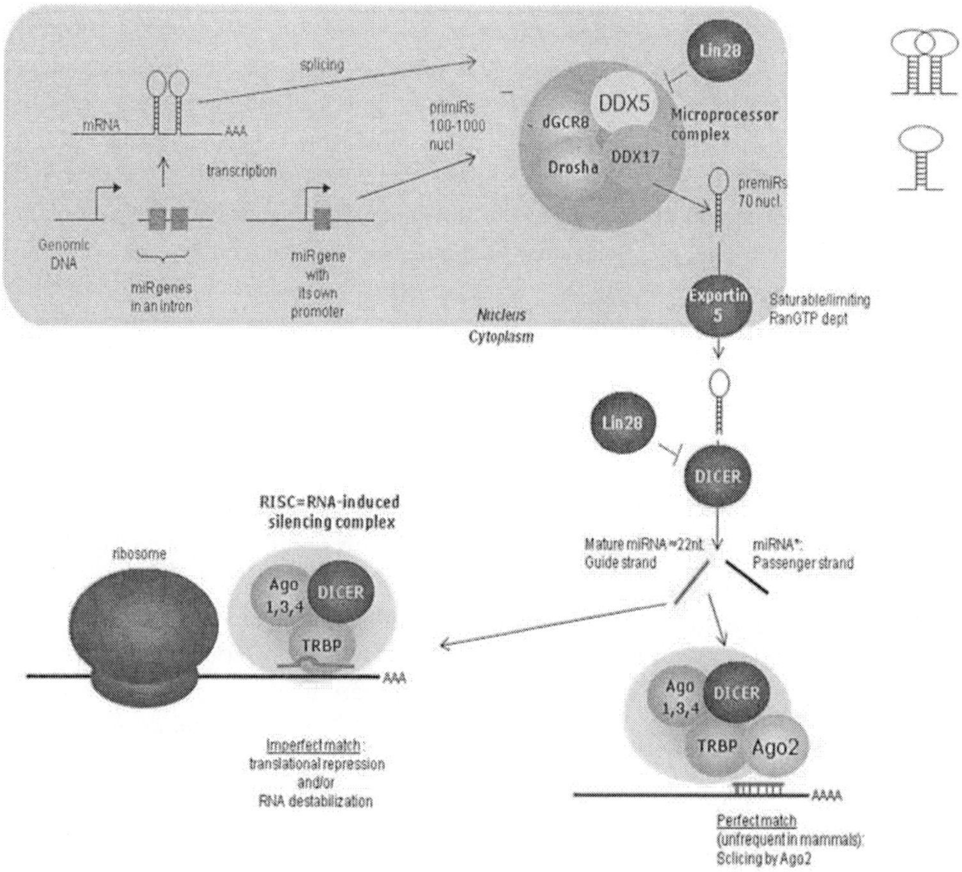

Figure 1. Major steps of miRNA biogenesis and activity.

The last class, microRNAs (21-24 nucleotides), on which this chapter will focus, represents a subset of nc small RNAs that recently attracted a considerable attention because of their role in development, physiology and diseases. microRNA repsent 1-5 % of all RNA expressed in mammalian cells.

MicroRNA Biogenesis Pathway

MicroRNAs are a family of single-stranded RNAs usually transcribed by RNA polymerase II (see Figure 1). MiRNAs genes have their own promoters when they are intergenic but the majority is mapping within introns. Following transcription, a series of biochemical steps will convert the primary miRNA transcript (pri-miRNA) to a mature miRNA. The first step takes place in the nucleus and is characterized by the recognition of the pri-miRNA by the microprocessor complex (composed of Drosha, a RNase and DGCR8) [13, 14]. The reaction results in the cleavage and removal of the sequences flanking the stem-loop structure of the pri-miRNA that is called from now pre-miRNA. The pre-miRNA is then exported from the nucleus according to a saturable and RAN-GTP dependant mechanism by

Exportin 5. The digestion of the bulge is then carried out by the ribonuclease Dicer. The guide strand of the loop i.e. the mature miRNA is subsequently loaded on the RNA-induced silencing complex (RISC) within the P-bodies (processing bodies) in the cytoplasm whereas the passenger strand (sometime named miRNA*) is usually degraded [14].

The RISC complex, containing argonaute proteins and TRBP, will interact with its target in the 3' untranslated region of messenger RNAs through a sequence specific base pairing that result in case of extensive annealing in an Ago2-catalyzed mRNA cleavage [15]. Alterations of major components of the miRNA processing machinery have been seldom described in hepatocellular carcinoma. Recently, it was shown that mice with hepatocyte-specific inactivation of DiGeorge syndrome critical region gene 8 (DGCR8) are miRNAs deficient and exhibit a delay in cell cycle progression after partial hepatectomy indicating that microRNAs exerts a significant control of liver regeneration. Another murine model emphasizes the crucial role of miRNA in hepatocyte homeostasy [16]. Liver conditional knock-out of Dicer-1 in mice triggers a strong apoptosis of hepatocytes. However, some Dicer-1 -/- cells survive and two thirds of the mice will develop spontaneous HCC at one year of age [17]. Recently, a series of consistent inhibitors of miRNA biogenesis were described. The most relevant in tumor process are embryonic proteins of the LIN28 family, commonly expressed in stem cells, they are usually absent from terminally differentiated cells. LIN28 messenger were found overpexressed in primary liver cancers. Their expression was inversely correlated with that of the lethal-7 (let-7) family of tumor suppressors miRNA. It seems that LIN28 proteins have the capacity to prevent the processing of miRNAs by DROSHA and DICER RNAses [18, 19].

Different Modalities of Messenger Repression

Each highly conserved mammalian miRNA targets mRNA of hundred of distinct genes. Most protein coding genes are, thus, regulated by this mechanism. Initially, mammalian miRNAs were thought to repress protein output essentially through translation inhibition [20, 21]. However, recent work indicates that the outcome of miRNA action in mammals is predominantly a mRNA « destabilization » less drastic than the exceptional Argonaute2-catalyzed slicing of the target [22]. Destabilization usually necessitates, in the first place, the base pairing to the 5' region of the miRNA, centered on nucleotides 2-7, known as the seed. This motif is the most highly conserved region of metazoan miRNAs. It has been noticed that mammalian protein-coding genes are submitted to selection pressure to maintain in their 3'UTR pairing to the seed of one or more miRNAs, an observation that strenghtens the importance of miRNAs in the fine tuning of gene expression. Recently, a novel class of miRNA target sites, the centered-sites, that use nt 4-15 of miRNAs have been described [23]. Molecular events driving to mRNA destabilization are currently poorly understood but plausibly linked to deadenylation or decapping [24].

Liver, Realm of miR-122

Before focusing on global miRNAs expression changes in primary liver cancer, it is necessary to describe a major player in liver cells: miR-122. Early work has shown that miR-122 is specifically expressed in the liver, where it constitutes around 70% of the total miRNA content [25]. It is one of the tissue-specific microRNAs thought to be important for establishing pattern of gene expression that may be responsible for maintaining the differentiated state of tissue. Mapping in 18q21.3, miR-122 expression was shown to follow a circadian rhythm in mice and to be primarily dependent on liver-enriched transcription factors (HNF1a, HNF4a, FOXA1 and FOXA2) [26, 27]. miR-122 is already highly expressed in embryonic liver at 9 weeks of age [28]. Unsurprisingly, miR-122 abundance is associated with a remarkable pleiotropy.

MiR-122 inhibition by antisense oligonucleotide in mice resulted in reduced plasma cholesterol levels, increased fatty acid oxidation and decreased liver synthesis of cholesterol and fatty-acid [29]. These effects were associated with a 2.5-fold increase of AMPK activity. Moreover, liver transcriptome analysis of mice depleted for miR-122 by antagomirs has shown that most of the genes induced are normally repressed in the liver, implying hepatocytes dedifferentiation in case of miR-122 decrease [30].

MiRNAs are considered as key determinants controlling virus infection in mammalian host. It has been demonstrated that miR-122 binds to the 5' nontranslational region of Hepatitis C virus (HCV) and is implicated in positively regulating the replication of HCV. Furthermore, antisense oligonucleotide depletion of DICER or miR-122 inhibits HCV replication and virion production [31, 32]. It seems that in contrast to the common action of miRNAs, HCV uses miR-122 in a way that enhances its efficiency of translation [33]. It was shown recently, that patients with chronic hepatitis C who have low miR-122 pretreatment levels will later poorly respond to interferon therapy [34].

Finally, it has been shown that miR-122 is repressed in a large subset (50-70%) of liver tumors [35, 36]. Samples with low miR-122 are generally associated with poor prognosis, the suppression of hepatocyte differentiation and the acquisition of invasive properties [37]. The stable restoration of miR-122 expression in hepatocellular carcinoma cell lines suppresses proliferation [27]. The position of miR-122 is however far to be settled as it has been reported to be overexpressed in HCV-associated HCC [38].

The role of other liver-enriched miRNAs as miR-192 and miR-194 is still poorly defined [28] [39].

Profiling Methods

Aberrations of microRNAs expression levels have been detected in every type of human tumors analyzed so far and represent the main mechanism of microRNAs alterations in cancer cells. MiRNAs are thus proposed to function as tumor suppressor genes or as oncogenes (called frequently oncomiRs) [40, 41].

The apparition of microRNAs among the majors concerns of scientists and clinicians corresponds fortunately to the genomics era. Thus, microRNAs analysis was from the onset submitted to unbiased approaches. MicroRNAs expression profiling already provided a great wealth of informations about the variations of microRNAs repertoire in diseases and in the refinement of molecular taxonomy of tumors. It is the case for human hepatocellular carcinoma for which different groups already defined miRNAs signatures. Uncertainties still remain, however, as the number of microRNAs present in human genome is still rising from 300-400 few years ago to around 1500 in 2010 [42, 43]. So far, no HCC profiling was performed an exhaustive set of miRNA (1500 are predicted and 1100 are in miRBAse v.16.0 in 2010) and therefore the exact picture of HCC miRNome remains to be taken [44, 45].

Various technologies were used from the onset to produce HCC microtranscriptome (or miRnome) analysis : hybridization of microbeads, high-density microarray, or large-scale real-time qPCR relying or not on microfluidic technologies [46-49]. More recently appeared the highly praised deep sequencing method that enables the production of unbiased transcriptomic data. This technology was applied to the sequencing of miRNA in 3 normal livers and two matching HCC/NT liver pairs [39].

Alterations of miRNAs Expression within HCC

The first systematic analysis of primary liver cancer samples for miRNAs (n=3) was a bead-based flow cytometric expression profiling [47]. The major interest of the study was that tumor from the gastrointestinal [50] tract were clustering together (liver between stomach and pancreatic cancers) suggesting that miRNAs expression is primarily driven by developmental origin. The second salient feature of the report was that most of the miRNAs had lower expression in tumours than in normal tissues irrespective of cell type suggesting that miRNAs expression reflects the state of cellular differentiation.

A major issue of initial miRNome analyses was the definition of a liver cancer signature from the comparison of tumors and matching non-tumor counterparts. [36, 38, 42, 51-55]. The first microRNAs expression profiling dedicated to HCC was published in 2006 by Murakami *et al.* [42]. Twenty-five couples of HCC and matching non-tumorous livers of various etiologies were hybridized on microarrays containing 180 mature and 206 precursor miRNAs. The microtranscriptome enabled the classification between tumor and non-tumorous samples with a remarkable accuracy (97%) implying that miRNAs may be used for early HCC detection. Since then, at least nine surveys reported microRNAs signature of HCC. A meta-analysis of these studies will be, of course useful, but rather difficult to perform as techniques, risk factors and populations studied are amazingly diverse. However, a set a miRNAs which expression is consistantly altered in HCC can be picked-up from the review of these studies.

Table 1. MiRNA species with a recurrently altered expression when compared to non tumor livers in large scale expression studies green arrows indicate decrease whereas red arrows signal increase of expression

MiRNA	Hou et al. T/NT	Gramantieri et al. T/NT	Su et al. T/NT	Ura et al. T/NT	Jiang et al. T/NT	Pineau et al. T/NT	Varnholt et al. T/NT	Huang et al. T/NT	Murakami et al. T/NT	Li et al. T/NT	Ladeiro et al. T/NT	**Score Transfo**
	deep-seq	custom array	Ohio custom ar	qPCR	qPCR	custom array	qPCR	custom array	custom array	custom ar	qPCR	
miR-101			↘		↘					↘		○○○
miR-122	↘	↘		↘							↘	○○○○
mir-125b-2	⑨		↘	↘								○○○
miR-130a		↘		↘		↘						○○○
miR-139				↘	↘							○○
miR-142		↘				↘						○○
miR-145		↘					↘					○○
miR-150		↘			↘	↘						○○○
miR-195		↘	↘						↘			○○○
miR-198							↘	↘				○○
miR-199a		↘	↘	↘	↘	↘			↘			○○○○○○
miR-199a*	⑨			↘	↘				↘			○○○○
miR-199b		↘	↘		↘	↘	↘					○○○○○
miR-200b		↘		↘	↘	↘						○○○○
miR-214		↘			↘	↘	↘			↘		○○○○○
miR-223		↘	↘	↘	↘							○○○○
miR-29c	⑨		↘				↘			↘		○○○○
miR-99a	⑨		↘	↘								○○○
miR-15a							↗	⑧				○○
miR-18			↗		↗							○○
miR-21	↗			↗	↗						↗	○○○○
miR-221		↗		↗	↗	↗		↗		↗		○○○○○○
miR-222			↗	↗		↗				↗	↗	○○○○○
miR-224			↗			↗			↗		↗	○○○○
miR-25			↗							↗		○○
miR-301				↗	↗							○○
miR-34a								↗		↗		○○
miR-93			↗					↗				○○

The analysis of currently available microRNAs profiling in HCC indicate that the most consistently repressed miRNAs are miR-214, miR-199a, miR-199b, and miR-223 (see Table 1) whereas miR-221, miR-222, miR-21 and miR-224 are found recurrently activated in HCC.

Alterations of miRNAs expression is apparently an early phenomenon. Varnholt and colleagues have shown a modest (2-3 fold) but systematic increase of expression of a large subset of miRNAs in hepatitic or cirrhotic livers of patients with HCC when compared to benign livers of patients without HCC or without chronic liver diseases [38]. Hepatitis B was associated with stronger changes of miRNAs expression in non-tumour livers than hepatitis C. The authors suggest that increased transcription of selected miRNAs represent a response to the cellular stress associated with inflammation and subsequent folate deficiency.

miRNAs and HCC Risk Factors

In their seminal study, Murakami and colleagues did not observed any differences of miRNAs expression between HBV-positive and HCV-positive tumors [42]. However, subsequent reports consistently found differential expression of selected miRNAs between HBV abd HCV-infected specimens. In a french series of HCC, miR-96 was associated with hepatitis B virus infection and miR-126* with alcohol abuse [56]. In a study performed in China, HBV-associated HCC were characterized by higher miR-122a and lower miR-210 expression [57]. Kaneko and colleagues report the differential expression of 19 miRNAs by comparing HBV(+) and HCV(+) HCCs or corresponding non-tumorous livers [55]. Differences of miRNAs expression were reproduced in HuH7 cells replicating HCV or HBV. Authors consider that it exists infection-specific subset of miRNAs controlling pathways in hepatocytes. The miRNAs repressed in HCV-associated tumors (e.g. miR-133b) were mostly associated with immune response whereas those repressed in the HBV group regulates primarily cell death and DNA damage (let-7a, miR-34].

miRNAs and Prognosis

Various prognostic signatures of HCC have been established for messenger RNAs [50]. Similar attempts using miRNAs profiling have been recently performed. In a survey on 241 HCC samples from China, Budhu et al. Identified those miRNAs differentially expressed in case of vascular invasion [58]. A supervised approach enables authors to define a 20-miRNAs metastatic signature that significantly coincides with survival as well. A striking feature, of the work is the narrow range of miRNAs variation levels (0.48 and 1.51 fold for the most repressed and activated respectively). In that survey, 16 out 20 miRNAs representing the metastatic signature were downregulated in the invasive form of HCC. Similar results were published by Varnholt et al. Who described a 19 miRNAs signature associated with disease outcome. Patients with reduced miRNA expression had a poorer survival than those with higher expression [38]. Only one candidate is associated with a majority of prognosis signatures [38, 57, 58)]. Inded, miR-125b is consistently found repressed in HCC patients with short survival. miR-125b is known for its ability to decrease lin28 and ERBB2-3 levels [59, 60]. In addition, a miR-125b isomir (miR-125b-2, 21q11-21) was found homozygously deleted in lung cancer cell lines [61]. Recurrent homozygous deletions represent highly significant events affecting primarily major oncosuppressors (CDKN2A-p16, TP53, PTEN, etc...) in cancer cells. However, as often observed for miRNAs the case of miR-125b is far to be settled. Indeed, consistent evidences showed that it can behave as an oncomiR and a resistance determinant in selected tumor types by targeting p53 and other proapoptotic genes [62, 63, 64].

Functional Analyses of miRNAs

Once identified, expression changes are usually followed by further exploration to decypher the biologial significance of these alterations within tumors. The analyses includes the panel of functional assays usually performed in cancer research (colony or foci formation, tumor formation in nude mouse xenograft model, luciferase reporter assay, etc...).

Another major aspect of most papers dealing with microRNA is the identification of relevant targets. Preliminary steps are dedicated to the manipulation of prediction programs that usually provide the scientist with an overwhelming list of potential targets. The choice of the relevant target that intervenes thereafter is dictated by the context but may appear in several instances as guided by personal intuitions of researchers [60-64].

Conclusion

The genetic pathology of HCC is still poorly known although tremendous efforts are currently produced to identify major somatic alterations governing liver tumor process. Recently, a high-resolution sequence identifying 11000 mutations in a single case of HCC was published [65]. However, despite the presence of mutation affecting the « usual suspects » as p53 or AXIN1 none of the other mutations found was apparently recovered from a validation set of 96 HCCs. Such a despairing situation suggests that the long awaited breakthrough in the domain of HCC genetics is still possibly bound to the characterization of the role of the small non coding RNA, one of the remaining « unexplored continent » in the field. Furthermore and with regard to the activity of microRNAs in particular, it will be necessary in a near future to broaden our conceptions. As shown in a recent paper, miRNAs are not always acting the way we think they do [66] and I cannot resist to quote *in extenso* a sentence from the outstanding review published by K. Breving : « Taken together, a single miRNA has the ability to regulate multiple targets in both negative and positive ways using miRNA-binding sites located throughout the mRNA transcript » [19]. This statement, althouth it is making our position significantly less confortable than previously thought, is merely recreational when we consider some lately published data that indicate a potential direct involvement of miRNAs in the control of gene expression [67].

References

[1] Burroughs A, Hochhauser D, Meyer T. Systemic treatment and liver transplantation for hepatocellular carcinoma: two ends of the therapeutic spectrum. *Lancet Oncol* 2004;5:409-18.

[2] Johnson P. Hepatocellular Carcinoma : is current therapy really altering outcome ? *Gut* 2002;51:459-62.

[3] Parkin D, Bray F, Ferlay J, Pisani P. Estimating the world cancer burden: Globocan 2000. *Int J Cancer* 2001;94:153-6.

[4] Pineau P, Marchio A, Battiston C, et al. In Human Hepatocellular Carcinoma, Chromosome Instability depends on p53 Status and Aflatoxin Exposure. *Mutat Res* 2008;653:6-13.

[5] Hoshida Y, Villanueva A, Kobayashi M, et al. Gene expression in fixed tissues and outcome in hepatocellular carcinoma. *N Engl J Med* 2008;359:1995-2004.

[6] Calvisi D, Ladu S, Gorden A, et al. Mechanistic and prognostic significance of aberrant methylation in the molecular pathogenesis of human hepatocellular carcinoma. *J Clin Invest* 2007;117:2713-22.

[7] Wiemer E. The role of microRNAs in cancer : no small matter. *European J Cancer* 2007;43:1529-44.

[8] Meli M, lbert-Fournier B, Maurel M. Recent findings in the modern RNA world. *Int Microbiol* 2001;4:5-11.

[9] Pezer Z, Ugarković D. Role of non-coding RNA and heterochromatin in aneuploidy and cancer. *Semin Cancer Biol* 2008;18:123-30.

[10] Calin G, Liu C, Ferracin M, et al. Ultraconserved regions encoding ncRNAs are altered in human leukemias and carcinomas. *Cancer Cell* 2007;12:215-29.

[11] Liu Q, Paroo Z. Biochemical principles of small RNA pathways. *Annu Rev Biochem* 2010;79::295-319.

[12] Choudhuri S. Lesser known relatives of miRNA. *Biochem Biophys Res Commun* 2009;388:177-80.

[13] Newman M, Hammond S. Emerging paradigms of regulated microRNA processing. *Genes Dev* 2010;24:1086-92.

[14] He L, Hannon G. MicroRNAs: small RNAs with a big role in gene regulation. *Nat Rev Genet* 2004;5:522-31.

[15] Schmittgen T. Regulation of microRNA processing in development, differentiation and cancer. *J Cell Mol Med* 2008;12:1811-9.

[16] Song G, Sharma A, Roll G, et al. MicroRNAs control hepatocyte proliferation during liver regeneration. *Hepatology* 2010;51:1735-43.

[17] Sekine S, Ogawa R, Ito R, et al. Disruption of Dicer1 induces dysregulated fetal gene expression and promotes hepatocarcinogenesis. *Gastroenterology* 2009;136::2304-15.

[18] Viswanathan S, Powers J, Einhorn W, et al. Lin28 promotes transformation and is associated with advanced human malignancies. *Nat Genet* 2009;41:843-8.

[19] Breving K, Esquela-Kerscher A. The complexities of microRNA regulation: mirandering around the rules. *Int J Biochem Cell Biol* 2010;42:1316-29.

[20] Baek D, Villén J, Shin C, Camargo F, Gygi S, Bartel D. The impact of microRNAs on protein output. *Nature* 2008;455:64-71.

[21] Bartel D. MicroRNAs: target recognition and regulatory functions. *Cell* 2009;136:215-33.

[22] Guo H, Ingolia N, Weissman J, Bartel D. Mammalian microRNAs predominantly act to decrease target mRNA levels. *Nature* 2010;466:835-40.

[23] Shin C, Nam J, Farh K, Chiang H, Shkumatava A, Bartel D. Expanding the microRNA targeting code: functional sites with centered pairing. *Mol Cell* 2010;38:789-802.

[24] Chekulaeva M, Filipowicz W. Mechanisms of miRNA-mediated post-transcriptional regulation in animal cells. *Curr Opin Cell Biol* 2009;21:452-60.

[25] Lagos-Quintana M, Rauhut R, Yalcin A, Meyer J, Lendeckel W, Tuschl T. Identification of tissue-specific microRNAs from mouse. *Curr Biol* 2002;12:735-9.

[26] Gatfield D, Le Martelot G, Vejnar C, et al. Integration of microRNA miR-122 in hepatic circadian gene expression. *Genes Dev* 2009;23:1313-26.

[27] Xu H, He J, Xiao Z, et al. Liver-enriched transcription factors regulate MicroRNA-122 that targets CUTL1 during liver development. *Hepatology* 2010;52:1431-42.

[28] Tzur G, Israel A, Levy A, et al. Comprehensive gene and microRNA expression profiling reveals a role for microRNAs in human liver development. *PLoS ONE* 2009;4:e7511.

[29] Esau C, Davis S, Murray S, et al. miR-122 regulation of lipid metabolism revealed by in vivo antisense targeting. *Cell Metab* 2006;3:87-98.

[30] Krützfeldt J, Rajewsky N, Braich R, et al. Silencing of microRNAs in vivo with 'antagomirs'. *Nature* 2005;438:685-9.

[31] Jopling C, Yi M, Lancaster A, Lemon S, Sarnow P. Modulation of hepatitis C virus RNA abundance by a liver-specific MicroRNA. *Scienc*e 2005;309:1577-81.

[32] Randall G, Panis M, Cooper J, et al. Cellular cofactors affecting hepatitis C virus infection and replication. *Proc Natl Acad Sci U S* A 2007;104:12884-9.

[33] Henke J, Goergen D, Zheng J, et al. microRNA-122 stimulates translation of hepatitis C virus RNA. *EMBO J* 2008;27::3300-10.

[34] Sarasin-Filipowicz M, Krol J, Markiewicz I, Heim M, Filipowicz W. Decreased levels of microRNA miR-122 in individuals with hepatitis C responding poorly to interferon therapy. *Nat Med* 2009;15:31-3.

[35] Kutay H, Bai S, Datta J, et al. Downregulation of miR-122 in the rodent and human hepatocellular carcinomas. *J Cell Biochem* 2006;99:671-8.

[36] Gramantieri L, Ferracin M, Fornari F, et al. Cyclin G1 is a target of miR-122a, a microRNA frequently down-regulated in human hepatocellular carcinoma. *Cancer Res* 2007;67:6092-9.

[37] Coulouarn C, Factor V, Andersen J, Durkin M, Thorgeirsson S. Loss of miR-122 expression in liver cancer correlates with suppression of the hepatic phenotype and gain of metastatic properties. *Oncogene* 2009;28:3526-36.

[38] Varnholt H, Drebber U, Schulze F, et al. MicroRNA gene expression profile of hepatitis C virus-associated hepatocellular carcinoma. *Hepatology* 2008;47:1223-32.

[39] Hou J, Lin L, Zhou W, et al. Identification of miRNomes in human liver and hepatocellular carcinoma reveals miR-199a/b-3p as therapeutic target for hepatocellular carcinoma. *Cancer Cell* 2011;19:232-43.

[40] Esquela-Kerscher A, Slack F. Oncomirs - microRNAs with a role in cancer. *Nat Rev Cancer* 2006;6:259-69.

[41] Hammond S. MicroRNAs as tumor suppressors. *Nat Genet* 2007;39:582-3.

[42] Murakami Y, Yasuda T, Saigo K, et al. Comprehensive analysis of microRNA expression patterns in hepatocellular carcinoma and non-tumorous tissues. *Oncogene* 2006;25:2537-45.

[43] Shao N, Hu H, Yan Z, et al. Comprehensive survey of human brain microRNA by deep sequencing. *BMC Genomics* 2010;11:409.

[44] Bentwich I, Avniel A, Karov Y, Aharonov R, Gilad S. Identification of hundreds of conserved and nonconserved human microRNAs. *Nat Genet* 2005;37:766-70.

[45] Ryu S, Joshi N, McDonnell K, et al. Discovery of novel human breast cancer microRNAs from deep sequencing data by analysis of pri-microRNA secondary structures. *PLoS One* 2011;6:e16403.

[46] Liu C, Calin G, Meloon B, et al. An oligonucleotide microchip for genome-wide microRNA profiling in human and mouse tissues. *Proc Natl Acad Sci U S A* 2004;101:9740-4.

[47] Lu J, Getz G, Miska E, et al. MicroRNA expression profiles classify human cancers. *Nature* 2005;435:834-8.

[48] Schmittgen T, Jiang J, Liu Q, Yang L. A high-throughput method to monitor the expression of microRNA precursors. *Nucleic Acids Res* 2004;32:e43.

[49] Yin J, Zhao R, Morris K. Profiling microRNA expression with microarrays. *Trends Biotechnol* 2007;26:70-6.

[50] Lee J, Heo J, Libbrecht L, et al. A novel prognostic subtype of human hepatocellular carcinoma derived from hepatic progenitor cells. *Nat Med* 2006;12:410-6.

[51] Jiang J, Gusev Y, Aderca I, et al. Association of MicroRNA expression in hepatocellular carcinomas with hepatitis infection, cirrhosis, and patient survival. *Clin Cancer Res* 2008;14:419-27.

[52] Pineau P, Volinia S, McJunkin K, et al. MiR-221 Overexpression contributes to liver tumorigenesis. *Proc Natl Acad Sci, USA* 2010;107:264-9.

[53] Huang Y, Dai Y, Yu X, et al. Microarray analysis of microRNA expression in hepatocellular carcinoma and non-tumorous tissues without viral hepatitis. *J Gastroenterol Hepatol* 2008;23:87-94.

[54] Su H, Yang J, Xu T, et al. MicroRNA-101, down-regulated in hepatocellular carcinoma, promotes apoptosis and suppresses tumorigenicity. *Cancer Res* 2009;69:1135-42.

[55] Ura S, Honda M, Yamashita T, et al. Differential microRNA expression between hepatitis B and hepatitis C leading disease progression to hepatocellular carcinoma. *Hepatology* 2009;49:1098-112.

[56] Ladeiro Y, Couchy G, Balabaud C, et al. MicroRNA profiling in hepatocellular tumors is associated with clinical features and oncogene/tumor suppressor gene mutations. *Hepatology* 2008;47:1955-63.

[57] Li W, Xie L, He X, et al. Diagnostic and prognostic implications of microRNAs in human hepatocellular carcinoma. *Int J Cancer* 2008;123:1616-22.

[58] Budhu A, Jia H, Forgues M, et al. Identification of metastasis-related microRNAs in hepatocellular carcinoma. *Hepatology* 2008;47:897-907.

[59] Wu L, Belasco J. Micro-RNA regulation of the mammalian lin-28 gene during neuronal differentiation of embryonal carcinoma cells. *Mol Cell Biol* 2005;25:9198-208.

[60] Scott G, Goga A, Bhaumik D, Berger C, Sullivan C, Benz C. Coordinate suppression of ERBB2 and ERBB3 by enforced expression of micro-RNA miR-125a or miR-125b. *J Biol Chem* 2007;282:1479-86.

[61] Nagayama K, Kohno T, Sato M, Arai Y, Minna J, Yokota J. Homozygous deletion scanning of the lung cancer genome at a 100-kb resolution. *Genes Chromosomes Cancer* 2007;46:1000-10.

[62] Zhou M, Liu Z, Zhao Y, et al. MicroRNA-125b confers the resistance of breast cancer cells to paclitaxel through suppression of pro-apoptotic Bcl-2 antagonist killer 1 (Bak1) expression. *J Biol Chem* 2010;285:21496-507.

[63] Klusmann J, Li Z, Böhmer K, et al. miR-125b-2 is a potential oncomiR on human chromosome 21 in megakaryoblastic leukemia. *Genes Dev* 2010;24:478-90.

[64] Le M, Teh C, Shyh-Chang N, et al. MicroRNA-125b is a novel negative regulator of p53. *Genes Dev* 2009;23:862-76.

[65] Totoki Y, Tatsuno K, Yamamoto S, et al. High-resolution characterization of a hepatocellular carcinoma genome. *Nat Genet* 2011;43:464-9.

[66] Lal A, Navarro F, Maher C, et al. miR-24 Inhibits cell proliferation by targeting E2F2, MYC, and other cell-cycle genes via binding to "seedless" 3'UTR microRNA recognition elements. *Mol Cell* 2009;35:610-25.

[67] Younger S, Corey D. Transcriptional gene silencing in mammalian cells by miRNA mimics that target gene promoters. *Nucleic Acids Res* 2011;Epub ahead of print.

In: Hepatocellular Carcionoma: A Global Challenge
Editor: Isabelle Chemin
ISBN: 978-1-61470-644-1

Chapter XII

The "omic" Approaches in Hepatocellular Carcinoma

Amelie Plymoth[*]
Department of Medical Epidemiology and Biostatistics, Karolinska Institutet, KI Campus, Solna, Sweden

1. Abstract

Hepatocellular Carcinoma (HCC) is a complex phenotypically and genetically heterogeneous polyclonal disease caused by a variety of risk factors. For a better understanding of the molecular mechanisms underlying the carcinogenesis, molecular profiling of genes, proteins, metabolites and other molecules are needed. The completion of the Human Genome Project changed the paradigm for large-scale biology projects and was critical for the development of the new era of "omics" research with the aim of understanding the complexity of a cell, tissue, and an organism in its entirety. Today, various physiological and pathological events can systematically be interpreted through the combination of comprehensive measurements of genomics (global gene analysis), epigenetics (global analysis of genetic modifications that are not attributable to changes in the primary DNA sequence), transcriptomics (global gene expression analysis), proteomics (global protein expression analysis), metabolomics (global metabolite expression analysis) and so on. Technological and bio-computing advances in large-scale omics analyses are providing researchers and doctors with an unprecedented capacity to capture and assess complex molecular information from biological samples. And importantly, large repositories of specimens collected in clinical or epidemiological studies are being developed, providing access to series of biospecimens with large statistical power for assessing complex sets of biomarkers.

In this chapter, systematic -omics approaches used in the study of HCC in the scales of genomics including chromosomal instability and epigenetic changes, transcriptomics and microRNAs, proteomics and also metabolomics are discussed. What are now needed

[*] PhD, MPH, MSc. E-mail: amelie.plymoth@ki.se; Phone: +46-(0)8-5248 2346.

are major integrative omics and systems biology efforts for a systematic understanding of the pathogenesis and pathophysiology of HCC. This will lead to discovery of new therapeutic targets, prediction of therapeutic response, personalized treatment regimens and ultimately to the prevention of HCC.

2. Introduction

Hepatocellular Carcinoma (HCC) is a complex disease associated with a variety of highly variable clinical phenotypes in affected individuals. During initiation, promotion, and progression of the disease an accumulation of genetic and epigenetic changes occur and a large number of genes, proteins, and other molecules are altered in HCC. The genesis and development of HCC cannot be derived to a single factor or a simple collection of single factors, but rather by interactions of multiple genes, miRNAs, proteins and metabolites in biological pathways.

Molecular profiling of genes, proteins, metabolites and other molecules are important for a better understanding of molecular mechanisms underlying carcinogenesis. The completion of the Human Genome Project changed the paradigm for large-scale biology projects and was critical for the development of the new era of "omics" research with the aim of understanding the complexity of a cell, tissue, and an organism in its entirety [1]. High-throughput omics technologies such as genomics, transcriptomics, proteomics and metabolomics provide powerful tools for molecular profiling of HCC and can be used for the discovery of candidate biomarkers for diagnosis, prognosis, and therapeutic selection for treatment of the cancer. Large amounts of data emerge from the omics world and the integration of this information together with clinical data is crucial for the systematic understanding of HCC.

2.1. Genomics

Analyses of somatic alterations and gene expression profiles in patients with HCC have provided important information about the genes involved in carcinogenesis. Activation of oncogenes and the role of tumor supressor genes such as retinoblastoma and p53 genes are well documented [2,3,4]. Recent observations indicate that free DNA originating from tumour cells is detectable in the plasma of liver cancer patients at an early stage. However, the most important molecular alterations in the initial stages of the disease are currently unknown [5].

The majority of the HCC patients contract the disease from the accumulation of genetic abnormalities, induced by exterior etiological factors such as HBV and HCV infections and the mycotoxin, aflatoxin B1 produced by moulds of the genus Aspergillus [6-8] (see Introduction to Section 1 of the book). Genomic studies on HCC focuses on DNA sequence changes, chromosomal aberrations, epigenetic abnormalities and micro RNAs, techniques which are presented below. These studies show that some of the major genomic alterations associated with HCC include chromosomal instability, CpG methylation, DNA rearrangements associated with HBV integration, DNA hypomethylation, and, to a lesser degree, microsatellite instability. Also, the altered transcriptome profiles in HCC have been correlated to several chromosome regions with amplification or loss of heterozygosity. Array-based comparative genomic hybridization analysis and allelic dosage analysis using genotyping arrays are useful for determining genetic factors involved in HCC [4].

The most common sequence variation in the human genome is the stable substitution of a single base, the single nucleotide polymorphism (SNP). With the development of genomics, a large number of SNPs, which reflect the maximum differences between humans, have been identified across the whole human genome. Since genetic variation plays an important role in many diseases, SNPs have been used to serve as tools in genetic studies of complex traits [9]. The results from a recently published genome-wide association study, where 440,794 SNPs in 355 chronic HBV carriers with HCC and 360 chronic HBV carriers without HCC were genotyped, provide evidence that the 1p36.22 locus confers susceptibility to HBV-related HCC, and suggests that KIF1B-, UBE4B- or PGD-related pathways might be involved in the pathogenesis of HCC [10].

The next stage of gene expression analysis will require systematic integration of expression profiles with locus information, which is effective in detecting structural genomic abnormalities, such as chromosomal gains and deletions.

2.1.1. Chromosomal Instability

Parts of the genome have been shown to be unstable in HCC (chromosomal instability). In these unstable regions gain or loss of the genomic DNA copy number can be seen [11] [12]. Regions of the genome that are amplified often harbor oncogenes whereas the chromosomal deletion regions often include tumor suppressor genes, which both present a growth advantage for tumorigenesis in HCC [13]. Different studies have reported chromosomal instability at the chromosomal regions, 1p, 1q, 3q, 4q, 5q, 6q, 8p, 8q, 10q, 11p, 16p, 16q, 17p, and 22q [14]. Gains of 1q21–23 and 8q22–24 have been associated with the early development of HCC in a genome-wide study of chromosomal aberrations of 158 HBV-associated HCC cases using comparative genomic hybridization [15]. Furthermore, the gain of 3q22–24 was identified as one of the late genomic events associated with tumor recurrence and poor overall patient survival.

Three HCC subgroups, organized in an evolutionary tree, have been identified based on the patterns of significant chromosomal aberrations [14]. These groups reflect the degree of tumor progression, including a number of chromosomal aberrations, tumor stage, tumor size, and disease outcome.

Different approaches are used to identify the chromosomal unstable regions of the genome in hepatocarcinogenesis. The approaches include cytogenetics [16], interphase fluorescence in situ hybridization (FISH) [17], Southern blot analysis [18], genotyping analyses [19], the conventional metaphasebased CGH [20] and array comparative genomic hybridization (aCGH). Array-based CGH is a technique that enables high-resolution, genome-wide screening of segmental genomic copy number variations (CNVs). This technique is becoming an essential and a routine clinical diagnostic tool which is gradually replacing cytogenetic methods [21]. With the widespread use of aCGH, different computational analyses methods are being developed to identify cytogenetic aberrations using aCGH data. An example of this is the LS-CAP algorithm.

2.1.2. Epigenetic Changes

Epigenetics may be defined as the study of all changes that are stably transmitted over many rounds of cell divisions, but that do not alter the nucleotide sequence in the genetic code. Further, epigenetic changes refer to changes in the DNA/chromatin that do not involve changes in the DNA sequence [22]. Epigenetic inheritance includes DNA methylation, histone modifications and RNA-mediated silencing, all of which are essential mechanisms that allow the stable propagation of gene activity states from one generation of cells to the next.

Epigenetics is a new and rapidly expanding field of cancer research. Over the past decade, the field has witnessed a remarkable progress in our knowledge of the importance of epigenetic events in the control of both normal cellular processes and abnormal events associated with tumour development and progression [23]. In addition to gene transcription, epigenetic mechanisms appear to play an important role in other cellular processes, including cell differentiation, DNA repair and replication as well as in stem cell biology. DNA hypomethylation, CpG island hypermethylation, and histone modifications represent epigenetic markers of malignant transformation [24]. DNA methylation is a major epigenetic mechanism which is intensively studied in the context of gene regulation and unscheduled silencing in cancer cells. Hypermethylation of gene promoters is associated with gene inactivation while the precise consequences of genome-wide hypomethylation are still debated. Recent studies have shed new light on the mechanisms underlying both promoter specific hypermethylation and global hypomethylation in cancer cells [ref zdenko curr opinion]. Epigenetic changes are stable and persistent during the development and progression of cancer and are therefore powerful cancer biomarker candidates [25]. Epigenetic deregulations seem to occur early in cancer development, consistent with the notion that epigenetic deregulations precede and promote malignant processes.

A number of epigenetic changes have been reported in HCC. Promoter methylation and subsequent loss of protein expression have been demonstrated in many oncogenes and tumor suppressor genes [8]. Promoter hypermethylation, and subsequent loss of protein expression, may be a key mechanism involved in the inactivation of some tumor suppressor genes in HCC. For example, frequent promoter hypermethylation and subsequent loss of protein expression has been demonstrated in HCC at tumor suppressor gene, p16, p14, p15, SOCS1, RIZ1, E-cadherin, and 14-3-3 sigma [4]. Promoter methylation also appears to be an early event, suggesting that this may precede cirrhosis.

In a recent study, DNA methylation signatures, able to distinguish hepatocellular carcinoma from surrounding tissues and from other tumour types were identified. Further, these DNA methylation signatures were correlated with survival after cancer therapy [26]. These studies provide compelling evidence that DNA methylation signatures can be exploited as biomarker in diagnosis and prediction of treatment outcome of HCC.

Bisulphite genomic sequencing is a standard technology used for detecting DNA methylation. This technique maps sites with the resolution of a single base-pair. The method utilizes the selective deamination of cytosine to uracil by incubation with sodium bisulphite and the sequencing subsequently generated PCR products. In contrast to cytosine, the 5-methylcytosine can be distinguished because it does not react with bisulphate [27,28]. The most widely used technique for mapping histone modification is chromatin immunoprecipitation assay [29]. Chromatin fragments are isolated using specific antibodies of histones and amplified DNA are used for PCR or microarray [30].

During the last decades, a collection of useful tools, both to design the experiments and to analyze the results, and databases for studying epigenetic changes have been developed [31]. PubMeth (http://www.pubmeth.org) is an annotated and reviewed database of methylation in cancer. It is based on automated textmining of literature and is afterwards manually curated and annotated [32].

2.2. Transcriptomics

Transcriptomics analyzes all RNA molecules, including mRNA, rRNA, tRNA, and other non-coding RNAs, transcribed from DNA in a cell, tissue or organ. High throughput profiling techniques used for detecting thousands of transcripts simultaneously include DNA microarray, SAGE (serial analysis of gene expression) and MPSS (massively parallel signature sequencing). Microarrays are among the most popular profiling methods used in cancer research and it is widely used to explore the molecular mechanisms of HCC and to find markers or patterns for early detection and diagnosis, stage classification and prognosis. By using microarrays researches can measure the mRNA expression of thousands of genes on a single chip by detecting their hybridization to the array of DNA probes on the chip. The bioinformatic processing of the transcriptome data is crucial and statistical and machine learning-based methods used include hierarchical clustering, linear discriminant analysis, Cox regression, support vector machines etc.

Differences in the transcriptomic platforms used and the experimental design, and also the underlying biological heterogeneity of HCC have led to inconsistency in identified expression signatures among studies. In order to describe a common molecular HCC classification, "biostatistical meta-analysis" analysis on microarray datasets from different transcriptome HCC studies have been performed [33]. Meta-analysis of transcriptomic studies can be an important way forward for constructing an international consensus defining common bases of a robust molecular classification of HCC [34].

A typical application of microarrays in cancer research is to classify patients with different disease status such as HCC tumor samples vs non-tumor samples, high histological grade vs low grade, early stage vs late stage, good prognosis vs poor prognosis, and HCC patients with HBV vs HCV infection etc [8]. Several transcriptomic studies on HCC have been published [35,36,(37,38,39,40,41,42,43,44,45] and a number of similar molecular subgroups of HCC tumours have been identified despite disparities among the studies in term of risk factors, geographical origin, grading of the tumours [34]. In a French study, where genome wide transcriptomic analysis was performed on 60 tumours of surgically treated HCCs, unsupervised transcriptomic analysis identified six robust subgroups of HCC (termed G1 to G6) associated with clinical and genetic characteristics (Figure 1). This 6-group classification has clinical application regarding the development of targeted therapies for HCC because specific pathway activations, particularly AKT and Wnt pathways, are closely associated to subgroups G1–G2 and G5–G6 respectively. Further, the research group identified and validated a robust 16-gene signature to classify HCC tumours into the 6-group transcriptomic classification. This signature should be very useful to determine alterations of specific pathways and to predict putative response to targeted drugs [37].

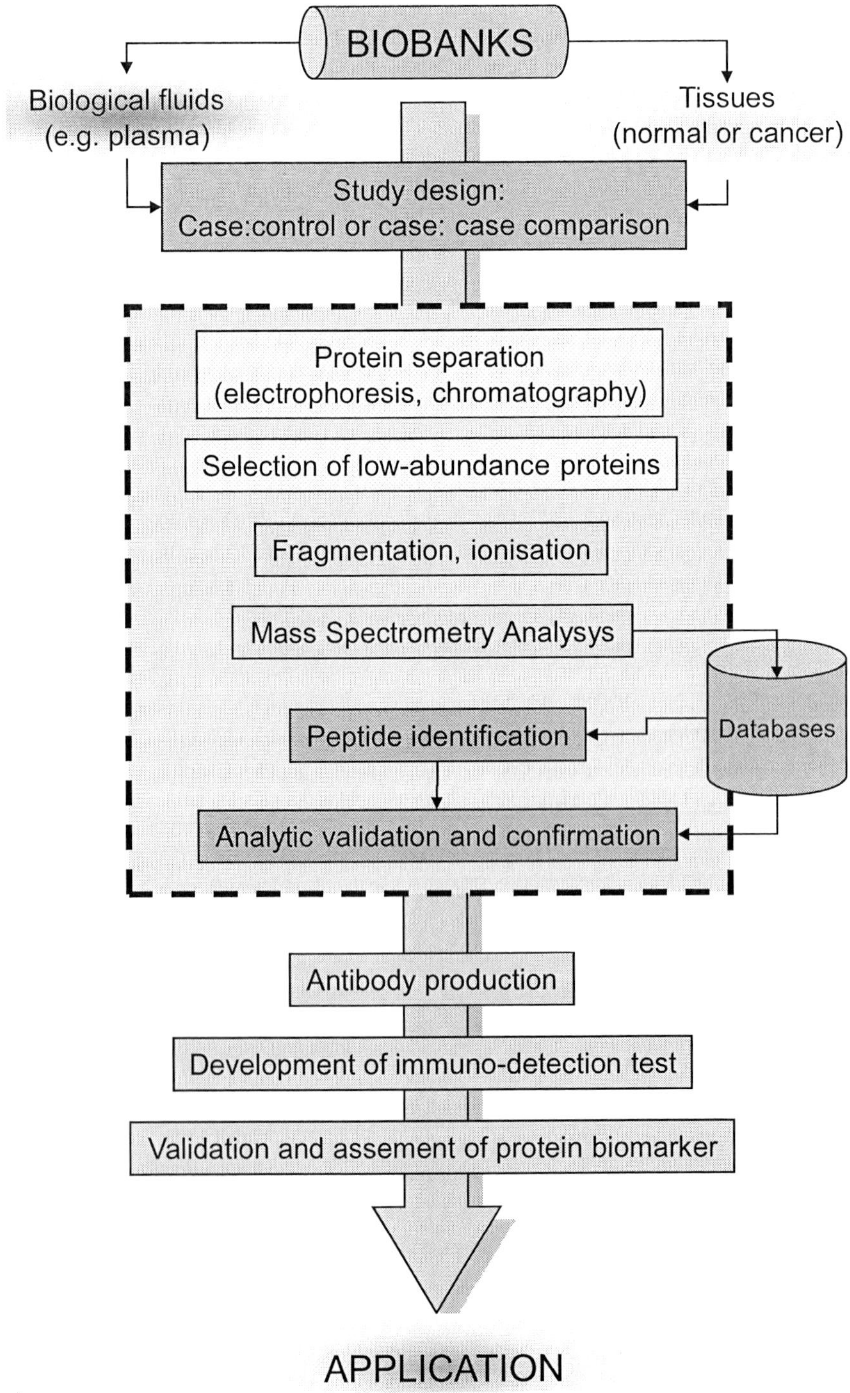

Figure 1.

A number of transcriptomic studies, comparing HBV and HCV associated HCC, have been performed. These studies show that the expression patterns of HBV and HCV associated HCC are different, implying that HBV and HCV cause hepatocarcinogenesis by different mechanisms [46, 47]. HBV induced hepatocarcinogenesis may involve the whole course from signal transduction, transcription, translation to protein degradation, which differs in some measure from HCV-induced hepatocarcinogenesis, and that exogenous transcription factor HBX and endogenous NF-jB are likely two key points of the course [9]. Research show that infecting virus type was the most weighted factor of gene expression in chronic hepatitis and that genes in pro-apoptotic and DNA repair responses especially those mediated by p53 and 14-3-3 were predominant in chronic hepatitis B [48].

2.2.1. MicroRNAs

Micro RNAs (miRNAs) are small non-coding RNAs that can regulate gene expression by binding to mRNA seed regions (nucleotides 2 to 8 relative to the 5' end of the miRNA) [49] [50,51]. Many studies show that miRNAs play essential physiological functions, particularly in cancer where they can act as oncogenes or tumour suppressors [52]. Specific alterations of miRNA expression have been identified as directly involved in carcinogenesis and several studies have identified a relationship between miRNA deregulation and the phenotype of HCC where miRNA deregulations seem to be associated to specific tumours subtypes [53,54,55,56,57,58,59,60,61,62,63,64,65,66,67]. In a study where the expression levels of 250 miRNAs in 46 benign and malignant hepatocellular tumours were compared to 4 normal liver samples using quantitative RT-PCR, miR-224was found over-expression in all tumors, miR-200c, miR-200, mir-21, miR-224, miR-10b and miR-222 specific deregulation was found in benign or malignant tumours [34]. Further, the expressions of miR-122, miR-221 and miR26 have been found to be associated with poor prognosis of HCC [56,63,68].

The fact that HCC tumours have distinct miRNAs expression fingerprints according to malignancy, risk factors and oncogene/tumour suppressor gene alterations, suggests that miRNAs can serve as promising HCC tumour biomarkers.

2.3. Proteomics

Proteomics is the study of the proteome, which is the protein complement of the genome in a biological system at a given point in time. Proteomics offers highly complementary information to genomics, epigenomics and transcriptomics. The proteome is dynamic; protein levels depend not only on the corresponding transcript levels but also on a multitude of translational controls and the regulation of protein degradation [69]. Proteomics, in contrast to genomics, has the potential to explore differences of several orders of magnitude in protein levels and to detect minute posttranslational modifications that are often just as important for protein activity as protein expression levels [70]. There is an increasing interest in the application of proteomics in all areas of the life sciences, especially in the area of biomedical research, and particularly for the analysis of biological fluids, which is very promising for biomarker discovery. Furthermore, proteomics is also providing essential insights into critical disease pathways, biomarkers relevant for risk identification and early disease detection, novel targets for therapeutics, molecular classification of diseases and monitoring of disease response to therapy and progression. For the cancer patient, biomarkers such as those identified by proteomics can aid in diagnosis and/or clinical management by allowing for early detection of clinically silent lesions, better defining subtypes of lesions and predicting or monitoring response to treatment [70,71,72,73,74].

The rapid development of proteomics as a field has depended upon major technological advances in many areas including gel-based or gel-free protein separation and sequencing techniques (shotgun sequencing), protein chips (surface-enhanced laser desorption ionization mass spectrometry, protein arrays, tissue arrays and antibody arrays), mass spectrometry (sensitivity, resolution, speed and throughput) and bioinformatics [75,76]. Currently, there is no technique that can cover on its own the huge diversity of single proteins contained in a complex sample and the wide dynamic range in the abundance of the individual protein species [77]. However, strategies for large-scale studies to measure all the proteins in model organisms and to study their complex interactions are emerging, providing a new layer to the knowledge of how cells deliver functions at the molecular level [78,79].

The plasma proteome is particularly challenging for in-depth proteomics analysis because of its complexity and because of the range of distribution of its protein constituents, which runs over 10 orders of magnitude. Before the advent of proteomics, mastering such a huge dispersion of concentrations was technically impossible. This is now within the reach of proteomics where in-depth analysis is made possible by three basic strategies: removal of high-abundance proteins, fractionation to reduce the sample complexity and targeted analysis of particular protein and peptide subsets such as glycoproteomics [73]. However, the dynamic range of detection by mass spectrometry is still a limiting factor that runs over three to four orders of magnitude for complex mixtures such as plasma [80].

Currently, clinical proteomics studies are increasingly shifting toward the parallel analysis of tissues and biological fluids to address the question of biomarker specificity. The main challenges that arise from such studies include tissue heterogeneity, abundance of the cell type of interest, marker quantitation, experimental design and choice of optimal analytic method selection, development of biological resource centers containing sufficient numbers of well documented biosamples of the correct type and in the correct state of physical preservation to support specific proteomics studies, validation of candidate biomarkers in large cohorts with long-term clinical follow-up, and reduction of validated proteomics-based bioassays to robust and efficient procedures that will work in the clinic [71,81] (Figure 1).

The most widely used protein biomarker for diagnosis of HCC is Alpha-1 fetoprotein (AFP), and others are AFP-L3 and des-gamma-carboxy prothrombin (DCP) that are all present in the blood. AFP has been used as a serum marker for many years and was already described in the 1960s [82]. However, AFP is not elevated in all patients with HCC, especially not in the early stages of HCC development, and some patients with cirrhosis and/or hepatic inflammation can have an elevated AFP, even without the presence of a tumor. Published studies have shown a sensitivity of 39%-65%, a specificity of 76%-94%, and a positive predictive value of 9%-50% for AFP for the presence of HCC [83]. Thus it is of great importance to identify novel HCC biomarkers for early detection and effective treatment of the disease, which will be of great value in high-risk population scanning, drug design and the mechanistic research of hepatocarcinogenesis.

A large number of proteomics based HCC biomarker discovery studies, from cell lines, tissue and plasma/serum, are continuously published in the literature. Important dysregulated proteins including isoforms or fragments, metabolic enzymes, proteins involved in calcium homeostasis, cytoskeleton and tumor suppression factors, and proteins that can increase the cell's resistance to apoptosis. Of them, the alteration of heat shock proteins and impairment of methylation cycle were found to be associated with clinical HBV-associated HCC [8,9]. Recently, several groups have also used proteomics approaches to analyze the highly homologous cytochrome P450 enzymes [84]. The pattern of gene expression in HCC is closely associated with the etiologic factor and the same is true for the protein expression [85,86]. Differential expression of the liver tissue proteome in HBV- and HCV-associated HCC indicates that the pathogenetic mechanisms of hepatocarcinogenesis may be different according to the viral factor, HBV and HCV.

Since HBV cannot infect common immortalized cell lines, the study of the molecular mechanisms of HBV infection was a great challenge until the establishment of the HepG2.2.15 cell line. The HepG2.2.15 cell line was established from HepG2 and it constitutively expresses HBV as a consequence of the integration of HBV genome [87]. Therefore, this cell line is used as an in vitro system to study the HBV life cycle and HBV-host cell interactions. Comparative proteomics analysis of HepG2.2.15 with HepG2 has shown revealed protein alterations in retinol metabolism, calcium ion-binding and protein degradation [88].

Plasma profiling of intact proteins, by protein multifractionation, is a useful method for the discovery of biomarkers for early detection and prediction of HCC. This method utilizes multidimensional separation of intact proteins according to their charge, hydrophobicity, and molecular mass, with particular attention to the isolation of low-abundance proteins and exhaustive liquid chromatography-tandem mass spectrometry (LC-MS/MS) analysis. This method has significantly improved the detection and allowed for an even deeper coverage of the liver and plasma proteomes and provides a powerful strategy for HCC biomarker discovery [89,90]. Paired HCC tumor and surrounding non-tumor tissues and sometimes also normal liver tissues is commonly studied in proteomic studies of HCC [91,92,93,94,95,96]. The techniques used for this includes 2DE, 2D-DIGE [92,96] and ICAT [97]. Before proteomics analysis, the hepatocytes are often separated by laser capture microdissection to decrease the heterogeneity in the liver tissue [97,98,99].

The glycosylation of proteins is known to change in tumor cells during the development of HCC as the result of alterations in the levels of glycosyltransferases, such as increased fucosylation of Golgi Protein 73 and alpha-fetoprotein [100]. Changes in both the total serum glycome and the glycosylation of specific IgG molecules have been observed in people with liver fibrosis and cirrhosis [101]. Therefore, proteomics based identification of HCC-related glycoprotein markers and analysis of glycan structural alterations might assist in the early detection of HCC.

To be able to identify liver disease related biomarkers it is very important to also have a good understanding of the "normal" liver proteome in healthy individuals. A major achievement in this direction has been made with the construction of the normal human liver proteome expression profile, with over 6,000 proteins identified in the Chinese as well as in the French Liver reference samples [84].

A number of candidate biomarkers for early detection of HCC have been identified by proteomics approaches but none of them have so far been fully validated in prospective studies. One of the factors explaining the slow progress of candidate proteomics biomarkers through the translational pipeline has been the difficulty to develop validation and standardization of procedures to improve reproducibility, sensitivity and specificity. This challenge has now largely been met by large, consortium efforts, leading to the discovery of drug-specific protein biomarker. Further progress in clinical proteomics will depend upon continued collaborative efforts and infrastructure development by the proteomic community.

2.3. Metabolomics

Metabolomics is the global analysis of metabolites, small molecules generated in the process of metabolism at a given time in a cell, tissue, organ or organism [102,103]. Metabolic disease phenotypes are studied and since metabolic pathways are downstream of gene expression and protein synthesis, the metabolites might reflect the biological activity of a cell at functional level more accurately [103]. Different methods are used for the study of the metabolites. They include nuclear magnetic resonance spectroscopy [104] direct infusion electrospray MS [105],gas and liquid chromatography, Fourier transform infra-red spectroscopy [106], and Raman spectroscopy [107].

Metabolomic studies on HCC are starting to emerge but the field is very young. In studies where 1H nuclear magnetic resonance (NMR) has been used, the metabolite profiles of extracts from tumor tissue, suggest that alterations in glycolysis and the metabolism of glycine and choline occur during HCC invasion and metastasis [108]. The serum metabolome profiles of liver cirrhosis and HCC showed higher concentrations of acetate, Nacetylglycoproteins, pyruvate, glutamine, alpha-ketoglutarate, glycerol, tyrosine, 1-methylhistidine and phenylalanine, together with lower concentrations of low-density lipoprotein, isoleucine, valine, acetoacetate, creatine, choline and unsaturated lipids compared to the serum metabolome profiles of healthy controls [109].

In another study the urinary endogenous metabolome was assayed using chemical derivatization followed by GC/MS, to investigate the urinary metabolic difference between hepatocellular carcinoma male patients (n=20) and normal male subjects (n=20). In this study 103 metabolites were detected and a diagnostic model was constructed with a combination of 18 marker metabolites which yielded a separation between the two groups with an area under the curve value of 0.9275 [110].

Conclusion

Hepatocellular Carcinoma (HCC) is a complex disease associated with a variety of clinical phenotypes with multiple underlying pathogenic mechanisms caused by a variety of risk factors. The majority of the HCC patients contract the disease from the accumulation of genetic abnormalities, induced by exterior etiological factors such as HBV and HCV and aflatoxin B1 and a large number of genes, proteins, and other molecules belonging to diverse cellular processes and pathways are altered in HCC. There have been many biomarkers proposed for early detection, diagnosis and treatment of HCC but none of them have so far made it into the clinic and the lack of good molecular markers present a major challenge in the health care.

Molecular profiling of genes, proteins, metabolites and other molecules are important for a better understanding of molecular mechanisms underlying carcinogenesis. Various physiological and pathological events can systematically be interpreted through the combination of comprehensive measurements of genomics (global gene analysis), epigenetics (global analysis of genetic modifications that are not attributable to changes in the primary DNA sequence), transcriptomics (global gene expression analysis), proteomics (global protein expression analysis), metabolomics (global metabolite expression analysis) and so on. The completion of the Human Genome Project changed the paradigm for large-scale biology projects and was critical for the development of the new era of “omics” research with the aim of understanding the complexity of a cell, tissue, and an organism in its entirety.

Large amounts of data emerge from the omics world. The integration and deciphering of the omics data by a systemsbiology approach data put individual omics data into a larger biological perspective which is needed for the systematic understanding of HCC. The high-throughput omics technologies such as genomics, epigenetics, transcriptomics, proteomics and metabolomics, discussed in this chapter, provide powerful tools for molecular profiling of HCC and can be used for the discovery of candidate biomarkers for diagnosis, prognosis, and therapeutic selection for treatment of the cancer. Examples of alterations associated with HCC identified by omics approaches, which are further discussed in this chapter, include amplification or deletion of chromosomal regions, copy number changes of genes and abnormal epigenetic alterations, corresponding changes seen at the mRNA, protein and metabolite level and noncoding miRNAs which have also been shown to have a roles in the disease.

Liver cancer is expansively studied with various high-throughput omics technologies and an increasing number of articles are being published. What are now needed are major integrative omics and systems biology efforts for a systematic understanding of the pathogenesis and pathophysiology of HCC. This will lead to discovery of new therapeutic targets, prediction of therapeutic response, personalized treatment regimens and ultimately to the prevention of HCC.

References

[1] Hood L, Heath JR, Phelps ME, Lin B. Systems biology and new technologies enable predictive and preventative medicine. *Science.* 2004 Oct 22;306(5696):640-3.

[2] Gouas D, Shi H, Hainaut P. The aflatoxin-induced TP53 mutation at codon 249 (R249S): Biomarker of exposure, early detection and target for therapy. *Cancer Lett.* 2009 Dec 1;286(1):29-37.

[3] Zhang X, Xu HJ, Murakami Y, Sachse R, Yashima K, Hirohashi S, et al. Deletions of chromosome 13q, mutations in Retinoblastoma 1, and retinoblastoma protein state in human hepatocellular carcinoma. *Cancer Res.* 1994 Aug 1;54(15):4177-82.

[4] Aravalli RN, Steer CJ, Cressman ENK. Molecular Mechanisms of Hepatocellular Carcinoma. *Hepatology.* 2008 Dec;48(6):2047-63.

[5] Le Roux E, Gormally E, Hainaut P. Somatic mutations in human cancer: applications in molecular epidemiology. *Rev Epidemiol Sante.* 2005 Jun;53(3):257-66.

[6] Pineau P, Marchio A, Battiston C, Cordina E, Russo A, Terris B, et al. Chromosome instability in human hepatocellular carcinoma depends on p53 status and aflatoxin exposure. *Mutat Res-Gen Tox En.* 2008 May 31;653(1-2):6-13.

[7] Saigo K, Yoshida K, Ikeda R, Sakamoto Y, Murakami Y, Urashima T, et al. Integration of hepatiti's B virus DNA into the myeloid/lymphoid or mixed-lineage leukemia (MLL4) gene and rearrangements of MLL4 in human hepatocellular carcinoma. *Hum Mutat.* 2008 May;29(5):703-8.

[8] Pei YF, Zhang T, Renault V, Zhang XG. An overview of hepatocellular carcinoma study by omics-based methods. *Acta Bioch Bioph Sin.* 2009 Jan;41(1):1-15.

[9] Sun W, Zhong F, Zhi LT, Zhou GQ, He FC. Systematic -omics analysis of HBV-associated liver diseases. *Cancer Lett.* 2009 Dec 1;286(1):89-95.

[10] Zhang H, Zhai Y, Hu Z, Wu C, Qian J, Jia W, et al. Genome-wide association study identifies 1p36.22 as a new susceptibility locus for hepatocellular carcinoma in chronic hepatitis B virus carriers. *Nat Genet.* 2010 Sep;42(9):755-8.

[11] Laurent-Puig P and Zucman-Rossi J. Genetics of hepatocellular tumors. *Oncogene* 2006, 25: 3778–3786.

[12] Luo JH, Ren B, Keryanov S, Tseng GC, Rao UN, Monga SP, et al. Transcriptomic and genomic analysis of human hepatocellular carcinomas and hepatoblastomas. *Hepatology* 2006;44:1012-1024.

[13] Huang J, Sheng HH, Shen T, Hu YJ, Xiao HS, Zhang Q and Zhang QH et al. Correlation between genomic DNA copy number alterations and transcriptional expression in hepatitis B virus-associated hepatocellular carcinoma. *FEBS Lett* 2006, 580: 3571–3581.

[14] Herath NI, Leggett BA, MacDonald GA. Review of genetic and epigenetic alterations in hepatocarcinogenesis. *J Gastroenterol Hepatol* 2006; 21:15-21.

[15] Poon TC, Wong N, Lai PB, Rattray M, Johnson PJ, Sung JJ. A tumor progression model for hepatocellular carcinoma: bioinformatic analysis of genomic data. *Gastroenterology* 2006;131:1262-1270.

[16] Lowichik A, Schneider NR, Tonk V, Ansari MQ and Timmons CF. Report of a complex karyotype in recurrent metastatic fibrolamellar hepatocellular carcinoma and a review of hepatocellular carcinoma cytogenetics. *Cancer Genet Cytogenet* 1996, 88: 170–174.

[17] Tjia WM, Hu L, Zhang MY and Guan XY. Characterization of rearrangements involving 4q, 13q and 16q in hepatocellular carcinoma cell lines using region-specific multiplex-FISH probes. *Cancer Lett* 2007, 250: 92–99.

[18] Tay N, Chan SH and Ren EC. Detection of integrated hepatitis B virus DNA in hepatocellular carcinoma cell lines by nonradioactive in situ hybridization. *J Med Virol* 1990, 30: 266–271.

[19] Wilkens L, Flemming P, Gebel M, Bleck J, Terkamp C, Wingen L and Kreipe H et al. Induction of aneuploidy by increasing chromosomal instability during dedifferentiation of hepatocellular carcinoma. *Proc Natl Acad Sci USA* 2004, 101: 1309–1314.

[20] Park SJ, Jeong SY and Kim HJ. Y chromosome loss and other genomic alterations in hepatocellular carcinoma cell lines analyzed by CGH and CGH array. *Cancer Genet Cytogenet 2006*, 166: 56–64.

[21] Shinawi M, Cheung SW. The array CGH and its clinical applications. *Drug Discov Today*. 2008 Sep;13(17-18):760-70. Epub 2008 Jul 17.

[22] Bird A. Perceptions of epigenetics. *Nature* 2007, 447: 396–398.

[23] Nino Sinčić; Zdenko Herceg. *DNA Methylation and Cancer: Searching for Ghosts and Angels above the Genes. Accepted for publication in Current Opinion in Oncology.*

[24] Lujambio A, Esteller M. CpG island hypermethylation of tumor suppressor microRNAs in human cancer. *Cell Cycle* 2007;6:1455-1459.

[25] Kanai Y: Genome-wide DNA methylation profiles in precancerous conditions and cancers. *Cancer Sci* 2010, 101:36-45.

[26] Hernandez-Vargas H, Lambert MP, Le Calvez-Kelm F, Gouysse G, McKay-Chopin S, Tavtigian SV, Scoazec JY, Herceg Z: Hepatocellular carcinoma displays distinct DNA methylation signatures with potential as clinical predictors. *PLoS One* 2010, 5:e9749.

[27] Frommer M, McDonald LE, Millar DS, Collis CM, Watt F, Grigg GW and Molloy PL et al. A genomic sequencing protocol that yields a positive display of 5-methylcytosine residues in individual DNA strands. *Proc Natl Acad Sci USA* 1992, 89: 1827–1831.

[28] Kondo Y, Shen L, Suzuki S, Kurokawa T, Masuko K, Tanaka Y and Kato H et al. Alterations of DNA methylation and histone modifications contribute to gene silencing in hepatocellular carcinomas. *Hepatol Res* 2007, 37: 974–983.

[29] Orlando V and Paro R. Mapping Polycomb-repressed domains in the bithorax complex using in vivo formaldehyde cross-linked chromatin. *Cell* 1993, 75: 1187–1198.

[30] Schones DE and Zhao K. Genome-wide approaches to studying chromatin modifications. *Nat Rev Genet* 2008, 9: 179–191.

[31] Ongenaert M. *Adv Genet.* 2010;71:259-95.

[32] Ongenaert M, Van Neste L, De Meyer T, Menschaert G, Bekaert S and Van Criekinge W. PubMeth: a cancer methylation database combining text-mining and expert annotation. *Nucleic Acids Res* 2008, 36: D842–846.

[33] Hoshida Y, Nijman SM, Kobayashi M, et al. Integrative transcriptome analysis reveals common molecular subclasses of human hepatocellular carcinoma. *Cancer Res* 2009;69:7385–92.

[34] Zucman-Rossi. Molecular classification of hepatocellular carcinoma. *Digestive and Liver Disease* 42S (2010) S235–S241.

[35] Lee JS, Chu IS, Heo J, et al. Classification and prediction of survival in hepatocellular carcinoma by gene expression profiling. *Hepatology* 2004;40:667–76.

[36] Lee JS, Heo J, Libbrecht L, et al. A novel prognostic subtype of human hepatocellular carcinoma derived from hepatic progenitor cells. *Nat Med* 2006;12:410–6.

[37] Boyault S, Rickman DS, de Reynies A, et al. Transcriptome classification of HCC is related to gene alterations and to new therapeutic targets. *Hepatology* 2007;45:42–52.

[38] Chen X, Cheung ST, So S, et al. Gene expression patterns in human liver cancers. *Mol Biol Cell* 2002;13:1929–39.

[39] Breuhahn K, Vreden S, Haddad R, et al. Molecular profiling of human hepatocellular carcinoma defines mutually exclusive interferon regulation and insulin-like growth factor II overexpression. *Cancer Res* 2004;64:6058–64.

[40] Kaposi-Novak P, Lee JS, Gomez-Quiroz L, et al. Met-regulated expression signature defines a subset of human hepatocellular carcinomas with poor prognosis and aggressive phenotype. *The Journal of clinical investigation* 2006;116:1582–95.

[41] Chiang DY, Villanueva A, Hoshida Y, et al. Focal gains of VEGFA and molecular classification of hepatocellular carcinoma. *Cancer Res* 2008;68:6779–88.

[42] Coulouarn C, Factor VM, Thorgeirsson SS. Transforming growth factor-beta gene expression signature in mouse hepatocytes predicts clinical outcome in human cancer. *Hepatology* 2008;47:2059–67.

[43] Yamashita T, Forgues M, Wang W, et al. EpCAM and alphafetoprotein expression defines novel prognostic subtypes of hepatocellular carcinoma. *Cancer Res* 2008;68:1451–61.

[44] Hoshida Y, Villanueva A, Kobayashi M, et al. Gene expression in fixed tissues and outcome in hepatocellular carcinoma. *N Engl J Med* 2008;359:1995–2004.

[45] Hoshida Y, Nijman SM, Kobayashi M, et al. Integrative transcriptome analysis reveals common molecular subclasses of human hepatocellular carcinoma. *Cancer Res* 2009;69:7385–92.

[46] M. Honda, S. Kaneko, H. Kawai, Y. Shirota, K. Kobayashi, Differential gene expression between chronic hepatitis B and C hepatic lesion, *Gastroenterology* 120 (2001) 955–966.

[47] C.F. Lee, Z.Q. Ling, T. Zhao, K.R. Lee, Distinct expression patterns in hepatitis B virus- and hepatitis C virus-infected hepatocellular carcinoma, *World J. Gastroenterol.* 14 (2008) 6072–6077.

[48] M. Honda, T. Yamashita, T. Ueda, H. Takatori, R. Nishino, S. Kaneko, Different signaling pathways in the livers of patients with chronic hepatitis B or chronic hepatitis C, *Hepatology* 44 (2006) 1122–1138.

[49] Moffett HF, Novina CD. A small RNA makes a Bic difference. *Genome Biol.* 2007;8(7):221.

[50] Ambros V. The functions of animal microRNAs. *Nature* 2004, 431: 350–355.

[51] Bartel DP. MicroRNAs: genomics, biogenesis, mechanism, and function. *Cell* 2004, 116: 281–297.

[52] Cullen BR. Transcription and processing of human microRNA precursors. *Mol Cell* 2004;16:861–5.

[53] Murakami Y, Yasuda T, Saigo K, et al. Comprehensive analysis of microRNA expression patterns in hepatocellular carcinoma and nontumorous tissues. *Oncogene* 2006;25:2537–45.

[54] Kutay H, Bai S, Datta J, et al. Downregulation of miR-122 in the rodent and human hepatocellular carcinomas. *J Cell Biochem* 2006;99:671–8.

[55] Meng F, Henson R, Wehbe-Janek H, Ghoshal K, Jacob ST, Patel T. MicroRNA-21 regulates expression of the PTEN tumor suppressorgene in human hepatocellular cancer. *Gastroenterology* 2007;133:647–58.

[56] Gramantieri L, Ferracin M, Fornari F, et al. Cyclin G1 is a target of miR-122a, a microRNA frequently down-regulated in human hepatocellular carcinoma. *Cancer Res* 2007;67:6092–9.

[57] Huang YS, Dai Y, Yu XF, et al. Microarray analysis of microRNA expression in hepatocellular carcinoma and non-tumorous tissues without viral hepatitis. *J Gastroenterol Hepatol* 2008;23:87–94.

[58] Wang Y, Lee AT, Ma JZ, et al. Profiling microRNA expression in hepatocellular carcinoma reveals microRNA-224 up-regulation and apoptosis inhibitor-5 as a microRNA-224-specific target. *J Biol Chem* 2008;283:13205–15.

[59] Jiang J, Gusev Y, Aderca I, et al. Association of MicroRNA expression in hepatocellular carcinomas with hepatitis infection, cirrhosis, and patient survival. *Clin Cancer Res* 2008;14:419–27.

[60] Varnholt H, Drebber U, Schulze F, et al. MicroRNA gene expression profile of hepatitis C virus-associated hepatocellular carcinoma. *Hepatology* 2008;47:1223–32.

[61] Connolly E, Melegari M, Landgraf P, et al. Elevated expression of the miR-17-92 polycistron and miR-21 in hepadnavirus-associated hepatocellular carcinoma contributes to the malignant phenotype. *Am J Pathol* 2008;173:856–64.

[62] Budhu A, Jia HL, Forgues M, et al. Identification of metastasis-related microRNAs in hepatocellular carcinoma. *Hepatology* 2008;47:897–907.

[63] Ji J, Shi J, Budhu A, et al. MicroRNA expression, survival, and response to interferon in liver cancer. *N Engl J Med* 2009;361:1437–47.

[64] Ji J, Yamashita T, Budhu A, et al. Identification of microRNA-181 by genome-wide screening as a critical player in EpCAM-positive hepatic cancer stem cells. *Hepatology* 2009;50:472–80.

[65] Ura S, Honda M, Yamashita T, et al. Differential microRNA expression between hepatitis B and hepatitis C leading disease progression to hepatocellular carcinoma. *Hepatology* 2009;49:1098–112.

[66] Huang XH, Wang Q, Chen JS, et al. Bead-based microarray analysis of microRNA expression in hepatocellular carcinoma: miR-338 is downregulated. *Hepatol Res* 2009;39:786–94.

[67] Su H, Yang JR, Xu T, et al. MicroRNA-101, down-regulated in hepatocellular carcinoma, promotes apoptosis and suppresses tumorigenicity. *Cancer Res* 2009;69:1135–42.

[68] Coulouarn C, Factor VM, Andersen JB, et al. Loss of miR-122 expression in liver cancer correlates with suppression of the hepatic phenotype and gain of metastatic properties. *Oncogene* 2009;28:3526–36.

[69] Gygi SP, Rochon Y, Franza BR, et al. Correlation between protein and mRNA abundance in yeast. *Mol Cell Biol* 1999; 19:1720–1730.

[70] Cox J, Mann M. Is proteomics the new genomics? *Cell* 2007; 130:395–398.

[71] Plymoth A, Hainaut P. Proteomics beyond proteomics: toward clinical applications. Accepted for publication in Current Opinion in Oncology.

[72] Pitteri S, Hanash S. A systems approach to the proteomic identification of novel cancer biomarkers. Dis Markers 2010; 28:233–239. *Recent review on proteomics-based identification of novel cancer biomarkers.*

[73] Hanash SM, Pitteri SJ, Faca VM. Mining the plasma proteome for cancer biomarkers. *Nature* 2008; 3:571–579.

[74] Dunn MJ. PROTEOMICS: ten years in the field. *Proteomics* 2010; 10:

[75] Aebersold R, Mann M. Mass spectrometry-based proteomics. *Nature* 2003; 422:198–207.

[76] Washburn MP, Wolters D, Yates JR. Large-scale analysis of the yeast proteome by multidimensional protein identification technology. *Nat Biotechnol* 2001; 19:242–247.

[77] Anderson NL, Anderson NG. The human plasma proteome: history, character, and diagnostic prospects. *Mol Cell Proteomics* 2002; 1:845–867.

[78] Picotti P, Rinner O, Stallmach R, et al. High-throughput generation of selected reaction-monitoring assays for proteins and proteomes. *Nat Methods* 2010; 7:43–46.

[79] Anderson NL. Libraries of specific assays covering whole proteomes: from yeast to man. *Clin Chem* 2010; 56:1521–1522.

[80] Mann M, Kelleher NL. Precision proteomics: the case for high resolution and high mass accuracy. *Proc Natl Acad Sci U S A* 2008; 105:18132–18138.

[81] Celis JE, Moreira JM. Clinical proteomics. *Mol Cell Proteomics* 2008; 7:1779.

[82] Abelev GI, Perova SD, Khramkova NI, Postnikova ZA, Irlin IS. Production of embryonal alpha-globulin by transplantable mouse hepatomas. *Transplantation* 1963; 1: 174-180.

[83] Daniele B, Bencivenga A, Megna AS, Tinessa V. Alphafetoprotein and ultrasonography screening for hepatocellular carcinoma. *Gastroenterology* 2004; 127: S108-S112.

[84] Beretta, L. HUPO's Effort To Define the Liver Proteome. *Journal of Proteome Research* Vol. 9, No. 2, 2010.

[85] *World J Gastroenterol.* 2008 Oct 21;14(39):6072-7.

[86] *Clin Cancer Res.* 2003 Nov 15;9(15):5493-500.

[87] M.A. Sells, M.L. Chen, G. Acs, Production of hepatitis B virus particles in Hep G2 cells transfected with cloned hepatitis B virus DNA, *Proc. Natl. Acad. Sci. USA* 84 (1987) 1005–1009.

[88] A. Tong, L. Wu, Q. Lin, Q.C. Lau, X. Zhao, J. Li, et al, Proteomic analysis of cellular protein alterations using a hepatitis B virus-producing cellular model, *Proteomics 8* (2008) 2012–2023.

[89] KK.Lai et al, Comprehensive and quantitative proteome profiling of the mouse liver and plasma; *Hepatology* 2008; 11;47(3):1043-1051.

[90] Beretta L. Comparative analysis of the liver and plasma proteomes as a novel and powerful strategy for hepatocellular carcinoma biomarker discovery. *Cancer Letters* 286 (2009) 134–139.

[91] S.O. Lim, S.J. Park, W. Kim, S.G. Park, H.J. Kim, Y.I. Kim, et al, Proteome analysis of hepatocellular carcinoma, *Biochem. Biophys. Res. Commun.* 291 (2002) 1031–1037.

[92] C.R. Liang, C.K. Leow, J.C. Neo, G.S. Tan, S.L. Lo, J.W. Lim, et al, Proteome analysis of human hepatocellular carcinoma tissues by two-dimensional difference gel electrophoresis and mass spectrometry, *Proteomics* 5 (2005) 2258–2271.

[93] D. Zhang, S.G. Lim, E.S. Koay, Proteomic identification of downregulation of oncoprotein DJ-1 and proteasome activator subunit 1 in hepatitis B virus-infected well-differentiated hepatocellular carcinoma, *Int. J. Oncol.* 31 (2007) 577–584.

[94] C. Li, Y.X. Tan, H. Zhou, S.J. Ding, S.J. Li, D.J. Ma, et al, Proteomic analysis of hepatitis B virus-associated hepatocellular carcinoma: identification of potential tumor markers, *Proteomics* 5 (2005) 1125–1139.

[95] X. Yi, J.M. Luk, N.P. Lee, J. Peng, X. Leng, X.Y. Guan, et al, Association of mortalin (HSPA9) with liver cancer metastasis and prediction for early tumor recurrence, *Mol. Cell Proteomics* 7 (2008) 315–325.

[96] W. Sun, B. Xing, Y. Sun, X. Du, M. Lu, C. Hao, et al, Proteome analysis of hepatocellular carcinoma by two-dimensional difference gel electrophoresis: novel protein markers in hepatocellular carcinoma tissues, *Mol. Cell Proteomics* 6 (2007) 1798–1808.

[97] C. Li, Y. Hong, Y.X. Tan, H. Zhou, J.H. Ai, S.J. Li, et al, Accurate qualitative and quantitative proteomic analysis of clinical hepatocellular carcinoma using laser capture microdissection coupled with isotope-coded affinity tag and two-dimensional liquid chromatography mass spectrometry, *Mol. Cell Proteomics* 3 (2004) 399–409.

[98] J. Ai, Y. Tan, W. Ying, Y. Hong, S. Liu, M. Wu, et al, Proteome analysis of hepatocellular carcinoma by laser capture microdissection, *Proteomics 6* (2006) 538–546.

[99] H.Y. Wang, Laser capture microdissection in comparative proteomic analysis of hepatocellular carcinoma, *Methods Cell Biol.* 82 (2007) 689–707.

[100] *Electrophoresis.* 2009 Sep;30(17):2957-66.

[101] Mehta A. and Block TM. Fucosylated glycoproteins as markers of liver disease. *Disease Markers* 25 (2008) 259–265.

[102] Goodacre R, Vaidyanathan S, Dunn WB, Harrigan GG, Kell DB. Metabolomics by numbers: acquiring and understanding global metabolite data. *Trends Biotechnol* 2004;22:245-252.

[103] Rochfort S. Metabolomics reviewed: a new "omics" platform technology for systems biology and implications for natural products research. *J Nat Prod* 2005;68:1813-1820.

[104] Wu H, Southam AD, Hines A, Viant MR. High-throughput tissue extraction protocol for NMR- and MS-based metabolomics. *Anal. Biochem.* 2008;372:204-212.

[105] Wickremsinhe ER SG, Ackermann BL, Gillespie TA, Chaudhary AK. A review of nanoelectrospray ionization applications for drug metabolism and pharmacokinetics. *Curr Drug Metab* 2006;7:913-928.

[106] Bergquist J, Palmblad M, Wetterhall M, Håkansson P, Markides KE. Peptide mapping of proteins in human body fluids using electrospray ionization Fourier transform ion cyclotron resonance mass spectrometry. *Mass Spectrom Rev* 2002;21:2-15.

[107] Seli E, Sakkas D, Scott R, Kwok SC, Rosendahl SM, Burns DH. Noninvasive metabolomic profiling of embryo culture media using Raman and near-infrared

spectroscopy correlates with reproductive potential of embryos in women undergoing in vitro fertilization. *Fertil Steril* 2007; 88:1350-1357.

[108] Wang J, Zhang S, Li Z, Yang J, Huang C, Liang R, Liu Z, Zhou R. (1)H-NMR-based metabolomics of tumor tissue for the metabolic characterization of rat hepatocellular carcinoma formation and metastasis. *Tumour Biol.* 2010 Oct 4.

[109] Gao H, Lu Q, Liu X, Cong H, Zhao L, Wang H, Lin D. Application of 1H NMR-based metabonomics in the study of metabolic profiling of human hepatocellular carcinoma and liver cirrhosis. *Cancer Sci.* 2009 Apr;100(4):782-5.

[110] Wu H, Xue R, Dong L, Liu T, Deng C, Zeng H, Shen X. Metabolomic profiling of human urine in hepatocellular carcinoma patients using gas chromatography/mass spectrometry. *Anal Chim Acta.* 2009 Aug 19;648(1):98-104.

Index

B

C

D

E

F

G

H

I

J

K

L

M

N

O

P

Q

R

S

T

U

V

W

Y

Z